Second Edition

Principles of
VEHICLE
EXTRICATION

Revised by: Carl Goodson
Edited by: Carol Smith

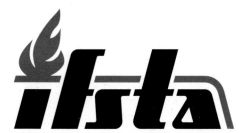

Validated by the International Fire Service Training Association
Published by Fire Protection Publications, Oklahoma State University

RECYCLABLE

The International Fire Service Training Association

The International Fire Service Training Association (IFSTA) was established in 1934 as a "nonprofit educational association of fire fighting personnel who are dedicated to upgrading fire fighting techniques and safety through training." To carry out the mission of IFSTA, Fire Protection Publications was established as an entity of Oklahoma State University. Fire Protection Publications' primary function is to publish and disseminate training texts as proposed and validated by IFSTA. As a secondary function, Fire Protection Publications researches, acquires, produces, and markets high-quality learning and teaching aids as consistent with IFSTA's mission.

The IFSTA Validation Conference is held the second full week in July. Committees of technical experts meet and work at the conference addressing the current standards of the National Fire Protection Association and other standard-making groups as applicable. The Validation Conference brings together individuals from several related and allied fields, such as:

• Key fire department executives and training officers
• Educators from colleges and universities
• Representatives from governmental agencies
• Delegates of firefighter associations and industrial organizations

Committee members participate because of their commitment to the fire service and its future through training. Being on a committee is prestigious in the fire service community, and committee members are acknowledged leaders in their fields. This unique feature provides a close relationship between the International Fire Service Training Association and fire protection agencies which helps to correlate the efforts of all concerned.

IFSTA manuals are now the official teaching texts of most of the states and provinces of North America. Additionally, numerous U.S. and Canadian government agencies as well as other English-speaking countries have officially accepted the IFSTA manuals.

ISBN 0-87939-176-6   Library of Congress Control Number: 99-69647

Second Edition

10   9   8   7   6   5   4   *Printed in the United States of America*

If you need additional information concerning the International Fire Service Training Association (IFSTA) or Fire Protection Publications, contact:

Customer Service, Fire Protection Publications, Oklahoma State University
930 North Willis, Stillwater, OK 74078-8045
800-654-4055   Fax: 405-744-8204

For assistance with training materials, to recommend material for inclusion in an IFSTA manual, or to ask questions or comment on manual content, contact:

Editorial Department, Fire Protection Publications, Oklahoma State University
930 North Willis, Stillwater, OK 74078-8045
405-744-4111   Fax: 405-744-4112   E-mail: editors@osufpp.org

Table of Contents

v

List of Tables

Preface

This second edition of **Principles of Vehicle Extrication** was written to update the information contained in the first edition. Since the first edition was published, there have been many changes in the design of land-based vehicles, and in the technology built into them. There have also been many improvements in the tools and techniques used to extricate victims from entrapment in crashed vehicles. This edition addresses those differences.

Acknowledgement and special thanks are extended to the members of the material review committee who contributed their time, wisdom, and knowledge to this manual:

Chairman
Robert H. Noll
Yukon Fire Department
Yukon, OK

Mahlon Greene
Central Mat-Su Fire Department
Wasilla, AK

Ed McManus
Saulsbury Fire Rescue Inc.
Endicott , NY

Mark Rabdau
Eagle Fire Protection District
Eagle, ID

David Stinnett
Holmatro Rescue Equipment
Forestville, CA

Secretary
Michael Ward
Fairfax County Fire & Rescue Dept.
Merrifield, VA

Merlin Klassen
Justice Institute Fire & Safety Division
New Westminster, BC

Robert Miller
Mesa Fire Department
Mesa, AZ

Eric Seeliger
Stillwater Fire Department
Stillwater, OK

Steven Taylor
Rescue Engineering Institute
Fort Wayne, IN

It would not be possible to develop a book of this scope without the assistance of many individuals and organizations. We thank all of the following for contributing photos, information, and/or their facilities and equipment.

Bryan Albee, Sonoma County (CA) Transit
Tony Alcocer, Santa Rosa (CA) Fire Department
Amkus Rescue Systems, Downers Grove, IL
Andreoli's Towing, Cotati, CA
Ajax Tools, Franklin Park, IL
B & N Auto Parts, Fort Wayne, IN
Steve Barker and Sons Towing, Decatur, IN
Barnett's Auto Parts, Portland, IN
Empire Equipment Co., Rohnert Park, CA
Terry Betts, Contra Costa County (CA) Sheriff's Office
Steve Bourne, Largo (FL) Fire Department

William Branter, California Highway Patrol, Rohnert Park, CA
Bob Brown, Holmatro Rescue Equipment, Cody, WY
Bryan (TX) Fire Department
Arthur Candenquist, National Railroad Passenger Corporation (Amtrak)
Canadian Automotive Rescue Society (C.A.R.S.)
Bill Chalgren, Holmatro Rescue Equipment
Champion Rescue Tools, Upland, CA
Crown Lift Trucks, Fort Wayne, IN
Ulrich Cimolino, Duesseldorf, Germany
Curtiss-Wright Rescue Systems, Fairfield, NJ
Jerry Denton, Amtrak Maintenance Facility, Oakland, CA
Discover Volvo Trucks, Fort Wayne, IN
East Allen County Schools, Fort Wayne, IN
Forestville (CA) Fire Protection District

Barry Gaab, Sonoma County (CA) Department of Fire Services
Allen Haggai, Thomas Built Buses, Highpoint, NC
Hale Products, Inc., Conshohocken, PA
Hough's Salvage Yard, Bryant, IN
Michael Hughes, Grosse Tete/Rosedale (LA) Fire Department
Insurance Institute for Highway Safety, Arlington, VA
Kari Kells, Indexer (Index West)
Laidlaw Transit, Inc., Santa Rosa (CA) Division
Tami Mann and the personnel of Jay County (IN) Rescue 19
National Association of Chain Manufacturers
National Highway Transportation Safety Administration, Washington, DC
National Interagency Fire Center, Boise, ID
National Safety Council, Itasca, IL
Pacific Gas and Electric Company, North Coast Division
Andy Pforsich, Santa Rosa (CA) Fire Department
Prestress Services, Decatur, IN
Todd Reynolds, Fire Protection Training Division/ TEEX
Mark Romer, Roseville (CA) Fire Department
Rincon Valley (CA) Fire Protection District Engine 7584, A-Shift
Vern Roof, Santa Rosa (CA) Fire Department

John Ryan, Fire Protection Training Division/TEEX
Tony Stimpson, Decatur (IN) Fire Department
Summit Coaches, Fort Wayne, IN
Dekevin Thornton, Marion (IA) Fire Department
Tom Turner, Blue Bird Corporation, Fort Valley, GA
Wayne Corporation, Richmond, IN
West-Cal Tractor, Santa Rosa, CA
West County (CA) Transportation Agency
Mike Wieder, Oklahoma State University

Last, but certainly not least, gratitude is extended to the following members of the Fire Protection Publications staff whose contributions made the final publication of this manual possible:

Cindy Brakhage, Associate Editor
Don Davis, Production Coordinator
Ann Moffat, Graphic Design Analyst
Desa Porter, Senior Graphic Designer
Tara Gladden, Editorial Assistant
Ben Brock, Graphics Technician
Susan F. Walker, Librarian
Kayla Moorman, Library Technician
Karen Flora, Support Specialist
Robert Crowe, Research Technician
Tim Frankenberg, Research Technician
Kris Kuehn, Research Technician
Lee Noll, Research Technician

Introduction

Vehicle extrication incidents occur everywhere that land-based vehicles operate — on streets and highways, on improved and unimproved rural roads, on railroads and light rail tracks, on farms and ranches, on industrial facilities and construction sites, and in remote wilderness areas. Statistically, motor vehicle crashes are the leading cause of death for Americans between the ages of 5 and 32, and are the leading cause of injury for all age groups. And, they are responsible for 13 percent of all firefighter deaths.

The majority of vehicle extrication incidents are handled by firefighters, either career or volunteer. Others are handled by members of dedicated rescue squads or rescue companies, either public or private. And some are handled by law enforcement personnel. The concepts and techniques described in this manual can be applied by any or all of these groups provided that they are properly trained and equipped. Within the pages of this manual, performing vehicle extrication safely and efficiently are recurring themes.

The term "extrication" means different things to different people, and in some jurisdictions it includes more or less than in others. According to NFPA 1670, *Standard on Operations and Training for Technical Rescue Incidents* (1999), extrication is defined as "the removal of trapped victims from a vehicle or machinery." However, because the IFSTA **Rescue** manual addresses freeing victims from entrapment in machinery, and the IFSTA **Aircraft Rescue and Fire Fighting** manual addresses extrication from aircraft, this manual focuses on extricating victims of entrapment in land-based vehicles. Some land-based-vehicle extrication incidents — those occurring on elevated or underground sections of light rail or subway systems — are considered to be technical rescue situations and are therefore beyond the scope of this manual.

Purpose

This edition of **Principles of Vehicle Extrication** is designed to provide rescue personnel with an understanding of the current challenges, techniques, and equipment available for the safe and effective extrication of victims trapped in land-based vehicles of all types. However, this manual only provides information — it does not provide training. In addition, the information in this manual deals only with the mechanics of freeing victims from entrapment in vehicles and related machinery. It *does not* include emergency medical information regarding the proper packaging of victims for extrication.

NOTICE

No one should expect to become proficient at vehicle extrication simply by reading this or any other book on the subject. The information contained in this manual must be combined with hands-on training delivered by qualified instructors and experience on extrication incidents.

The tools and techniques described in this manual represent the current state of the art as practiced by rescuers throughout North America, but they are not the only ways that extrication can be performed safely and efficiently. Since no single tool nor any single technique will be safe and effective in every situation, the readers are encouraged to master a variety of extrication tools and techniques.

Scope

This manual addresses Section 4-4.1 of NFPA 1001 (1997), Sections 3-1, 3-2, 3-3, 3-4, 3-5, all of Chapter 6 of NFPA 1006 (2000), and Chapters 2 and 6 of NFPA 1670 (1999), all published by the National Fire Protection Association.

The text begins with an introduction to vehicle extrication, scene management, and incident command. It continues with a review of extrication-related equipment and techniques. Extrication of victims trapped in passenger vehicles, buses, medium and heavy trucks, trains, and industrial and agricultural vehicles are also discussed. Finally, special situations and topics in vehicle extrication are discussed.

Notice on Gender Use

The English language has historically given preference to the male gender. Among many words, the pronouns, "he" and "his" are commonly used to describe both genders. Society evolves faster than language, and the male pronouns still predominate our speech. IFSTA/Fire Protection Publications has made great effort to treat the two genders equally, recognizing that a significant percentage of fire service personnel are female. However, in some instances, male pronouns are used to describe both males and females solely for the purpose of brevity. This is not intended to offend readers of the female gender.

Chapter 1

Introduction to Vehicle Extrication

Virtually every emergency response organization in North America, as well as those in most of the rest of the world, must at some time respond to incidents that involve persons, pets, or livestock trapped in vehicles. These incidents range from a baby or pet locked inside a parked automobile to severely injured passengers trapped in a wrecked automobile, truck, or bus. Some agencies respond to this type of incident on a regular basis, others less frequently. Regardless of the frequency with which the personnel in these organizations respond to vehicle extrication incidents, to do their jobs well they need to understand the challenges they face and have the training and equipment necessary to safely perform in these situations. In fact, the less experience the personnel have, and the less frequently they must extricate victims from vehicles, the more they need the best training and equipment available.

This chapter provides an overview of the vehicle extrication field, and it forms a foundation for the balance of the manual. Key vehicle extrication terms are defined, the organizations relevant to vehicle extrication in the United States and Canada are identified, and their respective roles and responsibilities are discussed. The critical knowledge, skills, and abilities necessary to safely and effectively perform vehicle extrication are identified. The factors involved in a successful extrication are discussed, along with the principles of vehicle extrication and vehicle anatomy. Also discussed are the roles and responsibilities of everyone involved in an extrication incident.

Definitions

In order to limit confusion about key terms used in this manual, the following definitions apply:

- *Extrication*—safely and efficiently freeing persons, pets, or livestock from entrapment in land-based vehicles of all types.
- *Disentanglement*—that part of vehicle extrication that relates to the removal and/or manipulation of vehicle components to allow a properly packaged victim to be removed from the vehicle. Sometimes referred to as removing the vehicle from the victim.
- *Rescue*—that part of vehicle extrication that relates to assessing, stabilizing, protecting, and removing a victim from entrapment.

Relevant Organizations

In both the United States and Canada, there are a number of governmental agencies and non-governmental organizations that have some responsibility and authority relevant to vehicle extrication. Some have the authority to legislate and regulate, others do not. In some cases, these organizations investigate transportation crashes and issue findings upon which new laws and regulations are based. In other cases, they may have authority to dictate design criteria to promote vehicle safety or broad authority to regulate how the highways are used, by whom, and under what conditions.

U.S. Organizations
In the United States, there are a number of organizations relevant to vehicle extrication. Among them are the following:

- National Highway Transportation Safety Administration (NHTSA)
- Insurance Institute of Highway Safety (IIHS)
- Transportation Emergency Rescue Committee (TERC)

- National Safety Council (NSC)
- American National Standards Institute (ANSI)

National Highway Transportation Safety Administration (NHTSA)

Established by the Highway Safety Act of 1970, the NHTSA is a part of the U.S. Department of Transportation. The NHTSA is responsible for reducing deaths, injuries, and economic losses resulting from motor vehicle crashes. The NHTSA does this by setting and enforcing safety performance standards for motor vehicle equipment and by funding state and local highway safety programs. Among its many services, the NHTSA investigates safety defects in motor vehicles and helps states and local communities reduce the threat posed by drunk drivers. The NHTSA also promotes the use of safety belts, child safety seats, and air bags. Highway safety information may be obtained from NHTSA on its web site at *www.nhtsa.dot.gov.*

Insurance Institute for Highway Safety (IIHS)

The IIHS is an independent research organization funded by a host of well-known insurance companies. The institute focuses on both crash avoidance and the crashworthiness of vehicles. At its state-of-the-art test facility, the institute conducts scientifically controlled crash tests on a variety of vehicles to test their safety performance (Figure 1.1). The institute also evaluates physical and environmental factors that may contribute to vehicle crashes. Evaluations are conducted on red-light cameras, traffic law enforcement technologies, and the elimination of roadside hazards. Information about IIHS programs can be obtained from its web site at *www.highwaysafety.org.*

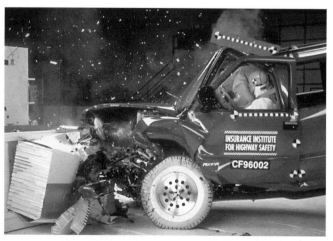

Figure 1.1 IIHS conducts scientifically controlled crash tests. *Courtesy of Insurance Institute for Highway Safety.*

Transportation Emergency Rescue Committee (TERC)

Sanctioned by the International Association of Fire Chiefs, the TERC was formed in 1986. Its mission is to serve as a competent source of guidance and information on transportation emergencies for those involved in providing emergency services. The committee is composed of members representing Great Britain, Canada, Europe, South Africa, and the United States. The members share their vehicle extrication expertise by conducting schools, seminars, and competitive exercises. The committee's goals are as follows:

- Develop a three-level system for vehicle extrication training.
- Develop guidelines to be met by vehicle extrication instructors.
- Develop safety guidelines for training.
- Disseminate information about vehicle extrication through a newsletter or other source.
- Develop a registration system for extrication judges.

Information about TERC and its activities can be found on the IAFC web site at www.iafc.org. (Sidebar: About IAFC, scroll down to TERC)

National Safety Council (NSC)

Although chartered by the U.S. Congress, the NSC is a nonprofit, nongovernmental, international public service organization dedicated to improving the safety, health, and environmental well-being of all people. Its mission is to educate and influence society to adopt safety, health, and environmental policies, practices, and procedures that prevent and mitigate human suffering and economic losses arising from preventable causes. Having no authority to legislate or regulate, the council serves as an impartial intermediary by building consensus among safety and health professionals from industry and labor on safety, health, and environmental issues. Information about NSC programs and activities can be found on its web site at www.nsc.org.

American National Standards Institute (ANSI)

Founded in 1918 by a small group of engineering societies and governmental agencies, ANSI is a private, nonprofit membership organization that facilitates the formulation of voluntary consensus standards and conformity assessment systems for the private sector. While ANSI does not develop standards, it facilitates that process and has approved more than 13,000 national and international standards to date. Information about ANSI and its activities can be found on its web site at www.ansi.org.

Organizations in Canada

In Canada, there are two leading organizations relevant to vehicle extrication, and each relates to this field in very different ways. These organizations are:

- Transport Canada
- Canadian Automotive Rescue Society

Transport Canada

Transport Canada, which is a part of the Canadian federal government, is the primary regulatory agency relevant to vehicle and highway safety in Canada. It is the agency responsible for most of the transportation policies, programs, and goals set by the Government of Canada to make sure that the national transportation system is safe, efficient, and accessible to all its users. The surface transportation section of Transport Canada works with other levels of government, the automotive industry, safety councils, consumer groups, and others to provide information pertinent to vehicle safety such as the risks and benefits of seat belts, air bags, child safety seats, and daytime running lights. Information about Transport Canada and its activities can be found on its web site at www.tc.gc.ca.

Canadian Automotive Rescue Society (C.A.R.S.)

The C.A.R.S. promotes safety within the vehicle extrication community. It does so by conducting realistic but highly controlled training exercises. The safety and health of all participants in these exercises are ensured by strict adherence to very specific safety rules. The rules require participants to be equipped with appropriate personal protective equipment and have a specified minimum level of training before they are allowed to participate. The rules also mandate the use of one or more safety officers to closely observe the training. Information about C.A.R.S. and its activities can be found on its web site at www.bordercity.com/cars/cars.htm.

Knowledge, Skills, and Abilities for Safe Vehicle Extrication

One of the most important skills for rescue personnel on vehicle extrication incidents is the ability to recognize the existing and potential dangers to themselves and others. Rescue personnel are trained and equipped to help those who cannot help themselves

and are willing to accept the risks involved in rescue operations. However, all on-scene rescue personnel must resist the urge to rush into the scene before it is safe to do so — and thereby add more victims to the incident.

> It is essential that all rescuers remember that they did not cause the problem, they are not responsible for the victims being in that situation, and they are not obligated to sacrifice themselves in a heroic attempt to save a victim — and especially not in an attempt to recover a body.

Therefore, during any emergency incident, the safety and survival priorities for emergency response personnel are — *self, fellow rescuers, bystanders, and victims.*

To safely and successfully extricate a victim trapped in a vehicle, rescuers must be able to:

- Assess the situation (perform size-up).
- Make informed decisions about how to stabilize the situation (stop it from getting worse).
- Devise and implement a plan of action that protects the rescuers and victim(s) from further injury and results in all victims being freed from entrapment.

To fulfill these general requirements, rescuers must have a significant amount of specific knowledge and a variety of skills and abilities. Although not listed in any order of importance or priority, rescuers should have an understanding of the following:

Capabilities and limitations of available resources. Section 2-2.1 of NFPA 1670 (1999) requires local jurisdictions to survey their response areas to assess the potential for rescue incidents, including extrication, and to make decisions about how these risks may be handled. Depending upon the jurisdiction's fiscal and political priorities, administrators may choose to train and equip their personnel to meet the identified levels of operational capability. They may choose to prepare for these contingencies by entering into mutual aid agreements with neighboring entities. They may contract with private providers for these services. Or, they may choose a combination of these approaches. In any case, local emergency response personnel should know the capabilities and limitations of all resources that would be immediately available, and those that would be available with some delay. One of the best ways of learning these capabilities and limitations — and of increasing the capabilities and reducing the limitations — is through realistic joint training exercises held on a regular basis.

How to activate the local emergency response system. Section 6-3.3 (i) of NFPA 1670 (1999) requires local jurisdictions to develop procedures for the procurement and utilization of the resources necessary to conduct safe and effective vehicle extrication operations. An important part of using the available resources to their fullest extent is knowing how to access those resources quickly when needed. Regardless of whether additional resources are available from within the primary agency, whether mutual aid units must be called, or whether private providers must be contacted, rescuers should be aware of how to activate the system.

Vehicle construction. A knowledge of how a variety of vehicles are constructed is critical to the safety of rescuers, trapped occupants, and bystanders. Knowing where air bags are located, how they may be activated accidentally, and how they may be safely deactivated, can protect both rescuers and trapped occupants. Knowledge of vehicle construction is also an important element in freeing trapped vehicle occupants in the most timely manner.

Dynamics of vehicle crashes. Knowing what happens to vehicles and their occupants when they collide with stationary objects or other vehicles is important to understanding the nature of the extrication problems involved. For example, knowing how vehicles designed with crumple zones react to impact compared to those without such features is important to assessing how occupants may be trapped in the wreckage. It may also indicate the types of injuries that occupants may have suffered.

How and why victims become entrapped in vehicles. Rescuers must combine their knowledge of vehicle construction with the dynamics of vehicle crashes to understand how and why vehicle occupants are entrapped in the wreckage of their vehicles. This knowledge can be obtained through years of experience or, more efficiently, by studying data and video footage of controlled crash tests conducted by research organizations.

Mechanisms of injury. Understanding how the inertial forces produced during vehicle crashes cause injuries to vehicle occupants helps rescuers determine the proper packaging and handling techniques in a given situation. Matching the packaging and handling techniques to the most likely victim injuries translates into less trauma for the victims and therefore a higher rate of survival.

Vehicle stabilization. Section 6-3.3(b) of NFPA 1670 (1999) requires that local jurisdictions develop procedures for making the rescue scene safe, including vehicle stabilization. Both rescuers and trapped vehicle occupants can be injured by sudden and unexpected movement of wrecked vehicles. Therefore, stabilizing wrecked vehicles is an important safety consideration. There are a variety of techniques and equipment commonly used to stabilize crashed vehicles, and rescuers should be well trained in their application.

Scene control and protection. Sections 6-3.3 (b) and (j) of NFPA 1670 (1999) require that local jurisdictions develop procedures for making the rescue scene safe, including controlling traffic. Controlling the perimeter of a crash scene is also of critical importance to the safety of rescuers, trapped victims, and bystanders. If the wrecked vehicles are still on the roadway, the scene must be protected from oncoming traffic. There may be other hazards, such as spilled fuel, other hazardous materials, or downed power lines, that threaten those at the scene. Vehicles that plunge into creeks, rivers, or other bodies of water add the dangers of hypothermia and drowning to the other hazards present for both the rescuers and victims. All these potential safety hazards must be identified and addressed if the extrication operation is to be conducted in safety.

Protecting rescuers. Sections 6-3.3 (h) and (j) of NFPA 1670 (1999 edition) require that procedures be developed for mitigating general and specific hazards at the scene and for maintaining traffic control. As mentioned earlier, these measures are necessary to protect everyone at the scene, including the rescuers. It is critically important that rescuers be protected so that they can provide the services for which they are responsible.

Safe and effective use of available tools and equipment. As mentioned earlier, rescuers should be well trained in the application of a variety of vehicle extrication techniques and equipment. This means being able to evaluate a given vehicle extrication problem, determine the best techniques to employ, and select and use the most appropriate tools and equipment according to the manufacturer's recommendations. Using tools and equipment safely requires hands-on training by qualified instructors and first-hand experience under the supervision of qualified supervisors (Figure 1.2).

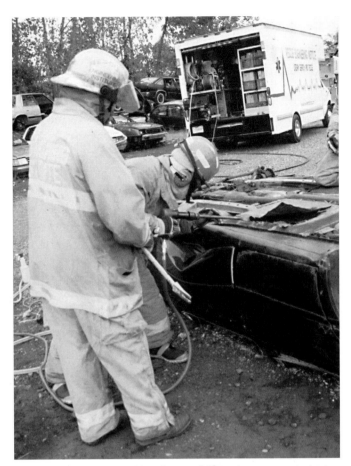
Figure 1.2 Rescuers need hands-on training to become competent.

Accessing trapped victims. Section 6-3.3 (f) of NFPA 1670 (1999) and Section 3-3.1 of NFPA 1006 (2000) require local jurisdictions to develop procedures for accessing victims trapped in a vehicle. Rescuers must know these procedures and be able to follow them in a way that results in the victims being freed from entrapment. This may involve the use of a variety of tools and equipment to manipulate and/or remove major vehicle components.

Assessing trapped victims. Section 3-3.2 of NFPA 1006 (2000) requires that rescuers be able to medically assess a trapped victim. Before trapped victims can be properly packaged, as required in the next section, they must be medically assessed to determine the nature and extent of any injuries they may have suffered during the crash. From the standpoint of victim survival, this can be one of the most critical steps in the entire extrication operation. If an injury is overlooked during this assessment, it can possibly develop into a life-threatening problem because of the movement and manipulation of the victim during extrication.

Protecting and packaging trapped victims. Sections 6-3.3 (d) and (e) of NFPA 1670 (1999) require

local jurisdictions to develop procedures for protecting and packaging victims for extrication from a vehicle. To meet these requirements, rescuers must have performed a thorough and complete medical assessment in order to determine how to properly package any injured victims trapped in wrecked vehicles.

Providing on-scene medical treatment. Sections 3-3.2 and 3-3.4 of NFPA 1006 (2000) require that rescuers stabilize and package injured or ill victims. This includes providing on-scene treatment of the injured to prepare them for transport.

Transferring injured victims to EMS personnel for transportation. Section 3-3.6 of NFPA 1006 (2000) requires that rescuers be able to transfer injured victims to EMS personnel for transportation to an appropriate medical facility. This includes properly preparing the victim for transfer as well as following local protocols and passing on critical information about the victim's condition.

Ensuring that the area and vehicles are left in a safe condition when command is terminated. Section 6-3.3 (h) of NFPA 1670 (1999) requires local jurisdictions to develop procedures for mitigating on-scene hazards associated with extrication incidents. Part of meeting the intent of this requirement is making sure that a vehicle extrication scene is left in a safe and environmentally stable condition. Wrecked vehicles must be removed from the scene, and any other hazards mitigated before the scene is abandoned. Any hazards that cannot be immediately mitigated must be isolated to prevent members of the public from inadvertently entering a hazardous area.

Obviously, obtaining all this knowledge and developing all these skills and abilities takes time, training, and experience. No one should expect to become proficient in vehicle extrication merely by reading this or any other text on the subject. Hands-on training delivered by highly qualified instructors and first-hand experience under the supervision of knowledgeable and conscientious company officers are absolutely necessary.

Success Factors

It could be argued that if a fire department puts out a fire, the operation must have been a success — regardless of how long it took, how many resources were used (or misused), or how many injuries were sustained or lives lost in the process. Likewise, it could be argued that if all occupants of a wrecked vehicle are removed from the vehicle, the extrication operation must have been a success — regardless of how long it took, how many resources were used (or misused), or how many occupants or rescuers were injured in the process or died as a result. Obviously, this simplistic view of emergency operations is not valid. To be successful, every emergency operation involves three factors:

- Personnel protection
- Incident stabilization
- Property conservation

Personnel Protection

This factor involves protecting both the victims involved in the incident, bystanders in the immediate area, and the emergency response personnel operating on the scene. Meeting this criterion involves a rapid but safe response by emergency personnel, controlling and protecting the scene from oncoming traffic or interference from curious bystanders, conducting the operation in a safe manner, and protecting trapped victims during the operation.

Incident Stabilization

This factor involves those steps necessary to prevent the situation from getting any worse than it was when emergency response personnel arrived. Meeting this criterion involves maintaining scene control and protection while the operation is being conducted, stabilizing the vehicles, stabilizing and removing trapped victims, eliminating sources of ignition, and providing fire protection and hazardous materials control as needed (Figure 1.3).

Property Conservation

This factor involves preventing *unnecessary* damage to property during and immediately after the operation. Meeting this criterion involves:

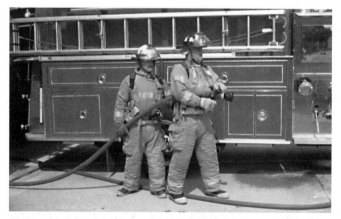

Figure 1.3. Providing fire protection is a part on incident stabilization.

- Developing procedures that result in as little property damage as possible — and no more — consistent with achieving incident objectives.

- Use of nondestructive techniques that accomplish the objective as fast or faster than other more destructive techniques.

- Providing security for unprotected property at the conclusion of the operation.

Extrication Principles

Depending upon which extrication reference is used, lists of extrication principles vary from as few as five to as many as thirteen. In this and the remaining chapters of this manual, the following principles will be discussed:

- Planning and Preparation
- Response
- Size-Up
- Scene Control and IMS
- Vehicle Stabilization
- Gaining Access
- Extrication Process
- Incident Termination

These principles include all the objectives listed in Chapter 6 of NFPA 1006 (2000), as well as additional principles deemed necessary by the IFSTA Vehicle Extrication committee.

Roles and Responsibilities of Extrication Personnel

Vehicle extrication incidents involve a number of separate and distinct functions that must often be performed simultaneously. These functions can be and sometimes are performed by members of a single response agency. However, to perform these functions most efficiently, groups of personnel from more than one agency are usually required. The following sections describe the roles and responsibilities of these various groups.

Extrication Team

This group is directly responsible for stabilizing crashed vehicles, accessing victims, stabilizing victims, disentangling victims, packaging victims for removal from wrecked vehicles, and transferring crash victims to EMS personnel.

Law Enforcement

This group is responsible for directing traffic around vehicle crash scenes, crowd control at these scenes, and investigating these incidents if they occurred on public streets or highways.

Emergency Medical Service (EMS)

This group is responsible for evaluating, treating, and transporting (if necessary) vehicle crash victims to appropriate medical facilities once victims are removed from wrecked vehicles. If local protocols permit, the EMS group may begin its work prior to the victims being extricated from the vehicles.

Fire Service

This group is responsible for protecting extrication teams, victims, EMS personnel, and any others working in and around crashed vehicles. Examples of hazards include fire, hazardous materials, and downed power lines.

Vehicle Anatomy

From an extrication standpoint, every vehicle can be considered to have eight sides with which rescuers must be concerned. Regardless of the type or size of vehicle, rescuers must observe, evaluate, and deal with the following aspects or "sides."

Top. Depending upon how the vehicle came to rest, the roof of the vehicle may or may not be the top aspect. If the vehicle is on its side, the roof may represent one side and one of its sides may be on top. If it is on its roof, the floor pan will be facing up. Regardless of which part of the vehicle is facing up, rescuers must be aware of what it means in terms of ease or difficulty of gaining access to the passenger compartment, or what it means in terms of fluids leaking into and contaminating the interior of the vehicle. In addition, rescuers must be aware of potential hazards such as broken power lines dangling above the vehicle.

Bottom. Normally, the floor pan will be the bottom side or aspect of the vehicle, and access to the passenger compartment may be relatively easy. However, this will not always be the case. Rescuers should be aware of what is and is not beneath the vehicle — leaking fuel, battery acid, or other potentially dangerous substances.

Driver's side. In most vehicles manufactured for the North American market, the driver's side is the left side. Obvious exceptions are vehicles used to deliver mail. More often than not, after vehicle crashes there is someone in the driver's seat, so this is the first place to look for vehicle occupants.

Passenger side. The passenger side is where occupants other than the driver are most likely to be found. Especially in the case of small children, they are often found wedged under the dashboard on the passenger side.

Front. Whenever a vehicle is moving forward, the front aspect or "side" usually arrives first and this translates into the front being damaged more often than any other part of a vehicle. With the exception of rear-engine vehicles, when vehicles suffer front-end damage, a number of engine-related hazards are created. Fuel lines may be broken and the electrical system damaged. This combination can result in serious fires starting in the engine compartment. In many cars, the battery is located near the front of the engine compartment. Damage to the battery can release highly corrosive acid.

Rear. In most front-engine vehicles, the fuel tank is located near the rear of the vehicle under the floor pan. While most rear-end collisions do not result in ruptured fuel tanks, some vehicles have design flaws that make fuel tank failure more likely. Rescuers must consider the potential for fuel leaks in rear-end collisions, and they should check this area as part of their initial size-up.

Interior. The interior of a wrecked vehicle is one of the most critical areas during vehicle extrication operations. In most cases, this is where trapped occupants will be found; therefore, the interior should be checked as soon as possible after arrival. This check may reveal the number of occupants and their condition, and possibly the presence of hazardous or unexpected cargo.

Exterior. Very often, but not always, the condition of the outside of a wrecked vehicle is a good indication of what may be found inside. But the outside may also provide other information — a commercial delivery van is most likely to contain a driver only, whereas a minivan may be a family vehicle occupied by both parents and several children. Obviously, seeing the outside of a wrecked school bus may indicate a multicasualty incident. In addition, the area surrounding the vehicle should be checked for pedestrians who may have been struck by the vehicle, and vehicle occupants who may have been thrown from the vehicle.

In addition, individual vehicle components are commonly described by specific terms. It is important that extrication personnel use the same terms for the door/roof posts and various other vehicle components.

Door/roof posts. Also called *pillars*, these are the structural members that surround the doors and support the roofs of vehicles. Door/roof posts are normally identified alphabetically from front to rear (Figure 1.4).

Quarter panels. Most automobiles have two quarter panels — from the trailing edge of the door opening to the rear bumper on each side. These panels often contain taillights, turn-signal lights, and backup lights (Figure 1.5).

Kick panels. While not technically correct, most extrication personnel refer to the side wall on each side of a vehicle that lies between the trailing edge of the front fender well and the lower half of the A-post as *kick panels.* Their upper limit is defined by the bottom of the dashboard and the top of the rocker panel (Figure 1.6).

Rocker panels. These are the usually rounded narrow body panels on each side of an automobile below the doors and between the kick panel and the quarter panel (Figure 1.7).

Summary

Vehicle extrication is a broad and diverse field, and one in which most emergency response organizations are involved. A number of national as well as state/provincial and local organizations relate in some way to the field. To be successful, those involved in vehicle extrication operations must possess a variety of skills, knowledge, and abilities. They must have a knowledge of vehicle anatomy, extrication principles, and the roles and responsibilities of those involved in extrication operations. Potential rescuers should be carefully selected for their physical and emotional strength and for their willingness and ability to learn the many aspects of safe and effective vehicle extrication operations.

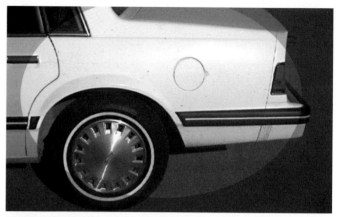

Figure 1.5 A typical quarter panel.

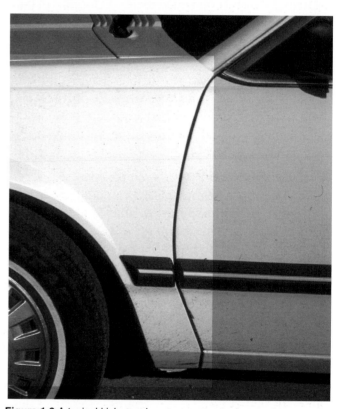

Figure 1.6 A typical kick panel.

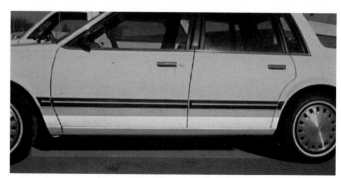

Figure 1.7 A typical rocker panel.

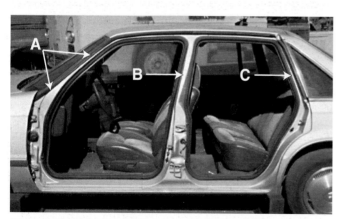

Figure 1.4 Vehicle door/roof posts are identified alphabetically.

Chapter 2

Scene Management and Incident Command

To a large extent, how an emergency scene is initially assessed and organized sets the tone for the remainder of the operation. If the initial assessment is performed inadequately, critical decisions can be delayed or even overlooked. This can put those involved in the operation at a serious disadvantage and perhaps put the victims in mortal jeopardy. On the other hand, if the initial scene assessment is properly done and an appropriate incident organization is established, the disposition of the problem is more likely to be carried out successfully.

This chapter discusses the emergency response to vehicle extrication incidents, the components of a vehicle extrication operation, and how to size-up a vehicle extrication incident. Also discussed are establishing control zones around the scene and implementing an incident management system. Finally, group/sector operations are discussed along with terminating a vehicle extrication incident.

Emergency Response

An agency's preparation for response to vehicle extrication incidents actually begins long before an emergency call is received. This preparation involves planning and decision making; in many cases, acquiring tools and equipment; and training agency personnel to deal successfully with this type of incident.

Planning

As discussed in the previous chapter, NFPA 1670 (1999) requires local jurisdictions to survey their response areas to determine the need for technical rescue capability, including vehicle extrication. Having made this determination, the jurisdiction must then decide how to provide the indicated level of response capa-

bility. They may choose to meet this need by entering into agreements with one or more outside agencies that are prepared to deliver this type of service, or they may choose to contract with a private provider. Finally, the jurisdiction may choose to purchase the needed tools and equipment and to train agency personnel to provide vehicle extrication services.

If the decision is to commit jurisdiction resources to training and equipping agency personnel to provide these services, the training must include those who will receive such calls and dispatch agency personnel to these incidents. Because this is one of the most critical elements in the agency's response to vehicle extrication incidents, communications personnel (dispatchers) must be carefully selected and thoroughly trained.

Receiving and Dispatching Information

Dispatchers (called *telecommunicators* by NFPA) are responsible for receiving vehicle extrication calls from the public and dispatching the appropriate emergency response units to the scene (Figure 2.1). To do

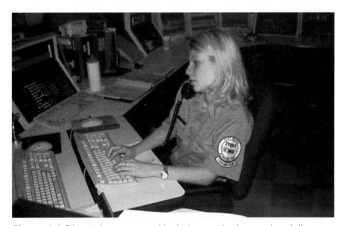

Figure 2.1 Dispatchers are a critical element in the service delivery system.

their jobs successfully, they must be trained to deal objectively and unemotionally with callers in order to obtain pertinent information from them. The pertinent information is as follows:

- Address or location of incident
- Nature and scope of incident
- Number and status of victims

Address or Location of Incident
Obtaining an accurate address or location of an emergency incident is obviously of critical importance. The advent of the 9-1-1 system has greatly simplified this process because it identifies the address from which the call is being made. However, not all emergency incidents — especially vehicle extrication incidents — occur at locations that have an assigned address. Many of these incidents occur on sections of highways that can only be identified by specifying direction and distance from landmarks such as highway interchanges or mileage markers.

Because many retail businesses and other commercial buildings are located along highway frontage roads, these structures can become easily identified landmarks, even to those who are not familiar with the area. For example, if a caller can tell the dispatcher that a car crash has occurred on I-40, westbound, in front of Southwest Plumbing Supply, the local dispatcher and emergency responders should be familiar enough with the area to know where that business is located and how to reach the incident scene. Also, a well-trained dispatcher should be able to determine the location of an incident by asking the caller the direction and distance to the nearest interchange.

Individuals being considered for employment as emergency dispatchers should be carefully screened. They should be intimately familiar with the response area in order to recognize when a caller is providing inaccurate information. For example, if an excited caller reports that the incident is located at the intersection of two parallel streets, the dispatcher should be able to recognize this discrepancy and elicit more information from the caller.

In addition to an intimate knowledge of the response area, dispatchers must have the maturity to be able to cope with callers who may be excited, angry, confused, or hysterical. Regardless of why a caller is excessively emotional, or what form that emotion takes, dispatchers must be able to remain unaffected by it and be able to function calmly and in a businesslike manner. They should also be able to maintain the proper attitude and focus — that is, to remain civil and courteous even when a caller is uncooperative or obstinate — and be willing to extend themselves on the citizens' behalf. This does not mean that dispatchers must endure the insults of an abusive caller, but it means that dispatchers should remember that they know the system far better than most callers. They should use that knowledge to help the agency provide the highest level of service possible. For example, if a caller reports an incident that is outside of the agency's area of responsibility, either geographically or functionally, the dispatcher should take the information from the caller and relay it to the responsible agency rather than telling the caller to contact the responsible agency himself.

Nature and Scope of Incident
The second piece of critical information that dispatchers must glean from callers is the type of emergency being reported and its magnitude. Is it a single vehicle rollover or a multiple-vehicle collision? Are only automobiles involved or are buses and heavy trucks involved also? Is the crash scene on a rural road, city street, or busy highway? Did the vehicle crash into a building or drive off a cliff? Is the crashed vehicle in a body of water or hanging from an overpass? All these variables affect the level and type of response.

Number and Status of Victims
Perhaps the most important information that dispatchers can glean from callers is the number of victims, if the victims are injured, and if so, how badly. In most cases, those who report emergencies do not have the background and training needed to accurately assess the condition of vehicle crash victims, nor should they be expected to do so. However, they may be able to provide general information about the number of obvious victims and what their conditions appear to be.

For the response to vehicle extrication incidents to be most effective, dispatchers must know the response system — in other words, what the most appropriate response to the reported incident is. In many jurisdictions, response levels to the most common types of incidents are predetermined and dispatchers need only be able to recognize the type of incident or when a particular call does not fit one of the scenarios on which the predetermined levels were based. In these cases, the dispatcher must know how to increase the response to the appropriate level. For example, if a call is to a multicasualty incident, the dispatcher must know how to increase the number of rescue units and ambulances. If hazardous materials are involved, the dispatcher must know how to include the appropriate haz mat units in the response. Ultimately, the lives of injured victims may depend upon the dispatcher's ability to send the most appropriate units to the scene in the shortest possible time.

Response to the Scene

Regardless of how well trained and equipped rescuers are, they cannot help vehicle crash victims if they do not reach the crash scene safely themselves. According to NFPA statistics, 13 percent of all firefighter deaths between 1989 and 1999 occurred while responding to or returning from alarms (Figure 2.2). Therefore, emergency response personnel must be trained to drive defensively. Apparatus drivers must always follow agency protocols and standard operating procedures, and driving defensively may mean coming to a complete stop before proceeding through intersections even though red lights and sirens are being used.

Personnel responding to the scene of a vehicle crash should begin to assess the overall situation. They should begin to create a mental picture of the incident based on the information they received in the initial dispatch — the day, date, time of day, weather, and the volume and type of vehicular traffic encountered during the response. All of these factors should be evaluated because they may affect the nature and

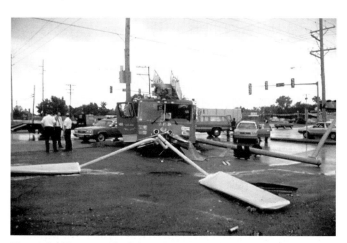

Figure 2.2 Too many firefighters become additional victims because of apparatus crashes.

extent of the incident, and they may or may not delay the response of other resources.

Taking Charge

On arrival, the first-in officer should take charge of the incident and attempt to accomplish three things. Listed in the order of their importance, these things are:

1. Protect himself, the members of his crew, and others at the scene.

2. Conduct an initial size-up of the incident.

3. Begin to organize and deploy the available resources to mitigate the incident.

In order to do these things successfully, the first-in officer must make some critical initial decisions.

Initial Decisions

The initial decisions required of anyone attempting to resolve an emergency of any type are generally the same. While keeping themselves and their crew out of harm's way, they must attempt to determine the nature and extent of the problem, and what will be required to isolate and mitigate that problem. These assessments are necessary to answer an extremely important question: Are the resources at the scene and en route sufficient to handle this incident? If not, the officer in charge must order the additional resources *immediately*. More about these initial decisions in the section on size-up.

Vehicle Extrication Components

The components of a vehicle extrication operation are generally the same as any other emergency operation, with some possible variations. The sequence of the following list from NFPA 1006 (2000) has been altered to more accurately reflect the order in which the steps are most often performed:

• Establish scene.

• Establish fire protection.

• Isolate potential energy sources (and other hazards).

• Stabilize vehicle.

• Determine vehicle access/egress openings.

• Create access/egress openings.

• Disentangle victims.

• Remove packaged victims.

In addition to the items in the previous list, it is important for those in command of vehicle extrication incidents to terminate the incidents in an orderly manner. This topic is discussed in detail at the end of this chapter.

Establish Scene

Establishing the scene means taking charge of the area immediately surrounding the incident in order to protect emergency responders, those involved in the crash, and bystanders. It also means creating a clear area in which emergency responders can function without interference.

Establish Fire Protection

Given the potential for fires at vehicle crashes, establishing fire protection is almost always indicated. Fire protection can range from someone standing by with a portable fire extinguisher to a number of fully charged hoselines being deployed and foam-making capability set up. Personnel must always follow local protocols, but it is recommended that at least one 1½-inch (38 mm) hoseline be charged and ready for use by at least two firefighters equipped with full PPE including SCBA.

Isolate Potential Energy Sources

In this context, energy sources include downed power lines, vehicle batteries, undeployed air bags, and energy-absorbing struts that may explode if overheated. Isolation includes identifying and cordoning off any downed wires, disconnecting vehicle batteries, deactivating undeployed air bags, and protecting shock absorbers and bumper struts from excessive heat and/or physical damage.

Stabilize Vehicle

Stabilizing a vehicle means preventing sudden and unexpected movement of the vehicle in any direction. In other words, keeping it from suddenly moving horizontally, vertically, rotationally, or from pitching or yawing. Stabilizing a vehicle can be done using a variety of chocks, cribbing, shoring, webbing, ropes, and/or chains.

Determine Vehicle Access/Egress Points

This means surveying the vehicles in which victims are trapped to determine how best to gain access to the victims and how to remove them once they are properly packaged. This may mean deciding to re-move one or more doors, remove or penetrate the roof, make entry/egress through a rear hatch, or any of several other possible actions.

Create Vehicle Access/Egress Points

Once the decisions regarding where and how to gain access to trapped victims have been made, all that remains is to create those openings. This may involve the use of a variety of manual and/or electric tools, pneumatic and/or hydraulic tools, and/or thermal cutting devices.

Disentangle Victims

Once access to trapped victims has been obtained, the work of safely freeing them from entrapment can begin. This may involve manipulating and/or removing the parts of the vehicle that prevent or restrict movement by the victims. Protecting the trapped victims during the disentanglement process is key to a successful operation.

Remove Packaged Victims

Once victims have been freed from entrapment, they can be safely removed from the wreckage provided that they have been properly packaged for movement. Packaging can include everything from simple bandaging to applying a C-collar with full spinal immobilization and traction devices.

Vehicle Extrication Components — Condensed

The preceding bulleted list represents the steps required to handle most vehicle extrication incidents. However, the following list includes all the items in that list, but with fewer steps. The balance of this manual will be based on safely and efficiently performing the following steps:

- Size-up
- Scene safety
- Command and control
- Groups/sector operations
- Incident termination

Size-Up

As in any other emergency incident, sizing up a vehicle extrication incident involves initial and ongoing assessments of the situation.

Initial size-up is intended to determine:

What has happened

What is happening

What is likely to happen

What hazards need to be mitigated

What resources are needed

The initial assessment is perhaps the most critical because it provides the information on which the incident action plan (IAP) is based. In addition, the decisions that are made and the actions that are taken or not taken at the beginning of an incident usually set the tone for the balance of the operation. If the initial size-up is thorough and accurate, and the initial decisions and actions resulting from it are effective, the operation is likely to be conducted safely and efficiently from start to finish. On the other hand, if the initial size-up and/or the resulting decisions and actions are flawed, the balance of the operation may be spent trying to overcome this deficit. As mentioned earlier, the size-up actually begins with the initial dispatch and continues during the response and throughout the incident.

One of the most important points in the size-up process occurs during the final approach to the scene. When the first-in unit approaches the scene, the officer in charge should be trying to see the "big picture," that is, to develop an overall impression of the nature and extent of the incident. Such things as the number of vehicles involved, their general condition, and their position in relation to other vehicles may be more apparent on approach than when actually at the scene. Downed power lines, smoke from incipient fires, and other actual or potential hazards may be seen during the approach to the scene.

On arrival, the officer should confirm the information gathered from the dispatch, during the response, and during the approach to the scene. This may require the first-in officer to walk around the perimeter of the scene. Or, depending upon the area involved, it may require that personnel be assigned to perform this duty and report their observations to the officer in charge. The most important things that need to be determined are as follows:

- How many people are in need of extrication?
- Are they injured or merely trapped?
- Do any victims require immediate intervention to preserve their lives?
- Are there life-threatening hazards such as fires, fuel leaks, downed wires?
- Are the resources on scene and en route sufficient for this incident?

If this initial scene survey confirms that an emergency exists, the first-in officer should formally assume command of the incident by calling the dispatch center and naming the incident, giving an initial report on conditions, and adopting one of the command modes discussed later in the section on command and control. In most cases, it is good practice to also specify the location of the command post and where later-arriving units should stage.

As mentioned earlier, size-up is an ongoing process that continues throughout the incident. A continuing size-up is necessary because the incident will not remain static — it will either continue to get worse or it will begin to get better, depending upon the situation, the number of resources available, and how effectively those resources were initially used. If the situation continues to deteriorate, additional resources may be needed and/or those on scene may need to be redeployed. If the situation begins to improve, some of the resources may be released to return to quarters.

After assuming command, or even before if the need is apparent, the incident commander (IC) should request any additional resources that may be needed. The sooner this is done, the sooner these additional resources will arrive at the scene where they are needed. If the IC is unsure about how many or what types of resources will be needed, he should request any that *might* be needed. Those that prove to be unnecessary can be returned to quarters while still en route or after they reach the scene. The IC's other immediate concern is how to protect those on the scene.

Scene Safety

There are a number of different aspects to scene safety at vehicle extrication incidents, and a number of different ways that safety can be provided. The first consideration is protecting the uninjured — emergency response personnel, uninjured vehicle occupants, and spectators. Some of the more common threats to the safety of those on the scene are other vehicular traffic, especially if the scene is in the traffic lanes of a busy street or highway; downed power lines that may or may not be readily visible; and spilled or leaking fuel or other hazardous materials (Figure 2.3). Less common, but not unusual, is the threat represented by irate and belligerent individuals who may have been involved in the incident or merely observed some aspect of it.

Apparatus Placement

To some extent, those at the scene can be protected by positioning emergency response vehicles between the scene and any oncoming traffic (Figure 2.4). Recent research has led many agencies to adopt a policy of shutting off all rear lights (except amber ones) on vehicles positioned in traffic lanes. This is done to avoid blinding and/or confusing oncoming drivers. In addition, Section 9-8.5 of NFPA 1901, *Automotive Fire Apparatus* (1996) requires lighting intended to alert motorists to the fact that the apparatus is blocking the traffic lane. But, in all cases, vehicle drivers should follow their agency's protocols regarding emergency lights on vehicles parked at the scene.

Control Zones

Another common way of protecting an emergency scene is to use barrier tape to cordon off the area into control zones. Usually, three zones are established — hot, warm, and cold (Figure 2.5). The *hot zone* is the restricted access area immediately surrounding the scene, and only those directly involved in the extrication operation are allowed in this zone. Surrounding that, the *warm zone* is established to create a space where those in support of the extrication operation may function. Surrounding the warm zone is another

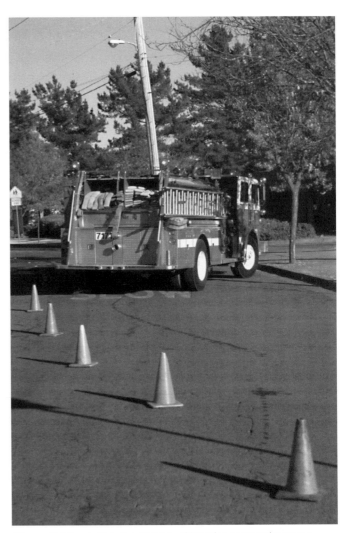

Figure 2.4 Apparatus should be positioned to protect the scene.

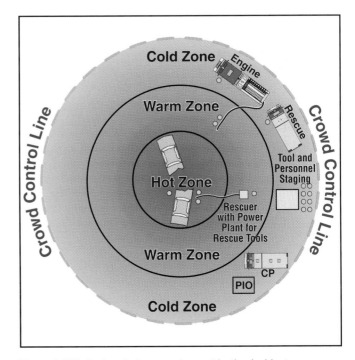

Figure 2.5 Typical control zones at an extrication incident.

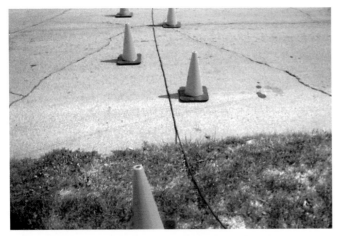

Figure 2.3 Hazards at the scene must be mitigated.

open area, the *cold zone*, in which incident command and related functions can be conducted. The outer limit of the cold zone is the *crowd control line* that creates a buffer between the public and the emergency operation. Only legitimate representatives of the media are allowed to cross the crowd control line, and then only when in accordance with local protocols. And, as mentioned earlier, one of the first actions needed is for someone to assume command of the incident.

Command and Control

While there is more than one incident command and management system in use in North America — and some jurisdictions are legally mandated to use a particular system — these various systems are much more alike than they are different. In general, there are only minor differences in terminology. Therefore, the Incident Management System (IMS) is the model that will be used in this manual.

In most jurisdictions, agency protocols require the first-in officer to assume command of any incident. Some incidents are clearly emergencies; this is apparent upon the arrival of the first-in unit. Other incidents require some investigation before the existence of a true emergency can be confirmed. Because of these differences in circumstances, the IMS provides for different command modes. Under IMS, the first-arriving officer has three optional modes available: nothing showing/investigating, fast attack, and command.

Nothing Showing/Investigating Mode

When the problem generating the response is not obvious to the first-in officer, he should assume command of the incident and announce that nothing is showing and that he is investigating. He should direct the other responding units to stage at Level I, accompany the crew on an investigation of the situation, and maintain command using a portable radio.

Fast Attack Mode

When the officer's direct involvement is necessary for the crew to take immediate action to save a life or stabilize the situation, the officer should take command and announce that the company is in the fast attack mode. Fast attack mode usually lasts only a short time. The crew will remain in a fast attack mode until one of the following occurs:

- The situation is stabilized.
- The situation is not stabilized, but the officer must withdraw to establish a command post. Depending upon the situation, the balance of the crew may be allowed to pursue their initial objective if they can function safely and effectively *and* if they have radio communications capability.
- Command is transferred.

Command Mode

Because of the nature and/or scope of some incidents, immediate and strong overall command is needed. In these incidents, the first-in officer should assume command as described earlier, and request any additional resources needed. In addition, the officer must decide how to use the balance of the crew. There are normally three options:

- Appoint one of the crew members as the acting officer, and give him a portable radio and an assignment (tactical objective).
- Assign the crew to work under the supervision of another officer.
- Use the crew members to perform staff functions in support of command.

When there is a need to transfer command of an incident to another officer, the transfer must be done correctly. Otherwise, there can be confusion about who is really in command of the incident. The officer assuming command must communicate with the officer being relieved by radio or face-to-face (face-to-face is preferred).

> Command may not be transferred to someone who is not on the scene.

When transferring command, the officer being relieved should brief the relieving officer on the following:

- Name of incident
- Incident status (number of victims, number of vehicles, hazard control, etc.)
- Safety considerations
- Action plan for the incident
- Progress toward completion of tactical objectives

- Deployment of assigned resources
- Assessment of the need for additional resources

Group/Sector Operations

Some of the most critical vehicle extrication operations are conducted at the group/sector level. In IMS, the terms "group" and "sector" are both used to designate functional units — scene control group, triage sector, etc. However, to avoid confusion, only one of these terms should be used within a particular agency. Once the agency has decided which term will be used, all agency personnel should be thoroughly trained using only that term to designate functional units. In most cases, all agencies within a county or region agree on which of these and other terms to use in order to reduce confusion during mutual aid operations.

In vehicle extrication incidents, the number of groups/sectors varies with the size and complexity of the incident. In some incidents, it may be possible for a single group/sector to perform all the necessary functions. In most incidents, however, several groups/sectors may be needed. The most commonly used groups/sectors are as follows:

Scene control. This group/sector is responsible for establishing and maintaining a safe environment in which the extrication operation can be conducted (Figure 2.6). As described earlier in this chapter, this normally involves traffic control, perimeter control, and hazard control. In particularly large incidents, traffic control and perimeter control may need to be separate groups/sectors. In some cases, hazard control will require a separate group/sector. If airborne contaminants were released in the crash, an evacuation group/sector may also be needed. They would be responsible for the orderly evacuation of those downwind of the incident.

Triage. This group/sector is responsible for checking the crashed vehicles and the surrounding area to locate all victims, determine their condition, and establish the priority in which they should be treated. Fulfilling these responsibilities may be relatively easy in a single-vehicle collision during the daytime and in good weather. Because triage may be extremely difficult in a multiple-vehicle collision at night in inclement weather, one or more lighting units may be needed to illuminate the scene.

Vehicle stabilization. This group/sector is responsible for protecting the rescuers and trapped victims from sudden and unexpected movement of the vehicles as described earlier in this chapter. This can range from the relative simplicity of stabilizing a single vehicle that is upright and resting on its wheels to dealing with multiple vehicles, vehicles on their sides or roofs, and/or vehicles teetering on the edge of a cliff or freeway overpass.

Victim access and disentanglement. Sometimes called the *extrication* group/sector, this group/sector is responsible for making entry into the crashed vehicle to allow the victims to be packaged for safe removal from the vehicle and to perform the required disentanglement of the victims.

EMS. This group/sector is responsible for packaging injured victims, safely removing them from the vehicle, and transferring them to the medical transportation provider.

Incident Termination

When all victims have been extricated and they have been treated and released or transported to a medical facility, all that remains is to terminate the incident. However, terminating an incident may be more complicated than it sounds. The objectives of terminating an incident are to restore the scene to as near normal as possible, make it safe for people to occupy, and make it safe for vehicles to drive through. Even after all victims have been dealt with, emergency responders may have to maintain control of the scene because of an ongoing investigation or if there are hazards that have not yet been mitigated.

Once the ranking law enforcement official releases the scene, all wrecked vehicles must be removed. If fuel or other hazardous materials have contaminated

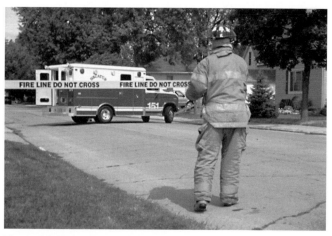

Figure 2.6 Scene Control Group/Sector cordons off the scene.

the scene, these hazards must be mitigated before the incident can be terminated. Likewise, if power lines and/or poles have been broken, utility company personnel will have to repair the damage (or at least remove the downed lines/poles) before the incident can be terminated. In some cases, such as when one or more vehicles burn during the incident, the roadway surface may have been so badly damaged that vehicles cannot safely drive on it. Appropriate barricades will have to be placed so that drivers will know to avoid these areas until the roadway can be repaired.

After all of these problems have been dealt with, the emergency responders must retrieve the tools and equipment they used during the incident. They must inspect them and make sure that they are ready for use at the next incident. Returning tools and equipment to the units from which they came can be made much easier if all items are clearly marked.

Finally, after all emergency responders have returned to quarters, the incident should be reviewed from a technical standpoint to see whether future performance can be improved because of anything learned from this incident. Also, personnel who had to deal directly with victims of horrific injuries should be required to attend a professionally conducted critical incident stress debriefing (CISD) session.

Everyone reacts to and deals with traumatic stress in different ways — some more successfully than others. Because emergency responders must train themselves to control their emotions during emergency situations, they sometimes lack an effective way of acknowledging and dealing with the effects of especially traumatic incidents — critical incident stress. Firefighters and other emergency responders sometimes use humor to defuse stress after traumatic incidents, but this is not always effective, and the effects of such stress can build up over time. Left untreated, the effects of critical incident stress can lead to a very serious condition known as post-traumatic stress disorder (PTSD). PTSD can produce some debilitating conditions that may be more than just career-threatening, they may be life-threatening. Finally, because firefighters and other emergency responders may feel that it is a sign of weakness to seek counseling for critical incident stress, those who have had close contact with dead or seriously injured victims should be *required* to attend CISD. They should not be required to participate, but they should be required to attend.

Summary

Responding to vehicle extrication incidents can be very challenging for everyone involved — the dispatcher taking the call, the emergency responders, the incident commander, law enforcement, EMS personnel, and, of course, the victims and witnesses. While the emergency response agency has no control over the victims and witnesses prior to an incident, it does have control over the emergency responders. The agency should train and equip its personnel to the highest level that agency resources will allow. Since more than one agency is often involved, cooperation, communication, and interagency training is extremely important. The lives of vehicle crash victims, and those of the emergency responders, may depend upon it.

Chapter 3

Extrication Equipment

The majority of vehicle extrication tools and equipment have remained virtually unchanged since their introduction. However, as in every other field of rescue technology, many have continued to evolve. Personal protective equipment and a number of traditional hand tools and power tools have been improved in recent years, or new ones introduced. Likewise, auxiliary equipment, such as generators, floodlights, and air compressors, that had to be added to basic rescue vehicles in the past are now standard equipment on many new vehicles.

This chapter discusses the personal protective clothing and equipment that rescuers need in order to perform vehicle extrication safely. Also discussed are various types of rescue vehicles and a variety of manually operated and power driven tools used in vehicle extrication incidents.

Personal Protective Equipment

The environment in which rescue personnel work dictates that they be provided with the best personal protective equipment (PPE) available. In many agencies, SOPs specify the most appropriate type and level of PPE to be used based on the hazards present, temperature and humidity, and other environmental factors. During an incident, the Incident Safety Officer (the IC on small incidents) enforces the applicable SOPs and dictates any changes in the type and level of PPE as necessary. In addition to wearing the most appropriate type and level of PPE, safety demands that personnel wear it properly — that is, with all openings closed and all fasteners fastened. Coveralls, street clothing, station uniforms, or even brush jackets worn by themselves are usually not acceptable at extrication incidents.

> Personnel not wearing appropriate PPE should not be permitted to operate on the scene of an emergency.

Special operations, such as extrication in a body of water or over a steep cliff, may require specialized personal protective equipment. For most extrication incidents, standard structure fire turnout gear is sufficient (Figure 3.1). In the following sections, the

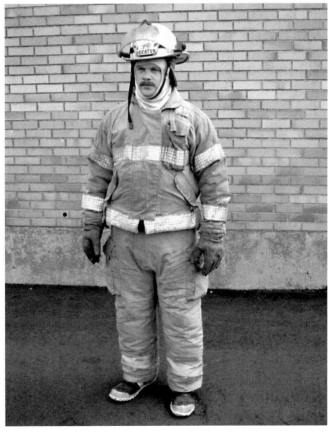

Figure 3.1 Standard turnout gear is appropriate for vehicle extrication.

basic types of turnout gear are described as well as other equipment that may be required.

Universal Precautions

Because rescue personnel must often work in close proximity to badly injured vehicle occupants, they must protect themselves from contact with blood and other bodily fluids. In addition to the other parts of the protective ensemble discussed next, rescue personnel should wear any other items necessary to isolate them from these substances. Additional items that may be necessary are medical exam gloves worn under their leather gloves, surgical masks if other respiratory protection is not being used, and perhaps Tyvec® gowns or sheets over their body protection.

Head and Face Protection

At all extrication incidents, proper protective headgear must be worn. Helmets protect the skull from flying objects, bumps into protruding objects, and head injuries due to falls or slips. All helmets should meet the requirements set forth by NFPA 1971, *Standard on Protective Ensemble for Structural Fire Fighting*, (1997).

The face and eyes must be protected from flying objects and spraying liquids that may cause severe injury. Unprotected, the eyes provide a pathway for infectious organisms. One of the most commonly used types of protection for the face is the protective shield of the helmet. The standard sizes of shields are 4 and 6 inches (100 mm and 150 mm). Generally, the 6-inch (150 mm) shield is more desirable for extrication personnel because it covers a larger portion of the face. This shield, *and* goggles or safety glasses, should be in place while extrication work is in progress (Figure 3.2).

> NFPA 1500 (1997) requires goggles or safety glasses to be worn in addition to the helmet faceshield when performing tasks such as those involved in extrication.

When agencies select head protection, fire-resistant, protective hoods should be considered. These hoods provide excellent heat protection for the neck, ears, head, and sides of the face. In addition to providing protection against radiant heat and direct flame impingement, they provide warmth during cold weather. They may also prevent some cuts and scratches caused by brushing against sharp objects (Figure 3.3). These hoods are recommended on all vehicle extrication operations.

Hearing Protection

Vehicle extrication operations can be extremely noisy. There may be generators, hydraulic power units, and all manner of power tools in use. The operators of these tools, and anyone nearby (including trapped victims), should wear appropriate hearing protection. This protection may be in the form of ear plugs inserted into the ear canal or external "ear muffs" worn along with all the other required PPE (Figure 3.4).

Body Protection

As mentioned earlier, appropriate protective clothing must be worn at all extrication incidents. Rescue com-

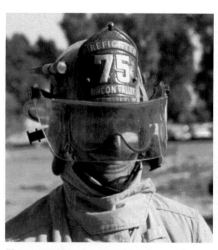

Figure 3.2 Goggles or safety glasses must be worn when using a faceshield.

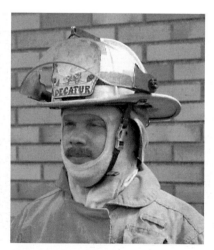

Figure 3.3 Flame-resistant hoods provide additional protection.

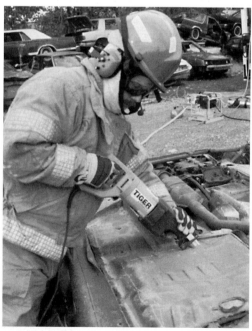

Figure 3.4 Hearing protection is necessary when noisy power tools are used.

pany members should be in complete gear upon arrival at the scene. If turnout gear is worn, it should conform to the standards set forth by NFPA 1971, *Standard on Protective Ensemble for Structural Fire Fighting*, (1997). In addition to providing protection against fire products, turnout gear protects rescuers from sharp objects, protruding or flying objects, and many other hazards found on the extrication scene. This protection reduces the chance of injury, thus making for safer operations.

It is also important that rescue personnel be visible on the incident scene. Therefore, when selecting protective clothing, consider visibility. Regardless of color, both pants and coats should have adequate reflective striping (Figure 3.5). NFPA 1971 gives specific requirements for the amount of striping necessary. Helmets can also be outfitted with reflective strips or patches.

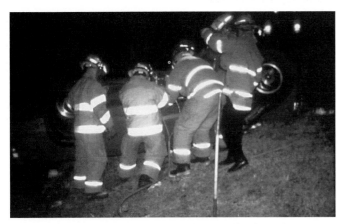

Figure 3.5 Both pants and coats should have reflective strips or patches. *Courtesy of Stillwater (OK) Fire Department.*

Foot Protection

Vehicle collision scenes are often strewn with broken glass and other potential hazards to the feet. Therefore, adequate foot protection is essential. When selecting foot protection, consider the hazards you will encounter — potential injuries from heat, punctures, and impact. All footwear should meet ANSI Z41-1991 *Standard for Men's Safety-Toe Footwear*, as well as NFPA 1971 (Figure 3.6). Because a proper fit is important in reducing foot fatigue and in preventing blisters or other sores, each rescuer should have his own pair of turnout boots.

Hand Protection

Gloves are an important part of personal protective equipment. The type of gloves worn by rescuers vary with the job they are doing and the type of protection required. If rescue personnel are fighting fire, they should be wearing gloves that meet the standards set forth by NFPA 1971. However, when personnel are performing extrication functions that do not involve fire, this type of glove may be too bulky and restrictive to allow for the needed dexterity.

When performing most extrication functions, rescuers need gloves that protect their hands but allow freedom of movement (Figure 3.7). Therefore, in most situations, rescuers should wear close-fitting leather gloves that are thin enough to allow dexterity but sturdy enough to protect their hands from cuts, punctures, and abrasions. In addition, NFPA 1500 requires that rescue personnel who are likely to come into contact with blood or other bodily fluids wear medical exam gloves inside their leather gloves (Figure 3.8). These gloves must meet the requirements of NFPA 1999, *Standard on Protective Clothing for Medical Emergency Operations* (1997 edition).

Figure 3.6 Sturdy boots are necessary for personnel safety.

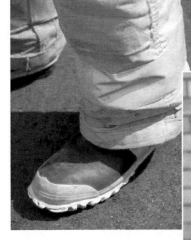

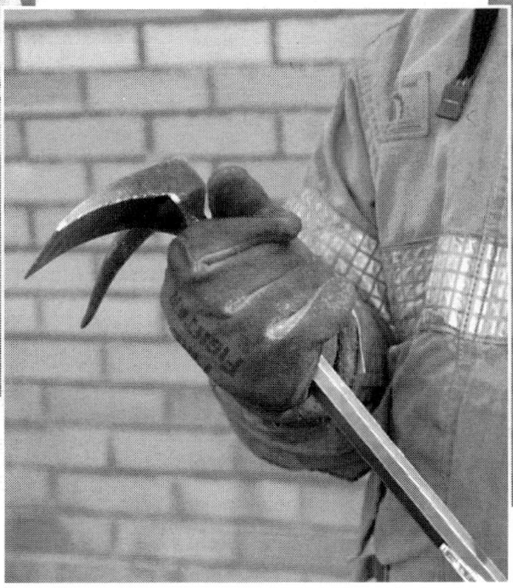

Figure 3.7 Gloves must provide protection and freedom of movement.

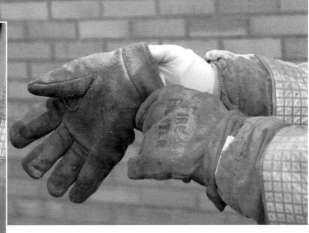

Figure 3.8 When working with injured victims, medical exam gloves are worn under the leather gloves.

Respiratory Protection

Although oxygen-deficient atmospheres are uncommon in vehicle extrication incidents, hazardous vapors, fumes, smoke, and dust are often present. Therefore, rescuers (and in some cases, trapped victims) often require respiratory protection. Rescue personnel should be well trained in the operation, use, capabilities, and limitations of all types of respiratory protection available to them. Achieving and maintaining this level of proficiency requires regular training and periodic testing.

Rescue personnel typically use either of three types of breathing equipment — positive-pressure, self-contained breathing apparatus (SCBA); airline breathing equipment; and filter masks.

Self-Contained Breathing Apparatus

The most desirable feature of self-contained breathing apparatus is that the wearer is independent of the surrounding atmosphere as long as the air supply in the tank lasts. All self-contained breathing apparatus must be of the positive-pressure type and should meet the requirements of NFPA 1981, *Standard on Open-Circuit Self-Contained Breathing Apparatus for the Fire Service* (1997).

The positive-pressure regulator is designed to produce a slight positive pressure inside the mask facepiece. The purpose of this design is to provide a constant positive pressure that is above atmospheric pressure, thereby keeping smoke and toxic gases outside the facepiece. This characteristic is extremely important because even trace amounts of some toxic gases can be injurious or fatal if inhaled.

Because facial contours vary from person to person, facepieces are designed in different sizes in order to obtain a proper fit. An ill-fitting facepiece can create a gap that cannot be closed even by fully tightening the straps. Therefore, it is recommended that each rescuer be issued his own personal facepiece. According to 29 CFR 1910.134 in the U.S., and the Workers Compensation Board (WCB) in Canada, all facepieces must be fit-tested at the time of issue and annually thereafter.

Facial hair (beards, moustaches, and long sideburns) may compromise the seal between the wearer's face and the facepiece. Even though the positive pressure within the facepiece will not allow contaminants in, an improper seal will allow air to escape and the air supply to be exhausted sooner. Obviously, this is unacceptable when operating in a contaminated atmosphere during an emergency.

> Facial hair that compromises the seal of a face mask should **NOT** be allowed on anyone whose job description requires them to wear self-contained breathing apparatus.

Most self-contained breathing apparatus in use today have either a 30-minute or 45-minute rating. These ratings are frequently misunderstood and personnel can be put in danger if the ratings are taken literally. These ratings are determined by timing a number of average, healthy individuals breathing at a relaxed, normal respiratory rate. When each person consumes the amount of air in the cylinder or unit, the time is recorded, the average is taken, and a rated time is assigned to the apparatus.

> The time-related ratings of SCBA cylinders represent the maximum amount of time the air supply will last under ideal circumstances.

The actual "duration of support" depends on the individual wearer's physiological and psychological conditioning. Protective breathing apparatus training should be frequent enough and of sufficient duration to allow personnel to become comfortable with having their faces covered by their masks and to overcome any tendency they may have toward claustrophobia. Given this type of training, rescuers who know their jobs well and who are in good physical condition can remain calm during emergencies and make maximum use of the air supply in each cylinder.

Airline Equipment

Another form of demand-type breathing apparatus is airline equipment. Air is supplied to the users by high-pressure hoses — up to 300 feet (90 m) long — from a bank of larger air supply cylinders or an air compressor. Rescuers using airline equipment wear a body harness to which the regulator and mask are attached. Also attached is a five-minute escape cylinder to give the wearer an emergency air supply should the airline fail. Some fire departments have adapted the breathing air systems on their aerial devices to airline systems. The same can be done to cascade systems on rescue vehicles or other apparatus.

While airline systems are most often used in the rescue of those overcome by toxic gases, fumes, or mists inside large industrial tanks, tank cars, and other confined spaces, it is possible that some vehicle extrication incidents will make the use of these systems necessary. If the scene has been or may be contaminated with airborne hazards, personnel may need to be provided with this type of air supply. Further information on self-contained breathing apparatus is available in the IFSTA **Self-Contained Breathing Apparatus** manual.

Filter Masks
According to NFPA 1500, when extrication personnel must work in close proximity to seriously injured victims, but in atmospheres that would not otherwise require SCBA or airline equipment, they should wear filter mask respiratory protection. These masks must be NIOSH-approved and meet the requirements for Type C respirators as defined in 42 CFR 84.

Special Protective Equipment

In a small number of vehicle extrication incidents, the IC may have to call in technical rescue personnel who are specially trained and equipped to operate in extremely hazardous environments. The special protective equipment that these teams wear may include hazardous materials suits, proximity or entry suits, and wet suits. However, if the trapped victims have been without benefit of respiratory protection in an extremely toxic atmosphere for some time, the IC must consider whether to conduct the operation as a rescue or as a body recovery.

> Rescue personnel should **NOT** be put in mortal danger to recover a body.

More information on special protective equipment may be found in the IFSTA **Fire Service Rescue** and **Hazardous Materials for the First Responder** manuals.

Care of Personal Protective Equipment
Proper care and maintenance of personal protective equipment is vital to maintaining its reliability. Each time equipment is used, clean and inspect it for defects that may limit its effectiveness the next time it is used. Care for all equipment — from protective clothing to breathing apparatus — according to the manufacturer's recommendations. Test breathing apparatus regularly. For more in-depth information

on personal protective equipment, consult the IFSTA **Essentials of Fire Fighting** (4th edition) manual.

Rescue Vehicles

The types of vehicles that fire departments and other emergency response organizations send to extrication incidents are many and varied. In this manual, however, they are classified as light, medium, and heavy rescue vehicles; rescue engines; standard engines; and ladder trucks. Obviously, the most sophisticated rescue vehicle is useless without trained personnel to staff it. Therefore, the term "*unit*" used in this chapter includes the vehicle and its crew.

Light Rescue Vehicles
Light rescue vehicles are designed to handle only basic extrication and life-support functions; therefore, they carry only basic hand tools and small equipment. Often, a light rescue unit functions as a first responder — that is, the unit attempts to stabilize the situation until more appropriate equipment arrives. The standard equipment carried by many ladder and engine companies also gives them light rescue capabilities.

Light rescue vehicles are generally built on a 1-ton or 1½-ton chassis. The rescue vehicle's body resembles a multiple compartment utility truck. The size of this vehicle limits the amount of equipment it can carry. A light rescue vehicle can carry a variety of small hand tools, such as saws, jacks, and pry bars, as well as smaller hydraulic rescue equipment and a small inventory of emergency medical supplies. These vehicles are generally capable of transporting two to seven personnel. Vehicles carrying more than three people require either a four-door cab or an enclosed crew compartment in the body of the vehicle.

Medium Rescue Vehicles
Obviously, medium rescue vehicles are designed to have a wider range of capabilities than the light rescue vehicles. These vehicles can carry as many as 8 to 10 personnel. In addition to basic hand tools, medium rescue vehicles may carry powered hydraulic spreading tools and cutters, pneumatic lifting bags, power saws, acetylene cutting equipment, and ropes and rigging equipment. Medium rescue units are capable of handling the majority of vehicle rescue incidents because they often carry a variety of fire fighting equipment, making them dual purpose units.

Specialized units are often considered medium rescue vehicles. Specialized units have specific uses, but they may carry generalized equipment that can be used in other types of incidents. Some types of specialized units are hazardous materials units, water rescue and recovery units, bomb disposal units, mine rescue units, technical rescue units, and lighting/power units.

Heavy Rescue Vehicles

Heavy rescue units must be capable of providing the support necessary to extricate victims from almost any entrapment. As their name implies, heavy rescue vehicles carry more and heavier equipment than do smaller vehicles. Heavy rescue vehicles also carry larger rescue crews — many have seating for 12 or more personnel. Additional types of equipment carried by the heavy rescue unit are A-frames or gin poles, cascade systems, larger power plants, trenching and shoring equipment, small pumps and foam equipment, large winches, hydraulic booms, large quantities of rope and rigging equipment, air compressors, and ladders.

Other specialized equipment may be carried according to the responsibilities of the rescue unit and the rescue exposures identified within the response district. Heavy rescue units are sometimes oriented more toward fire fighting than smaller units because they have more space available for fire fighting equipment.

Rescue Engines

Economic factors have forced many fire departments to use multipurpose or combination apparatus. One of the most popular of these multipurpose vehicles is the combination rescue/engine. This apparatus is designed to perform both the functions of a structural fire fighting pumper and a rescue vehicle. The result is an apparatus that is useful at almost any type of incident and that has sufficient rescue equipment to handle many vehicle extrication incidents. However, this versatility does not come without a price. Because they are dual-purpose units, they generally cannot provide the same level of service in either fire fighting or rescue as can the same size unit dedicated to one discipline or the other.

Rescue engines vary in size. Some fire departments use minipumpers or midipumpers (initial attack fire apparatus) with light rescue capabilities. Other departments use full-size engines that have been custom designed with extra-large compartments or other modifications for carrying rescue equipment. These larger apparatus are usually equipped with Class A fire pumps and large water tanks.

Standard Engines

In some departments, engine companies are expected to provide certain extrication services. Using the equipment carried on most standard engines, company personnel are able to perform many vehicle extrication tasks. In some cases, the first-arriving engine company can perform an extrication before other specialized equipment arrives. In other cases, the engine company can establish a perimeter, set up fire protection, and perhaps provide additional personnel to rescue companies working the incident.

Ladder Trucks

In many fire departments, ladder companies are better equipped to perform extrication operations than are their engine companies because most ladder trucks carry a greater quantity and variety of equipment than engines carry. Equipment that is normally used for forcible entry can often be used for vehicle extrication purposes. On large-scale incidents, ladder company personnel can be used to supplement rescue personnel when additional help is needed but additional rescue companies are not readily available.

In departments whose fiscal constraints preclude the establishment of a dedicated rescue service, ladder companies normally carry a full complement of rescue equipment, and they routinely do most of the vehicle extrication work. Because aerial apparatus typically have a large amount of compartment space, they lend themselves to carrying additional extrication equipment. Personnel who are already trained in ladder company operations are easily cross-trained to perform vehicle extrication operations.

Rescue Vehicle Bodies

Several types of bodies are used on rescue vehicles in various jurisdictions. The primary differences between the various types of vehicle bodies are in the amount of compartment space and its configuration.

Exclusive Exterior Compartmentation

Exclusive exterior compartmentation is most commonly found in smaller rescue units, although some larger units are also set up in this manner. These vehicles offer no walk-through area or interior storage. Tools and equipment are only accessible from outside the vehicle.

Exterior compartmentation is advantageous because personnel do not have to enter the vehicle to access needed equipment. However, there are also disadvantages to this design. One disadvantage, except on vehicles equipped with roll-up compartment doors, is that the compartment doors must have enough room to swing open. This can be a problem in situations where space is limited. Another disadvantage, even on vehicles equipped with roll-up compartment doors, is that the number of personnel transported to the scene may be fewer than in vehicles with other body styles because of limited space within the vehicle.

Exclusive Interior Compartmentation
Vehicles with exclusive interior compartmentation have all of their storage in an interior walk-through area. Some find this arrangement convenient because the entire inventory is accessible from the inside of the vehicle and out of the weather.

Vehicles designed with an interior walk-through area can sometimes transport more personnel inside the vehicle than vehicles with only exterior compartmentation. However, having to enter the vehicle for tools and equipment may slow procedures at an emergency scene. In addition, having to carry heavy tools and equipment from the walk-through level down to the ground level and back again can make the process more difficult.

Combination Compartmentation
Perhaps the most functional style of rescue vehicle body is one with a combination walk-through area and both exterior and interior compartmentation. Vehicles with this type of body offer the advantages of each design, and if equipped with roll-up compartment doors, few of the disadvantages of the less versatile designs. Having large compartments on the exterior promotes better ergonomics by allowing bulky and heavy pieces of equipment to be carried in a position where they are easily accessed. Likewise, protective clothing, medical supplies, and similar inventory items can be carried inside out of the weather.

Rescue Vehicle Chassis

Just as there are a number of different vehicle bodies, there are also different types of rescue vehicle chassis. The two primary types of vehicle chassis are commercial and custom. Each has certain advantages and disadvantages.

Commercial Chassis
Commercial chassis are built by commercial truck manufacturers, such as General Motors, Ford, Mack, Kenworth, and others. These truck chassis are typically used for commercial vehicles, such as plumber's trucks, garbage trucks, dump trucks, and delivery trucks. Commercial chassis are also the most commonly used chassis for rescue vehicles. All light and medium chassis units and a large percentage of heavy rescue chassis units are commercial chassis. Commercial chassis cost less initially than custom chassis and service is more readily available. The primary disadvantage is that commercial chassis, particularly smaller ones, may not last as long as custom chassis in the rigorous service that extrication responses involve.

Custom Chassis
Custom chassis are built by manufacturers who specialize in fire apparatus chassis, so they are designed to withstand the heavy use of the emergency service. Custom chassis often incorporate special design features specified by the agency purchasing them. Generally, the use of custom chassis is limited to heavy rescue vehicles. Their primary disadvantages are higher initial cost and the availability of service.

Special Rescue Vehicle Equipment and Accessories

Depending upon the topography within the response district and the availability of specialized apparatus from neighboring agencies, many emergency response organizations require special equipment and accessories to be incorporated into their rescue vehicles. Some of the most common of these special features are all-wheel drive capability, winches, gin poles and A-frames, stabilizers, cascade systems, air compressors, and power generating and lighting equipment.

All-Wheel Drive
The nature of the response area will determine the need for this capability. Rough terrain within the district, or the likelihood of snow and ice in the winter, may necessitate that rescue vehicles be equipped with all-wheel drive capability. All-wheel drive allows safer, more reliable vehicle operation during extreme conditions. Mountainous areas and large areas under cultivation are examples of areas where off-road capability may be necessary.

Winches
Many rescue vehicles, especially those that are designed as multipurpose vehicles, are equipped with bumper-mounted winches (Figure 3.9). A winch uses steel cable wound onto a rotating drum that is geared to give maximum pulling power. Winches may be

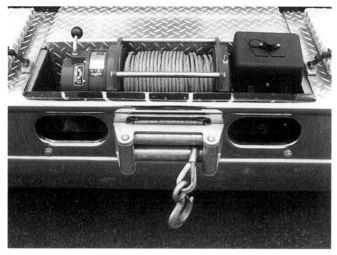

Figure 3.9 A typical bumper-mounted winch.

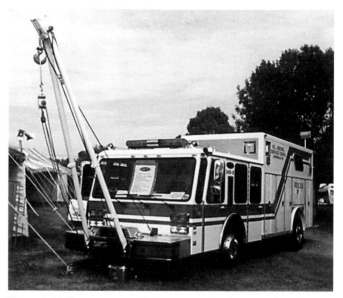

Figure 3.10 Some rescue vehicles have either a gin pole or an A-frame. *Courtesy of Mike Wieder.*

powered by the apparatus engine or an electric motor. Most vehicle-mounted winches are operated with controls located adjacent to the winch, or remotely by means of a long electrical cord. A drum brake prevents the drum from overrunning when the winch clutch is disengaged and the cable is being unwound. A vehicle-mounted winch should never be used in an attempt to move any object that is beyond the rated capacity of the winch.

Gin Poles and A-Frames

Gin poles and A-frames are vertical lifting devices that may be attached to the front or rear of the apparatus (Figure 3.10). Some of these devices have lifting capabilities in excess of 3 tons (2 721 kg). Both gin poles and A-frames have a pulley at the working end that is used with a vehicle-mounted winch when lifting capability is needed. A gin pole consists of a single pole that is supported by guy wires to both sides of the vehicle. A-frames consist of two poles attached some distance apart on the apparatus roughly forming the letter A. Stabilizers steady the rescue vehicle whenever A-frames are used.

Gin poles and A-frames are not designed to withstand lateral (sideways) stress, so take care to avoid such strains. Guy wires or guide ropes may be used to increase lateral stability. When gin poles or A-frames are used, it is important not to exceed the rated weight the apparatus chassis is designed to carry. Exceeding the gross vehicle weight limit may result in damage to the axles, chassis frame, or both.

Stabilizers

Also known as stabilizing jacks or outriggers, stabilizers are used to steady the rescue vehicle when a hydraulic lifting boom, gin pole, or A-frame is employed. *Stabilizers* reduce strain on the vehicle's suspension system when heavy loads are lifted and help to prevent the vehicle from rolling over when parked on a slope. Generally, there are two types of stabilizer systems: hydraulic, which is set using lever controls, and manual, which resembles a screw-type jack and is set by hand.

Cascade Systems

Some rescue vehicles are equipped with a bank of large capacity air tanks. They are called cascade systems because of how they are used to refill SCBA tanks. Their primary use is to refill SCBA tanks during an emergency operation and to refill tanks used to operate pneumatic tools such as air chisels. Most cascade systems consist of three to twelve 300-cubic-foot cylinders that are interconnected by high-pressure tubing. For more information on operating cascade systems, see the IFSTA **Self-Contained Breathing Apparatus** manual.

Air Compressors

The air compressors on rescue vehicles are one of two types: breathing air or nonbreathing air.

Breathing Air

Some rescue vehicles are equipped with air compressors that can generate breathing-quality compressed air. Air from these units can be used to fill cascade or SCBA tanks, to supply airline equipment in confined spaces, or for purging areas of nonflammable, oxygen-depleting gases. When operating, these compressors must be located in a clear atmosphere to avoid drawing contaminated air into the units and supplying it to the users. Generally, these units are placed upwind of any emergency scene to avoid such contamination.

Nonbreathing Air
Compressors that produce nonbreathing air are used to operate air chisels, pneumatic lifting bags, etc. Because of the many styles and sizes, as well as their relatively low cost, nonbreathing air compressors are found on many rescue vehicles. These compressors do not require a clear atmosphere for operation as do breathing air compressors.

Power Generating Equipment
Auxiliary power and lighting are often needed at extrication incidents. Power is needed to run electrical equipment, such as saws and other electric tools. Illuminating the scene during nighttime operations is obviously important for safety and efficiency. Power-producing equipment are usually either inverters or generators. When agencies select power-producing equipment, they should be certain that the equipment will produce sufficient power for the tools and appliances that are to be used during extrication operations.

Inverters
Also called alternators, inverters are used on rescue vehicles and ambulances when large amounts of power are not necessary. *Inverters* are step-up transformers that convert the vehicle's 12- or 24-volt DC current into 110- or 220-volt AC current. Advantages of inverters are fuel efficiency and little or no noise during operation. Their disadvantages include limited power-producing capacities and limited range from the vehicle.

Generators
Generators can be either portable or permanently mounted on the apparatus. They are the most common power sources used on emergency vehicles. Portable generators are powered by small gasoline or diesel engines and generally have 110- and/or 220-volt capacities. Most portable generators are designed to be carried by either one or two people — a two-person carry is recommended for safety. Portable generators are extremely useful when electrical power is needed in an area that is not within reach of the vehicle-mounted system.

Vehicle-mounted generators usually have a larger capacity than portable units. In addition to providing power for portable tools and equipment, vehicle-mounted generators provide power for the floodlighting system on the vehicle. Vehicle-mounted generators can be powered by gasoline, diesel, or propane engines or hydraulic or power take-off systems. Switch-controlled floodlights are usually wired directly to the generators, and outlets are also provided for other equipment. These power plants generally have 110- and 220-volt capabilities with capacities up to 50 kw and occasionally greater. Vehicle-mounted generators tend to be noisy during operation making it difficult to communicate near them. In addition, their exhaust fumes may contaminate the scene if they are not positioned downwind.

Lighting Equipment
Two types of lighting equipment — portable and stationary — are most often used in vehicle extrication incidents. Each type has certain advantages and disadvantages.

Portable Lights
Portable lights are used when the scene is beyond the effective reach of stationary lights or when additional scene lighting is necessary. Portable lights generally range from 300 to 1,000 watts. They may be supplied by a cord from the power plant or may have an attached power unit. 29 CFR 1910. 306 requires that all such cords be equipped with ground fault circuit interrupters. The lights usually have handles for safe carrying and large bases for stability. Some portable lights are mounted on telescoping stands.

Stationary Lights
These lights are mounted on the vehicle and their main function is to provide overall lighting of the incident scene. Stationary lights are usually not *fixed* because they are mounted on telescoping poles that allow them to be raised, lowered, or rotated to provide the best possible lighting. Some dedicated lighting units have hydraulically operated booms with banks of lights with capacities ranging from 500 to 1,500 watts per light. Scene lighting should not exceed the rated capacity of the power plant. Overtaxing the power plant will provide poor lighting, may damage the power generating unit, and electric tools will not function as designed.

Auxiliary Electrical Equipment
A variety of other equipment may be used in conjunction with power plants and lighting

equipment. Electrical cables or extension cords are necessary to conduct electric power to portable equipment. The most common size cable is a 12-gauge, 3-wire type. The cord may be stored in coils, on portable cord reels, or on vehicle-mounted automatic rewind reels. Twist-lock receptacles provide secure, safe connections. Electrical cable must be adequately insulated, waterproof, and have no exposed wires.

Junction boxes may be used when multiple connections are needed. The junction is supplied by one inlet from the power plant and has several outlets. Many junction boxes have a small light on top that stays on as long as power is being supplied to the unit.

In areas where mutual aid operations are common, some agencies may have different sizes or types of receptacles (for example, one has two prong; the other three). Adapters should be carried so that equipment can be interconnected when necessary. Adapters should also be carried to allow rescuers to plug their equipment into conventional electrical outlets.

Extraction Tools and Equipment

Acquiring the knowledge, skills, and abilities required to perform safe and effective vehicle extrication begins with learning the capabilities and limitations of the tools and equipment available. The tools and equipment procured by the response agency will depend upon the nature and extent of the rescue problems identified in the survey of the district required by NFPA 1670, *Standard on Operations and Training for Technical Rescue Incidents* (1999). The following sections discuss the tools and equipment most commonly used in vehicle extrication incidents.

> Personnel should be required to wear appropriate PPE when using any of this equipment.

Stabilization Equipment
One of the first and most important steps in performing vehicle extrication safely—for the rescuers and victims alike—is stabilizing the vehicle. As mentioned earlier, any sudden and unexpected movement of the vehicle while rescuers and victims are inside can be dangerous, even fatal. Therefore, rescuers must know how to use the resources available at the scene to quickly but securely stabilize the vehicle. The means used to stabilize vehicles most often include the application of cribbing, step chocks, shoring, and rigging.

Cribbing
In addition to the wooden cribbing that has been used in extrication operations for many years, some cribbing and other shoring devices available today are made of plastic, others are made of steel. Each type of cribbing has certain advantages and disadvantages, as well as certain capabilities and limitations.

Cribbing of all types is used along with wedges or shims. Wooden *wedges* are usually 4- x 4-inch material cut from corner to corner (Figure 3.11). The usual application for wedges is for two of them to be driven in from opposite sides to tighten cribbing or shoring. *Shims* are essentially of the same shape as wedges but may be cut from narrower stock. In addition, shims are used singularly to take up space between cribbing and the object being supported.

Wooden Cribbing. Much of the cribbing used in vehicle extrication is made of wood that is solid, straight, and free of major flaws such as large knots or splits. Various sizes of wood can be used, but the most common is 4- x 4-inch (100 mm x 100 mm) wood timbers (Figure 3.12). The length of the pieces may

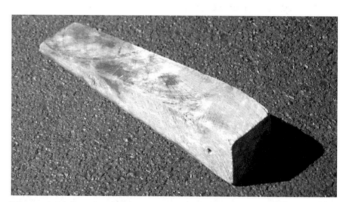

Figure 3.11 A typical wooden wedge.

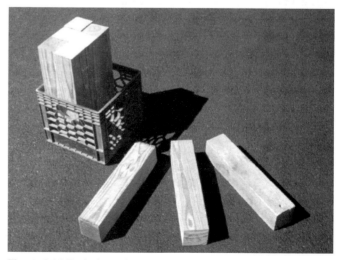

Figure 3.12 Typical wooden cribbing.

vary, but 18 to 22 inches (450 mm or 550 mm) is average. The ends of the pieces may be painted different colors for easy identification by length. Other surfaces of the cribbing should be free of any paint or finish because they can make the wood slippery, especially when it is wet. Cribbing pieces may have a hole through one end and a loop of rope or webbing tied through the hole to form a handle. Cribbing can be stacked in a compartment with the grab handles facing out for easy access, or it can be stored on end inside a plastic crate or other box.

Plastic Cribbing. A growing number of emergency response agencies are using cribbing made of recycled plastic (Figure 3.13). Plastic cribbing has the advantage of being impervious to oil, gasoline, and other substances that can soak into and contaminate wooden cribbing.

The most common application for cribbing in vehicle extrication is called a *box crib* (Figure 3.14). This cribbing arrangement is so named because of the box that is formed when the pieces are set. On a flat, level base, two pieces are set parallel approximately 13 inches (330 mm) apart. Two more pieces are then laid at right angles atop and across the ends of the first

two pieces. This process is continued until the desired height is reached. To maintain the stability of a box crib, the height of the cribbing stack should not exceed one and one-half times the length of the cribbing pieces being used.

A stack of cribbing seldom exactly fills the space between the base and the underside of the vehicle to be stabilized, but it is important that the cribbing fit that opening tightly to prevent any movement of the vehicle. Therefore, the gap between the top of the cribbing stack and the vehicle must be filled by driving a wooden shim into the gap atop each of the top cribbing pieces or by driving the shims beneath the stack. The shims are driven in until the fit is tight (Figure 3.15). Properly constructed, a box crib is a very stable support.

Another common application of the box crib is as a base for a pneumatic lifting bag. In this application, the top tier of cribbing must be solid — that is, with several pieces laid side by side so that there is no opening in the middle (Figure 3.16). Leaving an opening in the middle would allow the lifting bag to

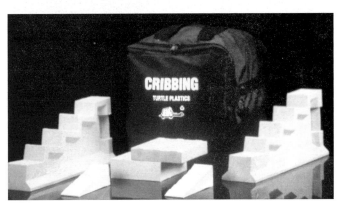

Figure 3.13 Typical plastic cribbing. *Courtesy of Turtle Plastics.*

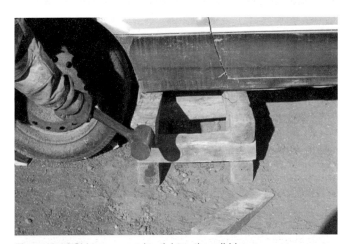

Figure 3.15 Shims are used to tighten the cribbing.

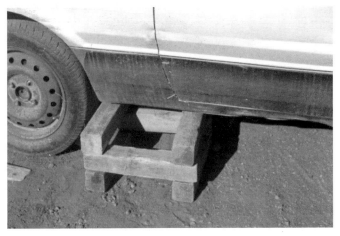

Figure 3.14 A properly constructed box crib.

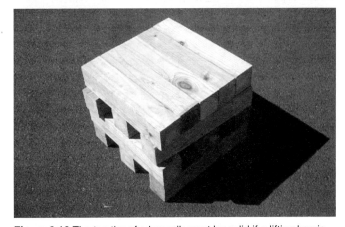

Figure 3.16 The top tier of a box crib must be solid if a lifting bag is used.

bulge into the opening, reducing its lifting efficiency and perhaps damaging the bag. The inflating bag might also push the top pieces off the side of the stack. To reduce the possibility of the pneumatic bag shifting atop the cribbing stack, some agencies place a mat

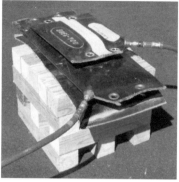

Figure 3.17 Placing a mat under the lifting bag increases safety.

made of foam rubber or belting material on top of the cribbing and under the lifting bag (Figure 3.17). However, regardless of the application, constructing box cribs can be a time-consuming process; therefore, it is usually faster to use ready-made steel cribbing or step chocks.

Metal Cribbing. Various equipment manufacturers now produce adjustable metal struts that can be used in place of box cribs. Some consist of a square steel tube attached to a base plate to spread the load and provide more secure footing. The lower tube houses another tube that telescopes from the first one. Both tubes are perforated with a series of holes along both sides that allow a pin to be inserted to hold the tubes at the desired length. Any space remaining between

the top of the tube and the bottom of the vehicle can be taken up with a screw jack in the end of the tube (Figure 3.18). Some innovative rescue agencies have fabricated their own versions of these devices (Figure 3.19). These devices can be extremely effective when applied to the right situation. However, as with any other tool or device, there are conditions that do not lend themselves to their use, and cribbing or step chocks may work better in these situations.

Step Chocks

Like box cribs, step chocks are so named because of the series of steps that are formed when they are fabricated. Some step chocks are made of recycled plastic; others are made of wood (Figure 3.20). Regardless of whether an agency purchases manufactured step chocks and other shoring materials or fabricates their own, they are advised to test these devices under controlled conditions that will allow them to identify the capabilities and limitations of each. Following that, SOPs can be developed for the safe and effective application of these devices.

Plastic chocks have the advantage of being impervious to fuel, oil, and other liquids that tend to soak into the wooden ones, and they are free of splinters. However, like wooden step chocks, plastic step chocks have certain disadvantages and limitations. It has been reported that until plastic step chocks and other shoring devices are worn by use or are intentionally abraded, their surfaces may have less purchase than wooden ones. This may allow them to slip under certain circumstances.

Wooden step chocks are constructed of a 2- x 6-inch (50 mm x 150 mm) base approximately 30 inches (762 mm) in length. Centered

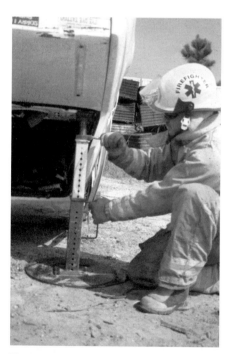

Figure 3.18 Metal cribbing is snugged up with a screw device. *Courtesy of Steve Bourne.*

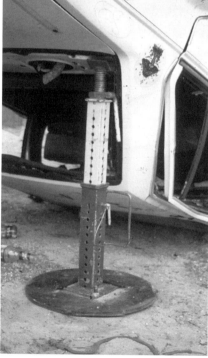

Figure 3.19 A homemade metal cribbing device. *Courtesy of Steve Bourne.*

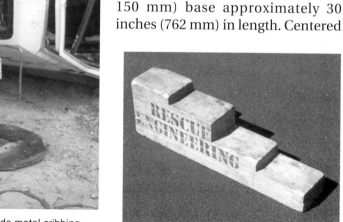

Figure 3.20 Typical step chocks.

on the base are progressively shorter lengths of 2- x 6-inch (50 mm x 150 mm) lumber stacked one upon the other. Each step is approximately 6 inches (150 mm) shorter than the one beneath. The total number of steps is limited only by the length of the base (Figure 3.21). Experience has shown that it is better to construct wooden step chocks by laminating the pieces together with wood glue and screws, rather than with nails.

A step chock is installed by placing it on a firm, level surface and pushing the entire unit under the vehicle until the entire device is under the vehicle or one of the steps makes contact with the side of the vehicle. However, the chock should not be installed where it would interfere with the swing of the vehicle's doors. Any space between the highest step under the vehicle and the underside of the vehicle is then eliminated by driving a shim under the step chock (Figure 3.22). In

some cases, especially when a vehicle is resting on its top, it is better to invert the chock and slide it under the vehicle like an oversized wedge (Figure 3.23). Plastic step chocks lend themselves to this technique.

Shoring

The term "shoring" is used interchangeably for both the process and the materials and equipment. Shoring is used in the same way as cribbing and step chocks when the opening to be spanned is too large to make either cribbing or chocks a practical way to stabilize the vehicle. Shoring may consist of 4- x 4-inch (100 mm x 100 mm) or larger timbers of any length (Figure 3.24). Or, manufactured pneumatic shores can be used (Figure 3.25). A third type of shoring system is one manufactured of square tubular

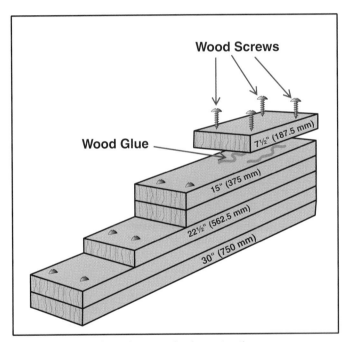

Figure 3.21 Typical wooden step chock construction.

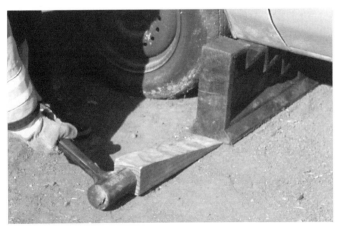

Figure 3.22 The chock is tightened with a shim.

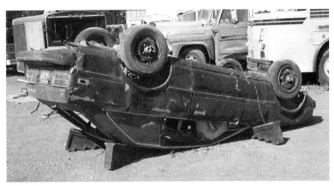

Figure 3.23 Another way to stabilize a vehicle.

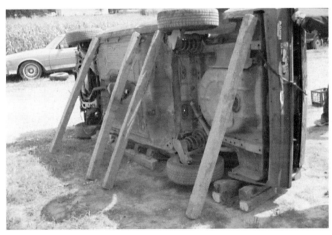

Figure 3.24 Typical wooden shoring.

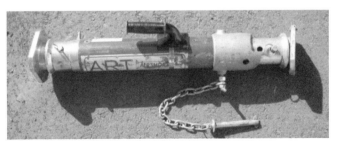

Figure 3.25 A typical manufactured air shore.

steel. The perforated steel sections telescope to the needed length, and the base is secured to the vehicle with one or more nylon straps (Figure 3.26).

Rigging

Rigging is a general term for some of the other tools and equipment that are used to stabilize vehicles. Rigging includes using rope, chains, and webbing.

Rope. Rope is one of the most versatile and useful items carried on fire apparatus and rescue vehicles. In vehicle extrication incidents, rope can be used for hoisting, lowering, rigging, and even crowd control, but its primary use is to secure and stabilize vehicles (Figure 3.27).

The rope used must be of high quality to withstand the stresses exerted on it, but it does not have to be life safety rope unless it is to suspend or support personnel. Rope rescue, including low-angle rescue, such as carrying an extrication victim up a slope in a basket litter, is beyond the scope of this manual. Therefore, the balance of this discussion will focus on the use of rope for securing and stabilizing vehicles.

Because non-life-safety rope is classified as "utility" rope, it may be made of manila fiber or any of the synthetics of which ropes are made. However, despite its great strength, nylon rope is not ideal for vehicle

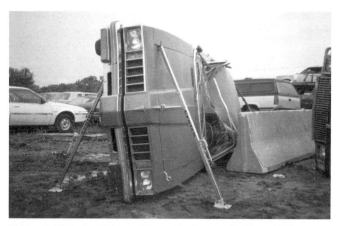

Figure 3.26 Typical telescoping metal shoring. *Courtesy of Steve Bourne*

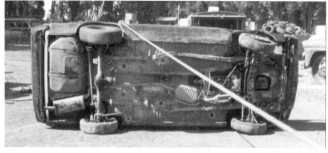

Figure 3.27 A vehicle stabilized with rope.

stabilization because it stretches under load. If a nylon rope must remain in place for an extended period, it may have to be retightened periodically. It is more efficient to use a different type of rope so that it can be applied and tensioned once and not have to be adjusted repeatedly during the operation.

Chains. With few exceptions, chain and webbing of the appropriate size and strength may be used interchangeably. However, because they are obviously different materials, they are discussed separately in this manual. From a safety standpoint, it is more important that rescuers know the capabilities and limitations of the chains and webbing available to them than which medium is used. Using chains and webbing beyond their limitations can result in their failure — perhaps catastrophically.

Only rescue-rated steel alloy chains should be used in vehicle extrication because they are strong and highly resistant to abrasion and chemical degradation. Special alloys are available that are resistant to corrosive or hazardous atmospheres. Proof coil chain, also known as common or hardware chain, is not suitable for use in vehicle extrication operations. The minimum chain size generally used for extrication operations is ⅜-inch (10 mm). For any operation, it is important to match the rated strength of the chain to the tools being used and the job being done. Table 3.1 lists the safe working loads for various sizes of chains.

Chain failures occur when the chain is abused or neglected in use or storage. Improper treatment of chain components leads to metal fatigue and chain failure. Regularly inspect chains link by link for signs of wear or damage. Remove defective chains from service. Table 3.2 lists the maximum allowable wear at any point of a link before the chain should be removed from service.

Hooks and attachments should be made of the same alloy material as the rest of the chain. All chains should have an attached tag that has the safe load weight stamped or printed on it. Hooks and attachments should have at least the same strength rating as, if not more than, the rest of the chain. In addition, observe the following safety rules when using chain:

- Do not drag a load with a chain under it.
- Do not cross, knot, or hammer a chain into position (for example, tying a knot in a chain to shorten it).
- Do not exceed the chain's listed safe working load.
- Do not use worn or damaged chains.

Table 3.1 Working Load Limits, Proof Test Loads and Minimum Breaking Loads for Alloy Steel Chain			
Nominal Size of Chain (in.)	Working Load Limit (lb)	Proof Test (lb)	Minimum Break (lb)
¼	3,250	6,500	10,000
⅜	6,600	13,200	19,000
½	11,250	22,500	32,500
⅝	16,500	33,000	50,000
¾	23,000	46,000	69,500
⅞	28,750	57,500	93,500
1	38,750	77,500	122,000
1⅛	44,500	89,000	143,000
1¼	57,500	115,000	180,000
1⅜	67,000	134,000	207,000
1½	80,000	160,000	244,000
1¾	100,000	200,000	325,000

Source: *Specification for Alloy Chain*, American Society for Testing and Materials, A-391-65. *Alloy Steel Chain Specifications, No. 3001*, National Association of Chain Manufacturers. Reprinted with permission.

- Do not impact load a chain.
- Do not connect chain hooks to anything but the chain itself.
- Do not weld links in alloy chain or otherwise expose them to excessive heat.
- Do not use chain appliances (hooks, pins, links, etc.) that are not of at least equal strength to the load being handled.
- Do not attempt to splice a chain by placing a bolt through two links.
- Do not apply force to a kinked chain — make sure that all the links are straight.

Webbing. Conventional webbing is made from the same materials used in synthetic ropes, so the same precautions and maintenance apply. The size of webbing varies with the intended use, but most webbing used for lifting and pulling operations starts at about 2 inches (50 mm) in width (Figure 3.28). The strength requirement for webbing is the same as for chain used in the same situation. One disadvantage of webbing is that it is susceptible to abrasion and chemical degradation. This makes it impractical for use in some extrication applications. If webbing must be used in a situation where it is susceptible to abrasion or chemical contamination, protect it with a salvage cover or similar material.

Table 3.2 (U.S.) Maximum Allowable Wear at any Point of Link	
Chain Size (in.)	Maximum Allowable Wear (in.)
¼	3/64
⅜	5/64
½	7/64
⅝	9/64
¾	5/32
⅞	11/64
1	3/16
1⅛	7/32
1¼	¼
1⅜	9/32
1½	5/16
1¾	11/32

Reprinted with permission from the National Safety Council: *Accident Prevention Manual for Industrial Operations: Engineering and Technology,* 9th edition, Chicago: National Safety Council, 1988.

Table 3.2 (Metric) Maximum Allowable Wear at any Point of Link	
Chain Size (mm)	Maximum Allowable Wear (mm)
6	1.2
10	2
13	2.8
16	3.6
20	4
22	4.4
25	4.8
29	5.6
32	6
35	7.1
38	7.9
45	8.7

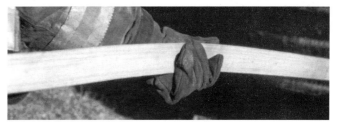
Figure 3.28 Typical webbing used in vehicle extrication.

There are two main types of webbing construction: flat and tubular. Both are similar in appearance except when viewed cross-sectionally. Tubular webbing is woven in two ways: spiral and chain. Generally, the spiral weave is stronger and more resistant to abrasion than the chain weave.

Hand Tools

The hand tools commonly used in vehicle extrication are many and varied. However, most of these tools are the same tools used for structural fire fighting and other emergency work. In general, these tools can be divided into three major categories: striking, prying, and cutting. The cutting tools category is further divided into subcategories including chopping tools, snipping tools, saws, and knives. Also often used in vehicle extrication are certain specialized hand tools and ordinary mechanic's tools — sockets and wrenches.

Striking Tools

The most common and basic hand tools are striking tools. Most striking tools have a heavy metal head mounted on one end of a relatively long handle. This category includes axes, battering rams, ram bars, punches, mallets, hammers, sledgehammers or mauls, and picks.

Striking tools can be dangerous and may cause serious crush or laceration injuries if used carelessly. High-velocity chips and splinters capable of piercing skin and eyes are sometimes produced when striking tools are used. Because of this danger, it is imperative that proper protective clothing be worn. Properly maintain all striking tools, with handles kept smooth and well set in the tool head. Keep the striking surface of the tool head free of chips and burrs. Keep axe blades clean and as sharp as their intended purpose and agency protocols dictate. Use striking tools with short, quick strokes. Long, sweeping strokes are more difficult to control and may strike anyone standing close by.

Prying Tools

Prying tools use leverage to provide a mechanical advantage. This means that using a prying tool properly can multiply the force applied. Prying tools are used to pry open doors, windows, hoods, and trunk lids of vehicles. These tools can even be used to lift vehicles or other heavy objects. The pry-axe, Halligan (Hooligan) tool, crow bar, claw tool, pry bar, Kelly tool, spanner wrench, and Quic-Bar® are examples of hand prying tools. Crowbars and other prying tools

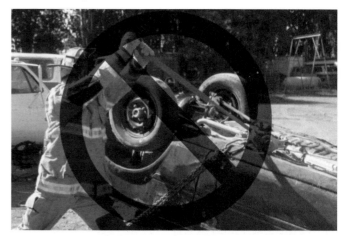

Figure 3.29 A "cheater" should never be used on a tool handle.

are excellent for widening a small opening for larger power tools to fit into.

When used correctly, prying tools are safer than are striking tools because of the absence of ballistic movement. However, prying tools can be just as dangerous as other types of tools if used incorrectly. For example, it is unsafe to strike the handle of a pry bar with another tool or to use a makeshift extension (sometimes called a "cheater") on the tool handle. A *cheater* is a piece of pipe slipped over the end of a prying tool handle to lengthen it, thus providing additional leverage (Figure 3.29). Using a cheater can exert forces on the tool that are greater than the tool was designed to handle. This can destroy the tool and perhaps cause serious injury to the operator or others. If a prying tool is inadequate for a particular application, use an additional tool or a larger one. Do not use prying tools as striking tools unless designed for that purpose.

Cutting Tools

Cutting tools are the most diversified of the tool groups. However, some cutting tools are designed to cut only specific types of materials. Misuse occurs when a tool is used to cut material that it was not designed to cut or to cut in a way for which the tool was not designed. Misuse can destroy the tool and endanger the operator. Manual cutting tools can be divided into the following four distinct groups:

- Chopping tools
- Snipping tools
- Saws
- Knives

Chopping Tools. These tools are characterized by a metal head with a cutting edge attached to one end of a relatively long handle. Chopping tools include the flat-head axe, pick-head axe, pry-axe, and various types of picks. To ensure maximum cutting efficiency of these tools, keep the cutting head free of paint and covered with a thin coating of light-grade machine oil. Keep the blade sharp, but not so sharp that the cutting edge chips when the tool is used. Check tool handles regularly for looseness, cracks, splinters, or warping. Maintain cutting tools according to agency protocols.

Snipping Tools. These tools are used in situations where the material must be cut in a controlled fashion or where space does not allow larger tools to be used. They are most effective on relatively thin material that can easily fit within the jaws of the tool. They are generally safer than other types of cutting devices when working close to the victim. Tools that fall into this category are various kinds of scissors or shears, tin snips, bolt cutters, and wire cutters.

Cutting tools that are often misused are the opposing-jaw metal cutters. The most common types of opposing-jaw metal cutters are bolt cutters and insulated wire cutters, sometimes called "hot wire" cutters (Figure 3.30). These tools are very similar in appearance, but they are not interchangeable. The most dangerous misuse is to use bolt cutters instead of insulated wire cutters; this can result in electrocution. Only cutting tools approved by a recognized agency, such as Underwriters Laboratories or Factory Mutual, and maintained according to the manufacturer's recommendations should ever be used to cut energized electrical wire.

> Rescuers must follow their agency's protocols, but using bolt cutters to cut downed power lines to facilitate a vehicle rescue is **NOT** recommended.

Saws. Handsaws are useful on objects that require a controlled cut but do not fit into the jaws of a manual opposing-jaw cutter. Using handsaws is usually more time consuming than using powered saws or shears. However, handsaws are safer to use when working close to the victim or when working in a hazardous atmosphere. Handsaws commonly used for extrication include carpenter's saws, hacksaws, coping saws, keyhole saws, and windshield cutters. The cutting efficiency of hacksaws can be increased by using two blades, installed in the same direction. However, this should only be done if the saw has an industrial quality frame. Keep all saw blades sharp,

clean, and lightly oiled. The cutting efficiency of any saw can be increased by periodically spraying the surface of the material being cut with a light oil or soapy water to reduce friction between the material and the saw blade.

The most specialized tool in this category is the windshield cutter or glass saw (Figure 3.31). This is a saw with a short, heavy blade having very coarse teeth. The windshield cutter is designed for one purpose only—to quickly and efficiently remove a windshield from a vehicle. When one of these devices is used, occupants in the front seat of the vehicle need to be protected from flying chips and splinters of glass.

Knives. Various types of knives may be useful in vehicle extrications. While a sharp pocket knife may be adequate in some situations, knives specially designed for vehicle rescue are usually more efficient. These specially designed knives include V-blade (seat belt) knives, linoleum knives, and utility knives (Figure 3.32). Sharpen or replace knife blades after each use to ensure that they are in optimum working condition for the next use.

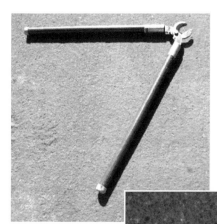

Figure 3.30 Approved "hot wire" cutters have nonconducting handles.

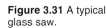

Figure 3.31 A typical glass saw.

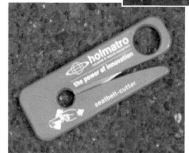

Figure 3.32 A typical seat belt cutter.

Specialized Hand Tools

Some of the hand tools used in extrication are so specialized that they are almost never used for anything else. The most common examples of this type of tool are spring-loaded center punches and glass hammers.

Center Punches. There are two basic types of center punches: standard and spring-loaded. A standard center punch is similar to a small chisel but with a pointed end. A spring-loaded center punch looks very similar to a standard punch but works much better for breaking tempered glass. A standard center punch can be used to break tempered glass, but it must be struck with another tool to provide the breaking force (Figure 3.33). A spring-loaded center punch provides its own breaking force when the tip is pressed against the glass (Figure 3.34).

Glass Hammers. Glass hammers consist of a pointed metal head attached to a plastic handle. They are used to break tempered glass by striking the glass with the point of the metal head. They are very effective at breaking glass, and some have a built-in seat belt cutter in the handle (Figure 3.35).

Lifting Tools

Except for pneumatic lifting bags, which are discussed later in this chapter, the primary lifting tools used in vehicle extrication are various forms of nonhydraulic jacks. The jacks most often used are various screw jacks and ratchet-lever jacks. Several types of nonhydraulic jacks are considered hand tools because they do not operate with hydraulic power. Although these tools are effective for their designed purposes, they do not have the same motive force as hydraulic jacks.

Screw Jacks. These are mechanical devices that can be elevated or depressed simply by turning a threaded shaft, making them among the easiest jacks to operate. Check screw jacks for wear after each use. Keep them clean and lightly lubricated, particularly the threaded shaft. The foot plates on which the jacks rest should also be checked for wear or damage. The two most common types of screw jacks used in vehicle extrication are the bar screw jack and the folding screw jack.

The *bar screw jack* is an excellent tool for stabilizing loads, but is considered impractical for lifting. The jack is extended or retracted by turning a threaded vertical shaft with a bar inserted into one of several holes in the jack's head.

The *folding screw jack*, also know as a *scissor jack*, is made up of a top and bottom plate separated by levers

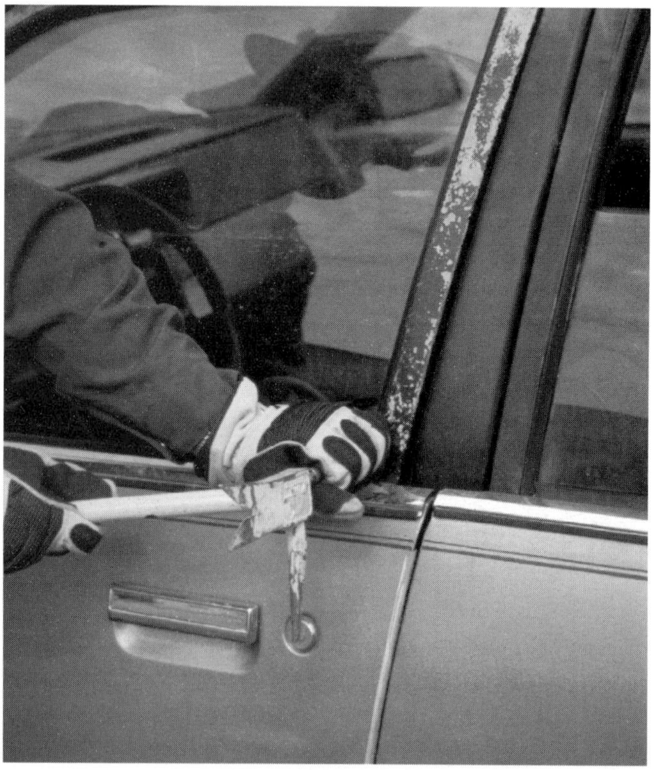

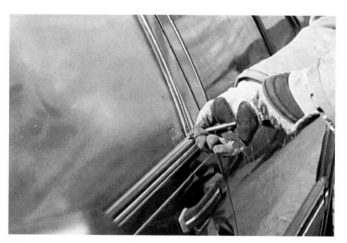

Figure 3.34 A spring-loaded center punch can be used alone.

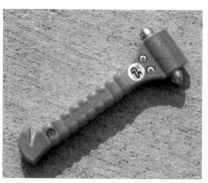

Figure 3.35 A typical glass hammer.

Figure 3.33 A standard center punch must be struck with another tool.

that are drawn together or pushed apart by the action of a threaded shaft being turned (Figure 3.36). The main advantage of folding jacks is that when fully collapsed they fit into relatively small spaces (4- to 6-inch [100 mm to 150 mm] clearance). Folding jacks are not always stable under load and are therefore considered safe only for light loads.

Ratchet-Lever Jacks. Sometimes called hi-lift jacks, these jacks consist of a vertical metal shaft, with notches or gear cogs along one side, that fits into a metal base plate. A movable jacking carriage fits around the shaft and has two ratchets on the notched side. One ratchet holds the carriage in position while the other works with a lever to move the carriage up or down. The ratchet jack is a good medium-duty jack but is the least stable under load (Figure 3.37). This type of jack can be used for limited spreading operations in the absence of hydraulic rams.

Mechanic's Tools
In some cases, especially when working very close to a trapped victim, it is better to disassemble a part of the vehicle rather than use a power saw or similar tool to cut it. This eliminates the noise, vibration, and sparks produced by powered cutting tools. Rescue vehicles should carry a basic set of ordinary mechanic's tools — primarily sockets, wrenches, pliers, and drivers.

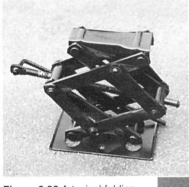

Figure 3.36 A typical folding screw jack.

Figure 3.37 A typical ratchet-lever jack.

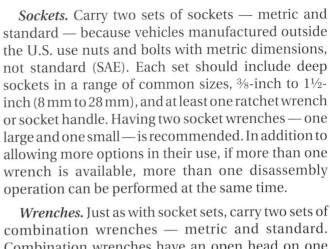

Sockets. Carry two sets of sockets — metric and standard — because vehicles manufactured outside the U.S. use nuts and bolts with metric dimensions, not standard (SAE). Each set should include deep sockets in a range of common sizes, ⅜-inch to 1½-inch (8 mm to 28 mm), and at least one ratchet wrench or socket handle. Having two socket wrenches — one large and one small — is recommended. In addition to allowing more options in their use, if more than one wrench is available, more than one disassembly operation can be performed at the same time.

Wrenches. Just as with socket sets, carry two sets of combination wrenches — metric and standard. Combination wrenches have an open head on one end and a closed head on the other end. This, too, allows more flexibility in their use. Obviously, both sets of wrenches should include a range of common sizes. In addition to the combination wrenches, also carry adjustable wrenches of various sizes.

Pliers. A variety of types and sizes of pliers should be part of the tool inventory of any rescue vehicle. Carry various sizes of conventional pliers, Channel-Lock® type pliers, Vise-Grip® pliers, and wire cutting pliers.

Drivers. The rescue vehicle's tool inventory should also include a variety of drivers — screw drivers and nut drivers. Include both Phillips head and straight screwdrivers in more than one size. Carry two sets of nut drivers — metric and standard — in a range of common sizes. Other drivers, such as Torx® drivers (sometimes called star drivers) should also be included.

Pneumatic (Air-Powered) Tools
Pneumatic tools use the energy of compressed air for power. Air pressure can be supplied by vehicle-mounted air compressors, apparatus brake system compressors, SCBA tanks, or cascade system cylinders. The most commonly used pneumatic tools in extrication are pneumatic chisels/hammers and pneumatic wrenches.

WARNING!
Never use compressed oxygen to power pneumatic tools. Mixing pure oxygen with tool lubricants can result in fire or violent explosion.

Pneumatic Chisels/Hammers
Most pneumatic-powered chisels (also called air chisels, air hammers, or impact hammers) are designed to

operate at air pressures between 100 and 150 psi (700 kPa and 1 050 kPa). Others operate up to 300 psi (2 100 kPa). In normal operation, they will use about 4 to 5 cubic feet (113 L to 142 L) of air per minute. Air chisels can be especially effective for auto extrication by cutting through the roof, roof support posts or doorjambs, seat bolts, and door lock assemblies (Figure 3.38). They are good for cutting medium- to heavy-gauge sheet metal and for popping rivets and bolts. However, cutting heavier gauge steel or other metals requires larger air supplies and higher pressures.

A variety of air chisel bits are available to fit many vehicle extrication situations. In addition to cutting bits, special bits for operations such as breaking locks or driving in plugs are also available. All bits should be kept sharpened and free of defects at all times.

CAUTION: Sparks produced when using air chisels in hazardous atmospheres may ignite flammable vapors.

Pneumatic Wrenches

Also known as impact wrenches, these tools are extremely useful for disassembling vehicle components (Figure 3.39). With an adequate air supply and the right size socket, these tools can remove nuts and bolts very rapidly. Their chief disadvantage is that they are quite noisy in operation.

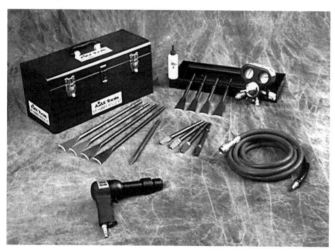

Figure 3.38 A complete air chisel set. *Courtesy of Ajax Tools.*

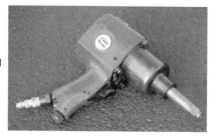

Figure 3.39 Impact wrenches are very useful for removing body components.

Pneumatic Lifting Bags

These devices allow rescuers to lift or displace objects that cannot be lifted with standard extrication equipment. There are three basic types of lifting bags: high pressure, medium pressure, and low pressure. A fourth type of bag is used for sealing leaks but has little or no application in vehicle extrication.

High-pressure bags are constructed of neoprene rubber reinforced with either steel wire or Kevlar® aramid fiber and have a rough, pebble-grained, surface to improve purchase. Before inflation, the bags lie virtually flat and are about 1 inch (25 mm) thick (Figure 3.40). They come in various sizes that range from 6 x 6 inches (150 mm x 150 mm) to 36 x 36 inches (914 mm x 914 mm). Depending on the size of the bags, they may inflate to a height of 20 inches (500 mm). The largest bags can lift around 75 tons (68 040 kg). The range of inflation pressure of the bags is about 116 – 145 psi (812 – 1 015 kPa).

Low- and medium-pressure bags are considerably larger than high-pressure bags and are most commonly used to lift or temporarily stabilize large vehicles or objects. Their primary advantage over high-pressure air bags is that they have a much greater lifting range. Depending on the manufacturer and the model, these bags may be able to lift an object upwards of 6 feet (2 m) (Figure 3.41). Low- and medium-pressure bags generally operate on 7 to 15 psi (49 kPa to 105 kPa), again depending on the manufacturer.

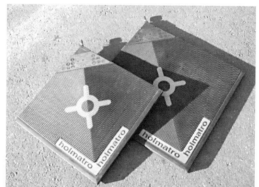

Figure 3.40 Typical high-pressure lifting bags.

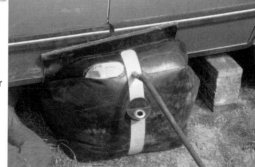

Figure 3.41 A low-pressure lifting bag under a vehicle.

Along with their accompanying hardware, leak-sealing bags are designed to be inserted into cracks or holes in low-pressure liquid storage containers or in the open ends of pipes. These bags are constructed much like high-pressure bags but are designed to be inflated at a much lower pressure, usually around 25 psi (175 kPa).

Pneumatic Lifting Bag Safety

Pneumatic lifting bags have a variety of applications in vehicle extrication incidents. They can be inserted into openings that are too small for other lifting equipment, and they are relatively quick and easy to use. However, their use is not without some risks. To minimize these risks, operators should observe the following safety rules when using pneumatic lifting bags:

- Plan the operation before starting the work.

- Be thoroughly familiar with the equipment, its operating principles, capabilities, and limitations.

- Consult individual operator's manuals and follow the recommendations for the specific system used.

- Keep all components in good operating condition and all safety seals in place.

- Have an adequate air supply and sufficient cribbing on hand before beginning operations.

- Position bags on or against a solid surface.

- Never inflate bags against sharp objects — use a protective mat.

- Never inflate bags fully unless they are under load.

- Inflate bags slowly and monitor them continuously for any shifting.

- Never work under a load supported only by lifting bags.

- Shore up the load with enough cribbing to support the load in case of bag failure.

- Interrupt the process frequently to increase shoring or cribbing — *lift an inch, crib an inch.*

- Ensure that the top tier is solid when using box cribbing and that a protective mat is used.

- Avoid exposing bags to materials hotter than 220°F (104°C). Insulate the bags with a nonflammable material. Bags should be removed from service if any evidence of heat damage is seen.

- Never stack more than two bags; center the bags with the smaller bag on top and inflate the bottom bag first (½ to ⅔ full), then inflate the top bag fully. If more height is needed, add more air to the bottom bag.

- Stacked bags can only lift the capacity of the lowest rated bag.

Electric Tools

In addition to the electrical lighting equipment discussed elsewhere in this chapter, a variety of electrically operated tools are used in vehicle extrication. The tools most often used are electric spreaders, electric saws, and electric wrenches.

Electric Spreaders

At least one manufacturer offers an electrically operated spreader that is similar in every other way to the hydraulic spreaders discussed later in this section (Figure 3.42). The electric spreader is lighter and more portable than many of the hydraulic units. Like the hydraulic units, the electric spreader can be equipped with conventional spreader arms for pushing and pulling, or with optional cutter arms. The electric spreader weighs approximately 40 pounds (18 kg) and is powered by a 12-volt DC power pack weighing 35 pounds (16 kg), which the operator can wear on his back. The electric spreader can also be converted to a straight cutting tool (Figure 3.43).

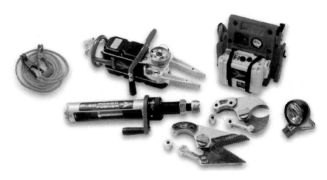

Figure 3.42 An electric extrication tool set. *Courtesy of Curtiss-Wright Rescue Systems.*

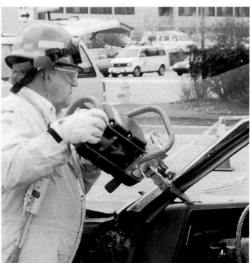

Figure 3.43
An electric shear cuts through a door post. *Courtesy of Curtiss-Wright Rescue Systems.*

Electric Saws

The electric saws used in vehicle extrication — except for reciprocating saws — are simply electrically operated versions of the other power saws discussed later in this chapter. There are electrically operated chain saws, reciprocating saws, and circular saws. Like all other tools, electrically operated tools have advantages and disadvantages. Among their advantages are that they are often lighter in weight and quieter in operation than gasoline-driven tools. However, their disadvantages include being tethered to a power supply by a power cord, and unless they are designed to be intrinsically safe, they cannot be operated in potentially flammable atmospheres.

Reciprocating Saws. These saws are easy to control and are well suited for cutting metal or wood because they produce far fewer sparks and airborne debris than does a rotary rescue saw. A reciprocating saw may be required when overhead cuts must be made or in areas where space is limited (Figure 3.44). This saw has a short, straight blade that moves forward and backward — an action similar to that of a handsaw. When equipped with metal-cutting blades, reciprocating saws are also extremely effective on bus and automobile extrication incidents. Other than the frame, these saws can easily cut almost any portion of a bus or automobile body to provide access to victims. Reciprocating saws are also much easier to control and are safer to use than circular saws.

Electric Circular Saws. Unlike the gasoline-powered circular saws (rotary rescue saws) discussed later in this chapter, the electrically operated circular saws used in vehicle extrication are usually the same as those used in construction. They are primarily designed for cutting wood, and they can be very useful when cutting shoring material on site. When equipped with a metal-cutting blade, they may also be used to make straight-line cuts in light-gauge sheet metal.

Electric Impact Wrenches

Electric wrenches are similar to the pneumatic impact wrenches discussed earlier in this chapter. They are used for the same purposes as the pneumatic versions (Figure 3.45). Depending upon the brand and model, they may or may not be as powerful as the pneumatic wrenches.

Electric Screwdrivers

Improvements in the batteries used to power electric screwdrivers have made these tools extremely useful in vehicle extrication incidents (Figure 3.46). With replaceable battery packs, these tools produce sufficient torque and rotational speed to be very effective for use in dismantling vehicle components.

Hydraulic Tools

There are two categories of hydraulic tools used for vehicle extrication: powered and manual. While most agencies that deliver vehicle extrication services use powered hydraulic tools and equipment on most extrication incidents, there are still situations that require the use of manual hydraulic tools and equipment. The following sections describe both types of tools.

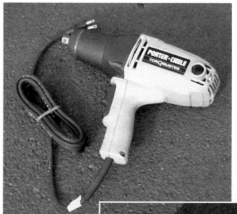

Figure 3.45 A typical electric impact wrench.

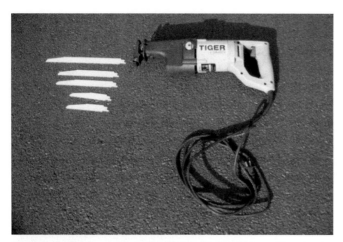

Figure 3.44 Reciprocating saws are excellent tools for cutting sheet metal.

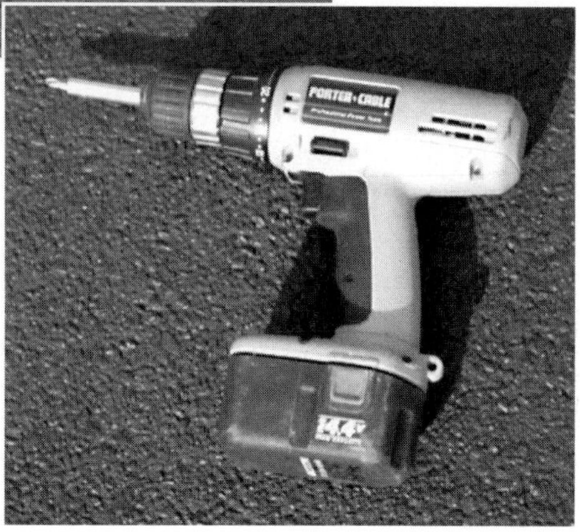

Figure 3.46 A typical cordless electric screwdriver.

Manual Hydraulic Tools

Manual hydraulic tools operate on the same principles as powered hydraulic tools except that the hydraulic pump is manually powered by someone operating a pump lever. The primary disadvantage of manual hydraulic tools is that they operate slower than powered hydraulic tools and with more limited range of operation. Two manual hydraulic tools are used most frequently in vehicle extrication: the porta-power system and the hydraulic jack.

Porta-Power®. The porta-power tool system is basically an auto body shop tool used for vehicle extrication. It operates by transmitting hydraulic pressure from a hand-pumped compressor through a hose to a tool assembly. A number of different tool accessories give the porta-power a variety of applications (Figure 3.47).

The primary advantage of the porta-power over the hydraulic jack is that the porta-power has accessories that allow it to be operated in narrow places in which the jack will not fit or cannot be operated. The primary disadvantage of the porta-power is that assembling complex combinations of accessories and actual operation of the tool are time consuming.

Hydraulic Jacks. Hydraulic jacks are excellent devices for many heavy lifting situations and for shoring or stabilizing operations. Hydraulic jacks operate on the principle that the pressure of liquids between two interconnected chambers of unequal size tends to equalize. A small chamber is used to pump fluid into a larger chamber. The energy applied is multiplied by the surface area differential to do more work in the large chamber. There is a check valve between the chambers that keeps the liquid from flowing back. Hydraulic jacks are available in capacities up to 20 tons (18 144 kg) or larger.

When using any kind of jack, hydraulic or otherwise, a good base is the primary consideration, followed by adequate blocking and cribbing. The load must be blocked or cribbed as it is lifted to reduce the chances of it falling. The weight of the load being lifted is transmitted to the base of the jack. Therefore, to prevent the jack from sinking into the surface, place it on a weight-distributing base. This spreads the force placed on the jack. The base may be a wide board or steel plate; it should be solid, flat, and level. If it is not level, it should be shimmed level, making sure enough room remains to place the jack.

> # WARNING!
> **Personnel should never work under a load supported by a jack only. If the jack fails, severe injury or death may result. Always make sure that the load is also supported by properly placed cribbing.**

Power-Driven Hydraulic Tools

The development of power-driven hydraulic extrication tools has revolutionized the process of removing victims from various types of entrapments. The wide range of uses, the speed, and the superior power of these tools have made them the primary tools used in most extrication situations. These tools receive their power from hydraulic fluid under pressure supplied through special hoses from a pump, commonly referred to as the *power unit* (Figure 3.48). Although a few hydraulic power units are operated by compressed air, most are powered either by electric motors or by two- or four-cycle gasoline engines. These power units may be portable and carried with the tool, or they may be permanently mounted on the vehicle and con-

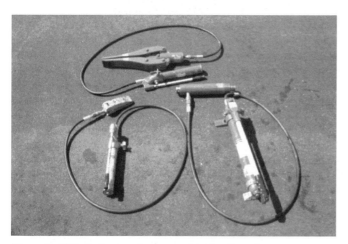

Figure 3.47 Typical manually-operated hydraulic tools.

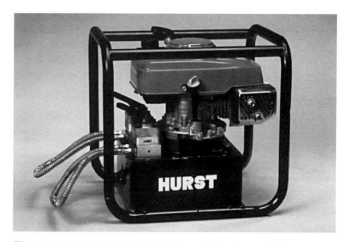

Figure 3.48 A typical hydraulic power unit. *Courtesy of Hale Products.*

nected to a hose reel. The tools powered by these units may be powered by manually operated pumps if the power unit fails. There are four basic types of powered hydraulic tools used in vehicle extrication: spreaders, shears, combination spreader/shears, and extension rams.

Spreaders. Powered hydraulic spreaders were the first powered hydraulic tools to become available for vehicle extrication. They are useful for a variety of different operations involving either pushing or pulling (Figure 3.49). Depending on the brand and model, some tools can produce more than 49,000 psi (343 000 kPa) of force. The tips of some tools may spread apart as much as 40 inches (1 016 mm), although many smaller, lighter units are also in use.

> Rescue personnel must know the capabilities and limitations of the extrication tools and equipment available to them.

Shears. When powered hydraulic extrication tools were first introduced, cutting was achieved by adding a cutting adapter to the tips of the spreader arms. Now, individual hydraulic shears are available for cutting roof support posts and other objects (Figure 3.50). These shears are capable of cutting almost any object (metal, plastic, wood) that will fit between their blades, although some models cannot cut case-hardened steel or high-strength low-alloy (HSLA) steel. Shears are typically capable of developing up to 100,000 psi (700 000 kPa) of cutting force and have an opening spread of up to about 9 inches (229 mm).

Combination Spreader/Shears. Several manufacturers of powered hydraulic extrication equipment now offer a combination spreader/shears tool. This tool consists of two arms equipped with spreader tips that can be used for pulling or pushing. The insides of the arms contain cutting shears similar to those described in the shears section (Figure 3.51). These tools are excellent for use on small initial response vehicles or in areas where limited resources prevent the purchase of larger and more expensive individual spreader and cutting tools. The combination tool's spreading and cutting capabilities may be more or less than those of the individual units, although the spreading capability is usually less.

Pedal Cutters. Originally designed for cutting reinforcing steel bars in construction, these powerful little devices cut pedal arms with ease (Figure 3.52). They can be used to cut virtually anything that will fit between the blade and the anvil.

Extension Rams. Extension rams are designed primarily for straight pushing operations, although they are effective at pulling as well (Figure 3.53). They

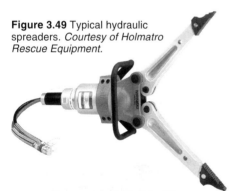

Figure 3.49 Typical hydraulic spreaders. *Courtesy of Holmatro Rescue Equipment.*

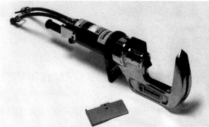

Figure 3.52 A typical pedal cutter shown with an optional crimping blade. *Courtesy of Champion Rescue Tools.*

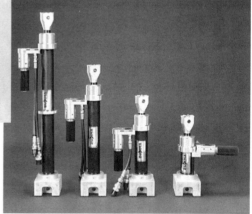

Figure 3.53 Typical hydraulic extension rams. *Courtesy of Amkus Rescue Systems.*

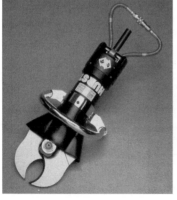

Figure 3.50 Typical hydraulic shears. *Courtesy of Hale Products.*

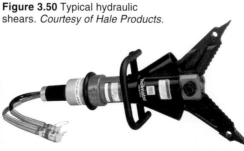

Figure 3.51 A typical spreader/shears combination tool. *Courtesy of Holmatro Rescue Equipment.*

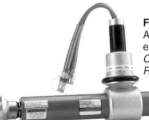

Figure 3.54 A telescoping hydraulic extension ram. *Courtesy of Holmatro Rescue Equipment.*

are especially valuable when it is necessary to push objects further than the maximum opening distance of the hydraulic spreaders. The largest of these extension rams can extend from a closed length of 36 inches (914 mm) to an extended length of nearly 63 inches (1 600 mm). They open with a pushing force of more than 48,000 psi (336 000 kPa). The closing force is about one-half that of the opening force.

Some manufacturers now offer telescoping extension rams (Figure 3.54). From a retracted length of as little as 12 inches (300 mm), some telescoping rams will extend to as much as 50 inches (1 250 mm). Unlike conventional hydraulic rams, telescoping rams cannot be used for pulling.

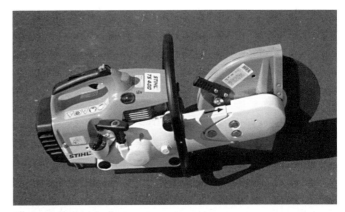

Figure 3.55 A typical rotary rescue saw.

Other Extriction Tools and Equipment

A variety of other tools and pieces of equipment are used in vehicle extrication. The categories discussed here are power saws, thermal cutting tools, and lifting/pulling tools.

Power Saws

Power saws are available in various designs, depending upon the purpose for which they are intended. It is important that the operator know the limitations of each type of power saw. When a saw (or any tool) is forced beyond the limits of its design and purpose, two things may occur: tool failure (including breakage) and/or injury to the operator. In addition, power saws of all types create sparks when cutting metal. They also create chips and splinters when cutting wood, plastic, glass, and other similar materials. Both the rescuers and victims need to be protected from this ballistic debris, as well as from the heat and noise generated by the cutting operation. Rescuers can be protected by wearing appropriate PPE. Trapped victims can be protected with a blanket or salvage cover spread over them and with ear plugs or other hearing protection.

Reciprocating Saws

These saws were discussed earlier in the section on Electric Tools.

Rotary Saws

Also called rotary rescue saws, these versatile tools may be used for cutting a variety of materials when equipped with the appropriate blade for the specific material being cut (Figure 3.55). In general, there are steel blades with carbide tips for cutting wood, and Carborundum® or other abrasive blades for cutting

masonry and metals. Because the abrasive blades can degrade when exposed to hydrocarbon vapors, these blades should not be stored in the same compartment with fuel containers.

Rescue saws must be used with extreme care to avoid injury to operators and trapped victims. Protect victims and rescue personnel in close proximity to the cutting operation from sparks when cutting metal and from chips and splinters when cutting wood. At least one charged hoseline should be standing by when metal is being cut. In addition to providing fire protection, water from the hoseline can be used to cool the saw blade by applying a fine mist to the blade while it is in operation. However, the cooling water must be started BEFORE cutting begins and continued throughout the cutting operation. Putting cold water on a hot blade may cause it to shatter and disintegrate. As with any other power tool, wear full protective clothing with face and eye protection when using circular saws.

CAUTION: The rotation of the blade of these saws creates significant torque that can cause the operator to lose control of the saw.

Chain Saws

Both electric- and gasoline-powered chain saws can be useful in some extrication situations. If chain saws are used, they should be powerful enough to penetrate dense material, yet lightweight enough to be easily handled in awkward positions. Chain saws equipped with carbide-tipped chains are capable of penetrating a large variety of materials, including light sheet metal. Although carbide-tipped chains cost almost four times as much as standard chains, they last twelve times longer.

While chain saws are capable of cutting the sheet metal and plastic parts of most vehicles, they often create more sparks, vibration, and noise than other saws. These characteristics can frighten trapped victims in close proximity to the cutting operation, and they are in danger of being struck by the cutting chain if it breaks while cutting. Therefore, chain saws are sometimes used to cut windshields, but are primarily used to cut timbers for shoring and cribbing material, or for cutting trees and heavy brush to clear the scene.

Power Saw Safety

Used improperly, power saws can be very dangerous for both rescuers and trapped victims. However, following a few simple safety rules will prevent most injuries from power saws:

- Match the saw to the task and the material to be cut. Never force a saw beyond its design limitations.

- Always wear appropriate protective equipment, including gloves, eye protection, and hearing protection.

- Do not use any power saw when working in a flammable atmosphere or near flammable liquids.

- Keep unprotected and nonessential people out of the work area.

- Follow manufacturer's guidelines for proper saw operation.

- Keep blades and chains well sharpened. A dull saw is more likely to malfunction than a sharp one.

Thermal Cutting Devices

To free trapped victims, it is sometimes necessary to cut through materials that are too dense to be cut with power saws. In these situations, a variety of thermal cutting tools can be used. The ones most commonly used are exothermic cutting devices, oxyacetylene cutting torches, and plasma cutters.

CAUTION: Before rescue personnel attempt to use any thermal cutting tool, they must be thoroughly trained in the safe operation of the tool to be used.

Exothermic Cutting Devices

Also known as burning bars, these devices are ultra-high-temperature burning tools that are capable of cutting through virtually any metallic, nonmetallic, or composite material (Figure 3.56). Most often used in railroad emergencies, they cut through materials, such as concrete or brick, that cannot be cut with an oxyacetylene torch, and they cut through heavy gauge metals much faster. The device produces temperatures in excess of 8,000°F (4 154°C). The cutting bars or

rods range in size from ¼- to ¾-inch (6 mm to 10 mm) in diameter and from 22 to 36 inches (550 mm to 900 mm) in length.

A similar exothermic cutting device is called an ARC-Aire®. This tool uses a hollow magnesium rod fitted into a handle that flows oxygen through the rod. The rod is ignited by an electric striker and burns down as the oxygen is increased. This tool produces temperatures from 6,000° to 10,000°F (3 298° to 5 520°C). The rods last between 15 and 30 seconds.

Plasma-Arc Cutters

Like burning bars, plasma-arc cutters are also ultra-high-temperature metal-cutting devices, generating temperatures of up to 50,000°F (28 000°C). In operation, up to 200 amperes of electrical power is fed to an arc rod that melts the metal being cut. A jet of extremely hot gas (usually air, nitrogen, or a mixture of argon and hydrogen or argon and helium) is used to blow the molten metal away from the cutting area.

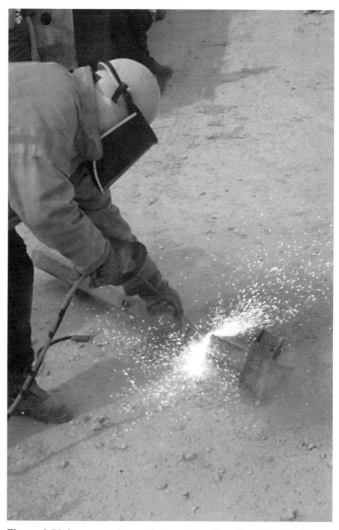

Figure 3.56 A rescuer demonstrates an exothermic cutting device.

Oxyacetylene Cutting Torches

Like the exothermic cutting device, the oxyacetylene cutting torch cuts by burning (Figure 3.57). It can be used for cutting heavy gauge metal that is resistant to more conventional extrication equipment. The torch preheats the metal to its ignition temperature, then burns a path in the metal with an extremely hot cone of flame caused by the introduction of pure oxygen into the flame.

Like all other cutting devices that operate with a highly flammable gas and produce a flame, use oxyacetylene cutting torches with extreme caution. Do not use cutting torches in any area in which the atmosphere may be flammable. It is also advisable to have charged hoselines in place before beginning cutting torch operations. Cutting torch operators should be experienced and efficient in using the tool in all situations. Anyone who uses a cutting torch should train regularly in exercises that present a variety of cutting problems.

Another hazard associated with cutting torches is the storage of oxygen and acetylene. Always keep oxygen and acetylene cylinders in an upright position,

whether they are in use or in storage. Acetylene is an unstable gas that is both pressure and shock sensitive. Acetylene storage cylinders, however, are designed to keep the gas stable and safe to use. The cylinders contain a porous filler of calcium silicate, which prevents accumulations of free acetylene within the cylinder. They also contain liquid acetone in which the acetylene is dissolved and stored in liquid form. When an acetylene cylinder's valve is opened, the gas leaves the mixture as it travels through the torch hoseline assembly.

> **WARNING!**
> Keep acetylene cylinders in an upright position to prevent acetone, a flammable liquid, from flowing through the cylinder valve and pooling in the work area.

Oxyacetylene cutting torches generate an extremely hot flame. For preheating metal, the flame temperature in air is approximately 4,200°F (2 316°C). When pure oxygen is added through the torch handle assembly, a flame of over 5,700°F (3 149°C) is created. This is hot enough to burn through iron and steel with relative ease.

Cutting Torch Safety. As mentioned earlier, oxyacetylene cutting torches are potentially dangerous tools. However, by observing the following safety rules, most malfunctions and injuries can be avoided:

* Store and use acetylene cylinders in an upright position to prevent loss of acetone. When an acetylene cylinder is "empty" of acetylene, it still contains acetone. Never place empty cylinders on their sides.

* Handle cylinders carefully to prevent damage to the cylinder or the filler. A dent in the cylinder indicates that the filler may be damaged. If the filler is damaged, voids are created where free acetylene can pool and decompose, creating a potentially explosive condition. Dropping a cylinder may also cause the fuse plug to leak, creating a dangerous condition. Mark dented acetylene cylinders, and return them to the supplier.

* Avoid exposing cylinders to excessive heat. This means that an ambient air temperature exceeding 130°F (54°C) is undesirable for storing or using acetylene cylinders.

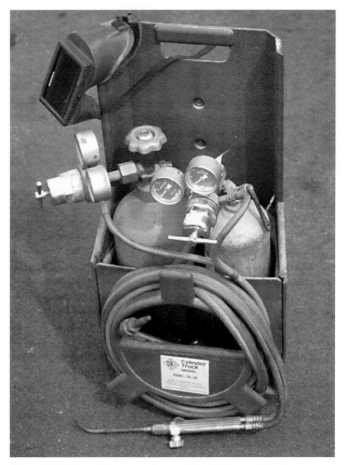

Figure 3.57 A typical oxyacetylene cutting torch used in vehicle extrication.

- Do not store acetylene cylinders on wet or damp surfaces. Cylinders rust at the bottom as protective paint is worn away.

- Store acetylene cylinders in an area physically separated from oxygen cylinders and other oxidizing gas cylinders. Segregate full acetylene cylinders from empty or partially full cylinders. Design storage areas to prevent acetylene cylinders from falling over.

- Perform a soap test (applying a solution of soap and water on fittings) to detect leaks after making regulator, torch, hose, and cylinder connections. Slow leaks in confined areas permit acetylene to accumulate in concentrations above the lower flammability limit. Acetylene has a wide flammability range: 2.5 percent to 81.0 percent by volume in air. Remove leaking cylinders to an open area immediately. Do not attempt to stop a fuse plug leak.

- Open acetylene cylinder valves no more than three-quarters of one turn. Do not use wrenches on cylinders that have handle valves. If the valve resists being turned, do not force it. Take the cylinder out of service immediately, and return it to the supplier for service.

- Do not use acetylene at pressures greater than 15 psi (103 kPa). Acetylene decomposes rapidly at high pressures and may explode as decomposition occurs.

- Do not exceed a withdrawal rate of one-seventh of the cylinder capacity per hour.

- Keep valves closed when not in use and when the cylinders are empty. After the valves are closed, bleed off the pressure in the regulator and in the torch assembly. Keep unconnected cylinders capped, whether they are full or empty, to prevent damage to fittings.

Lifting/Pulling Tools

Often, rescue personnel have to lift or pull a vehicle from a victim. The vehicle may weigh several tons (or tonnes), and the lift or pull may range from only 1 or 2 inches (25 mm to 50 mm) to several feet (meters). A variety of extrication tools have been developed to assist in this task. These include winches, come-alongs, and block and tackles.

Winches

Vehicle-mounted winches are excellent pulling tools. They can be deployed much quicker than a come-along and generally have a greater travel or pulling distance. The winch is usually mounted either on the front or rear bumper of the vehicle. The three most common drives for winches are electric, hydraulic, and power take-off. Either chain or steel cable wound on a drum is used for pulling. If a winch-equipped agency vehicle is not available at an extrication incident, the winch on a private tow truck can be used.

The rated capacity of winches varies; however, the winch is rated at its capacity when the first layer of cable is still on the drum. Winch and cable strength are strongest on the first wrap around the drum. As more cable is wrapped around the drum and the cable becomes layered, the strength decreases. As more cable is taken off the drum, the strength capacity increases. For safety reasons, do not remove the last layer of cable.

Many winches are equipped with hand-held, remote-control operating devices. These devices allow the operator to get a better view of the operation and, more importantly, allow the operator to remain outside of the winch danger zone. The *winch danger zone* is a circle around the winch with a radius equal to the length of cable or chain from the winch to the load (Figure 3.58). Staying outside of this circle protects the winch operator in case the cable or chain breaks.

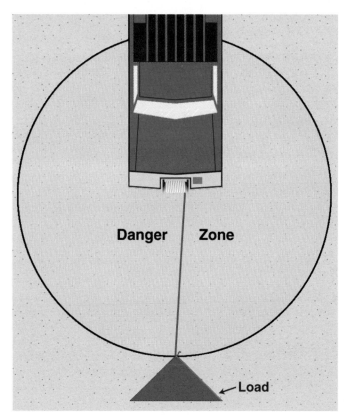

Figure 3.58 The danger zone in a vehicle-mounted winch operation.

In operation, the winch should be positioned as close to the load as possible in order to limit the length of cable or chain between the winch and the load. This reduces the size of the danger zone and, therefore, the chances of the operator or anyone else being struck by a broken cable or chain.

Like all other extrication tools and equipment, inspect winches periodically and after each use to ensure that they are in proper working condition. Inspecting the cable or chain for wear or damage and following the manufacturer's recommended preventive maintenance schedule should be all that is necessary.

Come-Alongs

Another lifting or pulling tool often used is the come-along (Figure 3.59). The most common sizes or ratings of come-alongs are 1 to 10 tons (907 kg to 9 072 kg). This tool uses leverage and a ratchet/pulley mechanism to increase pulling capacity. The come-along has a drum that is rotated by a lever handle directly or through gear action. A cable or chain is attached to the drum which makes the effective pull of the come-along equal to the length of the cable. The come-along is anchored to a secure object, and the cable is run out to the load to be moved. Once both ends are attached, the lever handle is operated to pull the load toward the anchor point. The lever handles on some come-alongs are designed to bend before the chain or cable reaches the breaking point.

Block and Tackle

Because of their mechanical advantage in converting a given amount of pull to a working capacity greater than the pull, blocks and tackle are useful for lifting or pulling heavy loads. A *block* is a wooden or metal frame containing one or more pulleys called sheaves. *Tackle* is the assembly of ropes and blocks through which the line passes to multiply the pulling force.

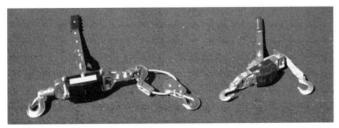

Figure 3.59 Typical come-alongs.

Block and tackle is not considered to be sufficiently reliable for life safety applications.

In vehicle extrication incidents, block and tackle may be very useful for stabilizing vehicles and similar applications. When using block and tackle, observe the following safety rules:

- Ensure that the rope is the right size for the weight being lifted and the blocks being used.
- Exert a steady, simultaneous pull on the fall line, and hold onto the gain.
- Ensure that the anchor to which the standing block is attached is strong enough to hold the load and the pull.
- Pull in a direct line with the sheaves.
- Pull downhill whenever possible.
- Allow no one to stand under or near the load in case the assembly fails.
- Lower suspended loads gradually, without jerking.
- "Mouse" open hooks to prevent slings or ropes from slipping off.

Summary

The tools and equipment required to perform safe and efficient vehicle extrication vary from the conventional manual and power tools carried on most fire apparatus to highly specialized and highly sophisticated devices. Likewise, the vehicles used by fire departments and other organizations that respond to vehicle extrication incidents also vary. Some are conventional municipal and wildland fire apparatus (engines and trucks); others are very specialized, dedicated rescue vehicles. To be most effective, rescue personnel must be thoroughly familiar with the tools and equipment available to them. They must know the capabilities and limitations of extrication tools and equipment, and know how to operate them safely.

Extrication Techniques

Once emergency responders are at the scene of a reported vehicle collision, they must first confirm that a collision has occurred and that there is a need for one or more vehicle occupants to be extricated. If the initial size-up confirms the need for extrication, then a variety of tools and techniques can be used to safely and efficiently extricate the victim. How these tools and techniques are applied determine whether the operation is successful, and, in some cases, whether the victim survives.

This chapter expands on the earlier discussions of initial size-up and vehicle anatomy, stabilization, and lifting. Also discussed are the use of hand and power tools for glass removal, door and side panel removal, roof removal, and dashboard and steering column roll-ups. Finally, dealing with vehicle seats and pedals are discussed along with special techniques for making entry at unusual points on the vehicle.

Initial Size-Up

As discussed in Chapter 2, size-up is an ongoing process that starts when the first unit is dispatched and continues throughout the incident. As the first unit approaches the scene, the officer in charge can begin to clarify the information supplied in the initial dispatch and add information based on what he observes.

One of the first decisions an officer in charge must make is where to position the emergency vehicles as they arrive. The first concern is to protect the scene from oncoming traffic, so emergency vehicles should initially be positioned to form a barrier between the involved vehicles and other approaching traffic. In addition, the driver of the first-arriving unit should set out bright orange traffic cones to warn other drivers of the incident scene and direct them around it.

Emergency vehicles should be positioned close enough to the scene to make their tools, equipment, and supplies readily available, but not so close that they interfere with on-scene activities. If possible, at least one traffic lane in each direction should be left open for other emergency and nonemergency traffic. However, the safety of those on scene is far more important than maintaining traffic flow. At least one lane in addition to those occupied by the involved vehicles should be closed to form a safety buffer between the scene and any oncoming traffic (Figure 4.1). If it is not possible to close an additional lane, the entire road should be closed and traffic detoured around the scene. (**NOTE:** The need for these lane and road closures should be discussed with law enforcement officials during pre-incident planning for extrication incidents.)

Agency protocols regarding vehicle emergency lights must always be followed; however, experience and testing have shown that during night operations, apparatus headlights and emergency lights tend to blind and confuse the drivers of oncoming vehicles.

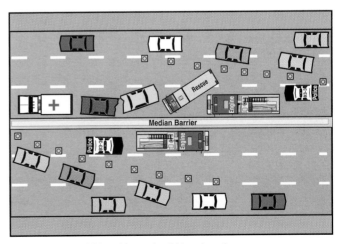

Figure 4.1 An additional lane should be closed.

Therefore, it is now SOP in some departments for the drivers of all emergency vehicles parked on the roadway during nighttime operations to shut down their headlights (except those being used to illuminate the scene) and red lights, leaving only their amber flashers on. Emergency vehicles parked off the roadway are to shut down all exterior lights.

Forming a protective barrier with emergency vehicles helps to isolate the scene and allows the first-in officer to quickly but carefully assess (size up) the situation. A thorough initial size-up is necessary to confirm that an emergency exists, avoid confusion, clarify required tasks, protect rescue personnel and prevent further injuries to victims, and to provide the information on which to base an incident action plan. During the initial size-up, the following questions should be answered:

- What are the traffic hazards?
- How many and what types of vehicles are involved?
- Where and how are the vehicles positioned?
- Is there a fire or potential for a fire?
- Are there any hazardous materials involved?
- Are there any utilities, such as gas or electricity, that may have been damaged? If so, are they posing a hazard to the victims and rescue personnel?
- Is there a need for additional resources?

If the initial size-up confirms that an emergency exists, the first-in officer should establish command by giving the communications center a brief report on conditions and naming the incident. For example:

Rescue 8: "Communications, Rescue 8."

Dispatcher: "Go ahead Rescue 8."

Rescue 8: "Communications, I am at the scene of a two-car collision at the corner of 5th and Maple. There are three trapped and injured victims. Rescue 8 is Maple Command. Dispatch one additional ambulance for a total of two, and assign an incident channel."

Dispatcher: "Communications copies; Rescue 8 is Maple Command, and you need one additional ambulance for a total of two. All units on the Maple incident switch to Orange-2 as the incident channel."

This brief exchange informs all who are monitoring the primary channel of the location, nature, and scope of the incident. It also transfers the incident radio traffic to another channel leaving the primary channel available for other traffic.

Assessing the Need for Extrication

At the scene, rescue personnel should be assigned to conduct a more thorough size-up of the situation. Ideally, one rescuer should be assigned to assess each vehicle involved in the incident, and one or more to assess in more detail the immediate area surrounding the vehicles. Those assigned to assess each vehicle should attempt to determine the number of injured or trapped victims and the severity of their injuries. Those assigned to survey the surrounding area should attempt to determine whether there are additional victims, such as pedestrians, who may have been struck by a vehicle or occupants who may have been ejected from a vehicle. They should also check for additional vehicles involved but not readily apparent (over an embankment, for example), any damage to structures or utilities that present a hazard, or any other circumstances that warrant special attention. Both groups should report their findings to the incident commander (IC) as soon as possible.

Medically qualified rescue personnel should be assigned to triage the victims to determine the extent of injury and entrapment. The IC needs this information to determine the order in which the victims should be removed. Obviously, those with the most serious injuries get a higher priority than those with lesser injuries. Victims who are injured but not trapped should be removed first to make more working room for rescuers trying to remove those who are trapped in the vehicle. The results of the medical assessment should also be communicated to the IC as soon as possible. As mentioned earlier, the IC uses this information as the basis for the incident action plan.

Vehicle Anatomy

In this context, *vehicle anatomy* refers to the condition of a particular vehicle after a collision. The anatomy of each vehicle involved in an incident must be assessed in terms of its center of gravity, mass, structural integrity, restraint systems, and energy absorbing features.

Center of Gravity

Whether a vehicle is upright, on its side, on its top, or teetering on the edge of some precipice, its stability is greatly affected by its center of gravity. In general terms, half the total weight of a vehicle is on each side of its center of gravity. A vehicle's center of gravity acts as a pivot point around which the vehicle will move unless prevented from doing so. The higher a vehicle's center of gravity, the more susceptible the vehicle is to rolling over. Therefore, the essence of vehicle stabilization is to support the vehicle on all sides of its center of gravity to prevent any movement.

When most automobiles and light utility vehicles are empty, the center of gravity is slightly forward of the front door in the center of the vehicle. However, given fuel in the fuel tank, objects in the trunk, and occupants inside, the center of gravity is likely to be somewhere aft of that point. Determining exactly where the center of gravity is on a particular vehicle may be especially difficult if the vehicle was significantly deformed by the collision. Therefore, every vehicle in which there are injured and trapped occupants should be stabilized using either a four-point or six-point crib, discussed later in this chapter.

Mass

The mass or weight of a vehicle also affects its stability after a collision. The heavier the vehicle, the greater its tendency to settle toward the stability of the ground. When a vehicle has come to rest on a slope, its mass makes it susceptible to sliding or rolling down slope. Therefore, the challenge for rescue personnel is to safely and effectively counteract this potential movement. Depending upon the situation, shoring installed on the down slope side of the vehicle may stabilize it, or ropes, chains, or webbing may be attached to the vehicle and an anchor point up slope. The anchor point may be a solid object, such as a large mature tree or a massive boulder, but it can also be the winch on a rescue vehicle or tow truck (Figure 4.2).

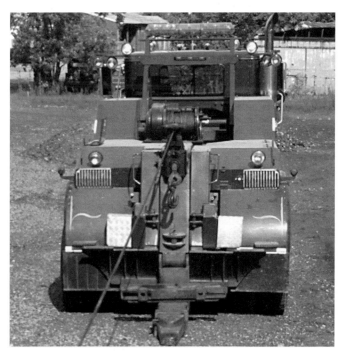

Figure 4.2 A large vehicle can be an anchor point.

Vehicle Integrity

The structural integrity of a vehicle is how strong the vehicle's chassis remains after a collision. The structural integrity of rigid frame vehicles may be less affected by a collision than that of vehicles with unibody or space-frame construction. Also, the structural integrity of rigid frame vehicles is less affected than vehicles with unibody construction when rescuers remove doors and/or the roof of the vehicle. Older vehicles tend to retain more of their structural integrity because they contain more steel and less aluminum, magnesium, and plastic in their construction.

When rescue personnel remove a vehicle's doors, roof, and side panels, the chassis is weakened to a greater or lesser degree. When the chassis is weakened, it tends to collapse in on itself. This creates unwanted and perhaps dangerous movement that must be prevented if rescuers and those trapped in the vehicle are to be protected.

Restraint Systems (Air Bags)

Modern technology has added increased collision protection for vehicle occupants by means of front impact air bags called Supplemental Restraint Systems (SRS), Side Impact Protection Systems (SIPS), Head Protection Systems (HPS), and knee bolsters, all commonly called *air bags*. In addition, a growing number of vehicles are equipped with seat belt pretensioners. Because restraint system technology is evolving so rapidly, all rescue personnel are encouraged to make every effort to stay current on what systems are being installed in new vehicles. One of the best ways to do this is to frequently visit the NHTSA web site listed in Chapter 1.

Although air bags have saved many lives, they have also added a potential safety hazard for both rescuers and vehicle occupants — accidental activation of one or more of these systems during extrication operations. Some modern vehicles have as many as eight separate airbags (Figure 4.3). For their own safety and that of the trapped occupants, rescue personnel must know where these bags may be located and how to disarm them. All restraint systems can be identified by either words or initials displayed at various points on the vehicle (Figure 4.4).

> ## WARNING!
> Front-impact air bags deploy at speeds of up to 200 mph (322 km/h) and exert a tremendous force — potentially lethal under the right conditions.

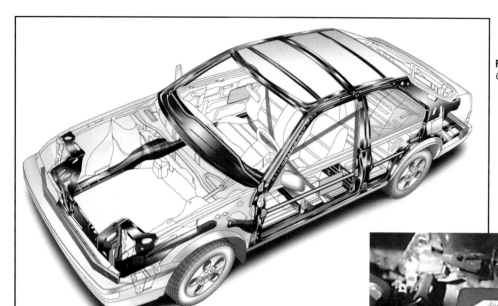

Figure 4.3 Possible air bag locations.
Courtesy of Holmatro Rescue Equipment.

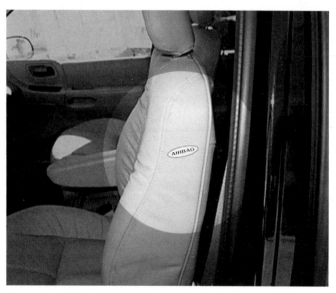

Figure 4.4 Restraint systems are identified by words or initials.

Figure 4.5 Typical air bag control unit.

Supplemental Restraint Systems (SRS)

Front-impact air bags are called supplemental systems because they are intended to *supplement* seat belts, not replace them. Electrically operated restraint systems receive their energy from the vehicle's battery. They are designed to activate through a system of inertia switches located forward of the passenger compartment and by microelectronic controls that may be located under the front seats or in the console between the front seats (Figure 4.5). These systems have a reserve energy supply that is capable of deploying an air bag even if the battery is disconnected or destroyed in the collision. When the battery is disconnected, the reserve energy supply will eventually drain away, disarming the restraint

system. Vehicle manufacturers list different time estimates on how long it takes for the reserve to deplete entirely. These estimates range from as little as 1 second to as much as 30 minutes. Most air bags are deactivated after about 10 minutes.

Both fire suppression and extrication activities are capable of accidentally activating either electrical or mechanical restraint systems. In electrically operated systems, an electrical impulse as small as .5 volts (such as a static discharge from an extrication tool) during the extrication process may cause the air bag to deploy. In mechanically operated systems, a sharp blow to the sensor or excessive pressure on the inside surface of the vehicle door can accidentally activate them. According to NHTSA, *"Even after a battery disconnect, it is possible that static electricity can deploy the air bag. Static electricity can be generated by the use of hydraulic shears and rams, rescue personnel sliding across the seat, and the cutting of safety belts. After a crash it is not possible to determine how much static electricity is present around the vehicle and specifically what wires [that] individuals and extrication equipment may contact. Also, the use of rams and the prying open of [vehicle] body parts can trigger the deployment of mechanically-*

activated side air bags. This is why it is always best to treat air bag systems as if they were <u>live</u>."

On many vehicles, the only way to deactivate electrically operated air bags is to turn the ignition switch to the "off" position, disconnect both battery cables (*negative* cable first), and wait for the reserve power supply to drain down (Figure 4.6). In addition, it is good practice to tape the ends of the battery cables after they have been disconnected from the battery (Figure 4.7). Some agencies also advocate grounding the vehicle (Figure 4.8). Some vehicles that have only a front seat are equipped with a key-operated switch that disables and drains the reserve power from the passenger-side air bag (Figure 4.9). (**NOTE:** Before disconnecting a vehicle's battery, it may be desirable to use its power to operate adjustable seats, electric door locks, and electric windows in the vehicle.)

Finding a vehicle's battery in order to disconnect it may be a significant challenge. Batteries are located in any of several places depending upon the make and model of the vehicle. In some models, the battery is located in the engine compartment (perhaps hidden by other components). In others, it is in the right or left front wheel well. In some vehicles, the battery is located in the trunk. In still others, it is located under the rear passenger seat (Figure 4.10).

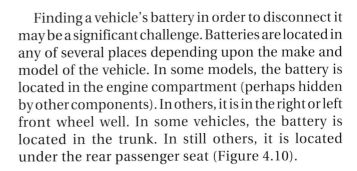

Figure 4.8 Some agencies advocate grounding the vehicle.

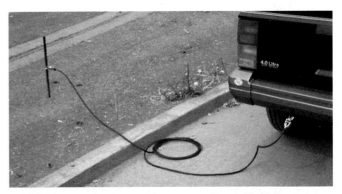

Figure 4.9 A typical air bag switch.

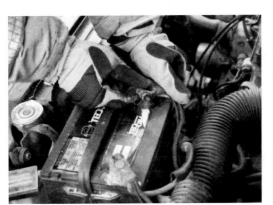

Figure 4.6 The negative cable should be disconnected first.

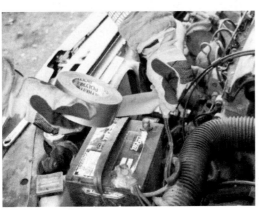

Figure 4.7 The cable ends should be taped.

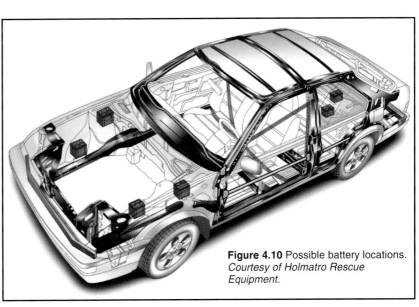

Figure 4.10 Possible battery locations. *Courtesy of Holmatro Rescue Equipment.*

Side-Impact Protection Systems (SIPS)

Most side-impact protection systems are mechanically operated and do not require power from the vehicle's electrical system to activate. Therefore, these air bags may deploy even if the battery has been disconnected. In these systems, disarming or preventing air bag deployment may require that the connection between the sensor and the air bag inflation unit be cut. How and where this is done is specific to each vehicle make and model.

Head Protection Systems (HPS)

A growing number of vehicles have head protection systems (HPS) installed. These air bags deploy from a narrow opening between the headliner and the top of the door frame. Unlike SRS and SIPS that deflate immediately after deployment, HPS bags remain rigidly inflated after activation. However, they are easily removed by cutting the nylon straps or deflated by being punctured with a sharp object or being cut with a knife. A slightly different type of HPS curtain is inflated by a high-pressure cylinder located in the C-post (Figure 4.11). This curtain deflates automatically shortly after deployment.

One danger with both of these systems is that if a rescuer is working through the window opening, he is in the deployment path of the air bag. This danger can be mitigated by a complete roof removal. However, when cutting the C-posts for the roof removal, rescuers must be careful not to cut into either of the high-pressure cylinders.

Knee Bolsters

Some vehicles are equipped with restraint devices that are intended to protect the lower legs of the driver. They are also intended as "antisubmarine" devices — that is, they are intended to help prevent the driver from sliding forward and becoming wedged under the dashboard. The same precautions apply as with other front-impact restraints.

Seat Belt Pretensioners

Some vehicles are equipped with seat belt pretensioners. Because seat belts are most effective when they are adjusted tightly across the torso of the people wearing them, pretensioners have been added to tighten the belts as the front-impact air bags deploy. These pyrotechnic devices are operated by the ignition of nitrocellulose that drives a piston to instantaneously eliminate any slack in the belt. In some cases, the belts may be tightened to the point that they restrict the

wearer's ability to breathe normally. Simply releasing or cutting the seat belts will relieve this pressure.

Because the pyrotechnic activating devices for seat belt pretensioners are usually located inside the B-post next to the seat, rescuers must be careful about cutting these posts. To avoid accidentally activating the pretensioner, cuts into the B-post must be made well above or well below the external seat belt retractor (Figure 4.12). Another way of handling those situations where the pretensioners are located in the B-post is to cut the seat belt and remove the buckle and excess belt so that they cannot strike anyone if the system suddenly activates. If the pretensioners are located between the front seats, all that is necessary is to unbuckle the belts.

Energy-Absorbing Features

Since the early 1970s, automobiles manufactured in North America have been equipped with energy-absorbing bumpers. Many cars and light trucks have also been equipped with reinforced door and dashboard structures to increase side impact protection. All these features are intended to reduce

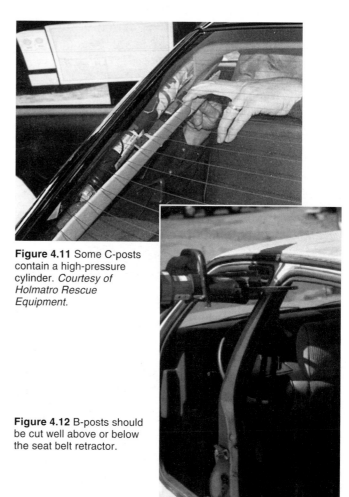

Figure 4.11 Some C-posts contain a high-pressure cylinder. *Courtesy of Holmatro Rescue Equipment.*

Figure 4.12 B-posts should be cut well above or below the seat belt retractor.

the monetary and human costs of vehicle collisions. However, they also add some potentially lethal hazards for emergency response personnel, and they can increase the difficulty of performing vehicle extrication.

Energy-Absorbing Bumpers

A number of different designs were used by vehicle manufacturers to meet federal standards intended to reduce the monetary costs of low-speed collisions — those at 5 mph (7.5 km/h) or less, later reduced to 2.5 mph (3.75 km/h). The two most prevalent designs, and the ones with which rescue personnel need be most concerned, are those with crushable bumpers and those that use energy-absorbing bumper struts.

Crushable Bumpers. One type of energy-absorbing bumper with which emergency response personnel must be careful is the crushable bumper. Some of these bumpers are made of polystyrene foam molded into an egg crate structure, covered by a flexible rubber shell. Others are made of fluoroelastomer molded into a honeycomb structure covered with a flexible shell (Figure 4.13). These bumpers are designed to absorb energy by flexing when struck. Unlike the bumpers with gas-filled struts discussed next, crushable bumpers are not a hazard in a fire — *until the fire is out.* As these bumpers cool after being exposed to the heat of a fire,

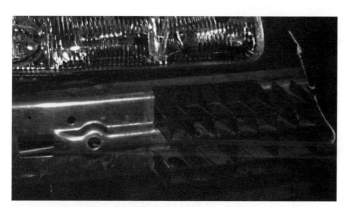

Figure 4.13 A typical crushable bumper.

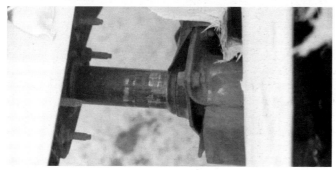

Figure 4.14 Typical energy absorbing bumper struts.

beads of a clear liquid form on the surface of the bumper. This liquid may appear to be water but it is actually concentrated hydrofluoric acid (HF), a highly corrosive substance.

> # WARNING!
> **Avoid skin contact with the clear liquid (hydrofluoric acid [HF]) that forms on the surface of crushable bumpers after a fire. Hydrofluoric acid is absorbed through the skin and will attack the bone. Flush these bumpers with copious amounts of water.**

Bumper Struts. Many automobiles on the road today are equipped with bumpers that incorporate energy absorbing struts to make them less vulnerable to damage in low-speed collisions. Two struts are mounted between the front bumper and the vehicle frame or chassis, and two more are mounted in the rear of the vehicle (Figure 4.14). Similar to conventional shock absorbers, these sealed units contain hydraulic fluid and compressed gas. When these struts are exposed to the heat of a fire, they can explode with tremendous force. If both struts attached to a bumper explode simultaneously, they can launch the bumper and/or the struts 100 feet (30 m) or more from the vehicle. If only one strut explodes, the other acts as a pivot point and the bumper can swing in an arc across the front or rear of the vehicle. Obviously, anyone in the path of a bumper attached to an exploding strut is in serious jeopardy. Therefore, when the front or rear bumper of an automobile is exposed to heavy flame impingement, all personnel should stay out of the danger zone — directly in front of the bumper and to each side a distance equal to the length of the bumper (Figure 4.15).

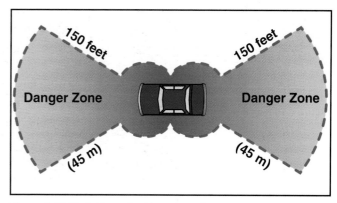

Figure 4.15 Firefighters should stay out of the danger zone.

WARNING!

When automobile bumpers are exposed to direct flame impingement, do not approach from directly in front or within the length of the bumper on each side.

Another hazard of which firefighters should be aware are the gas-filled struts used to support the hoods and hatchbacks (when open) on some vehicles (Figure 4.16). When exposed to the heat of a fire, these struts can explode and launch parts many yards (meters) from the vehicle at speeds sufficient to cause fatal injuries.

Side-Impact Beams

Because more than 40 percent of all vehicle fatalities are the result of side-impact collisions, passenger cars manufactured in North America have been equipped with side-impact beams since the late 1960s. Early designs were several layers of ordinary mild steel formed into a corrugated beam about 7 inches (178 mm) wide and about 2 inches (50 mm) thick, installed across each side door (Figure 4.17). Because mild steel has a tensile strength of about 20,000 to 23,000 psi (140 000 kPa to 161 000 kPa), these beams were relatively easy to cut with hydraulic shears. However, newer designs have made two major changes — the construction of the door beams and the addition of a dashboard support beam.

Newer designs of side-impact protection incorporate stronger materials such as high-strength low-alloy (HSLA) steel and micro-alloy (MA) steel (Figure 4.18). HSLA steel has a tensile strength of 40,000 to 70,000 psi (280 000 kPa to 490 000 kPa). MA steel has a tensile strength of 110,000 to 215,000 psi (770 000 kPa to 1 505 000 kPa). These new alloys may be too hard for the blades of available power shears. If this is the case, rescuers may have to make relief cuts above and below the bar and use a power spreader to move the end of the bar.

These new alloys add significantly to the structural integrity of any vehicle, and reduce the likelihood of the vehicle folding in the middle when struck from the side. They are also used in the construction of some dashboard support beams. These beams span the width of the vehicle from A-post to A-post (Figure 4.19).

Figure 4.16 A typical gas-filled strut.

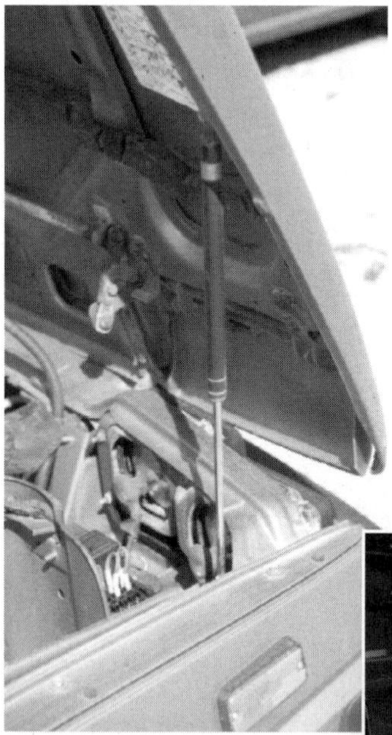

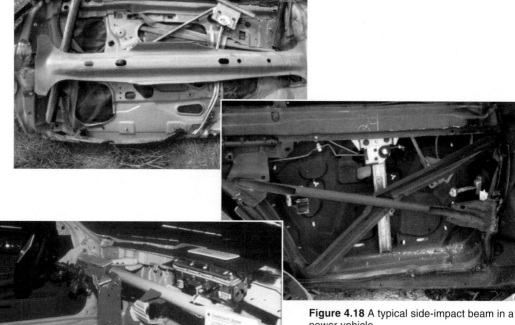

Figure 4.17 A typical side-impact beam in an older vehicle.

Figure 4.18 A typical side-impact beam in a newer vehicle.

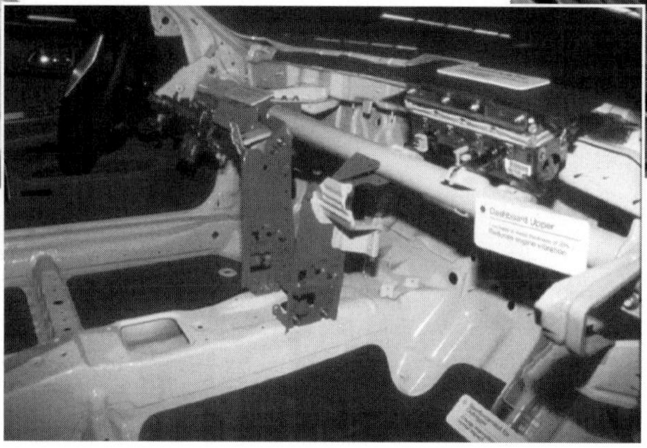

Figure 4.19 A typical dashboard support beam. *Courtesy of Dekevin Thornton.*

Vehicle Stabilization

Following scene assessment, rescue personnel must stabilize each vehicle involved in the collision. This is necessary to prevent further injury to the victims, possible injuries to rescue personnel, and further degradation of the vehicle's structural integrity. Stabilization refers to the process of providing additional support at key points between the vehicle and the ground or other solid surface. The primary goal of stabilization is to maximize the area of contact between the vehicle and the ground to prevent any sudden or unexpected movement of the vehicle. Generally, a combination of cribbing, ropes, webbing, and chains are used to accomplish these types of stabilization tasks. These techniques are discussed in the following sections.

Vehicles may be found in a number of different positions following a collision. Inexperienced rescuers may be tempted to test the stability of the vehicle as it is found — they must be trained to resist this temptation. This is particularly true of vehicles that are on their side, teetering on the edge of a cliff or embankment, or resting atop another vehicle.

WARNING!
The slightest push in the wrong place may cause a vehicle to move significantly, perhaps compounding the victims' injuries.

Vehicle Upright

Most vehicles involved in collisions remain upright. Even though all wheels are on the ground, some stabilization is required to ensure maximum stability for extrication operations. Vehicles should be stabilized to prevent movement in any direction.

The most common form of horizontal movement involves the vehicle rolling forward or backward on its wheels. This movement can be prevented by chocking the wheels with conventional wheel chocks, pieces of cribbing, or other suitable objects. If the vehicle is on flat ground, the wheels should be chocked fore and aft (Figure 4.20). If it is on a slope, the wheels should be chocked on the downhill side (Figure 4.21). The vehicle's mechanical systems, such as parking brake and transmission, can also be used to help prevent horizontal movement. Automatic transmissions should be placed in "park." Depending upon the relationship of the vehicle to the slope, manual transmissions should be placed in reverse gear to

prevent forward movement or placed in the lowest forward gear to prevent backward movement. The vehicle's parking brake should also be set. (**CAUTION:** Do not rely on mechanical systems — even if they are operable — as the sole means of stabilization. They should be used only with other stabilization measures.)

The standard operating procedure (SOP) in some departments is to deflate all four tires to stabilize an upright vehicle. This is done by either removing the valve core, snipping off the valve stems with wire cutters, or pulling the stems out with pliers. However, this action also allows the vehicle to move as it settles onto its rims, so not all departments advocate this practice. Again, agency protocols must be followed.

Deflating the tires does prevent the vehicle from rising as it gets lighter when the roof and other components are removed. However, if the tires are to be deflated, it should only be done after cribbing has been installed to support the weight of the vehicle.

WARNING!
Do not deflate any tire mounted on a split rim, nor deflate any tire before adequate cribbing has been installed to support the vehicle's weight.

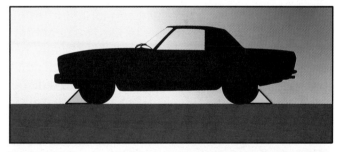

Figure 4.20 On a level surface, wheels should be chocked front and rear.

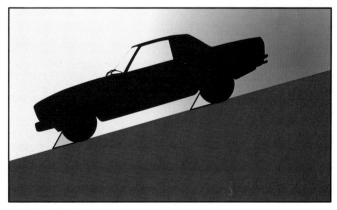

Figure 4.21 On a slope, wheels should be chocked on the downhill side.

There are numerous ways to prevent a vehicle from moving vertically — that is, to prevent it from settling or suddenly dropping. Step chocks, cribbing, jacks, and pneumatic lifting bags are most often used for this purpose.

Both wooden and plastic step chocks can be used when vehicles are upright. They are effective and quick and easy to install. At least four step chocks are usually needed to provide adequate stabilization (Figure 4.22). As described in the previous chapter, step chocks can be installed upright or upside down as a form of wedge. The situation will dictate which is the better way in any particular incident.

Cribbing, especially when used with wooden or plastic wedges, is relatively easy to install. However, installing cribbing usually takes longer than using step chocks. Cribbing is most often installed in a box formation until enough cribbing is installed to support the vehicle (Figure 4.23).

Different types of hydraulic and mechanical jacks can be used to support the frame of the vehicle (Figure 4.24). Their primary advantage is that they can be adjusted to the required height without the need for wedges. Their disadvantages are that they can be time-consuming to install, have limited range of motion, and are not as reliable as some other forms of stabilization.

Although they are designed primarily for lifting, pneumatic lifting bags can also be used for temporary support — *if no other means is available.* Usually, two or more bags are needed and may be installed along one side or in opposing positions on both sides or front and rear of the vehicle. Lifting bags take time to set up, and they allow some vehicle movement even when the bags are fully inflated. Therefore, pneumatic lifting bags should only be used in conjunction with appropriate cribbing.

When using any of these stabilization methods, rescue personnel must be careful to avoid placing their heads, hands, or any other part of their bodies under the vehicle while installing the stabilizing device. There is always the possibility of the vehicle dropping suddenly and unexpectedly, injuring or even killing anyone beneath it. To prevent any crushing hand injuries should a sudden drop occur, each piece of cribbing should be grasped from the sides, set outside of the vertical plane of the vehicle, and pushed into position under the vehicle with a tool or another piece of cribbing.

> Regardless of what equipment is used for vehicle stabilization, the goal is to create a stable foundation for extrication operations.

As in all extrication operations, the simpler the stabilization operation the better, as long as the technique used is safe and effective. Experience has shown that for stabilization most vehicles require support at a minimum of four points and perhaps six. Obviously, it takes less time to install support at four points than six, but the situation will dictate how much support is needed and where it should be installed.

Four-Point Support. Although commonly called a four-point crib, the means employed may involve the use of cribbing or any of the other equipment described in this chapter. Regardless of what equipment is used

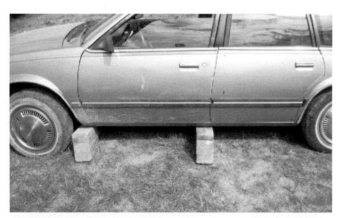

Figure 4.22 Chocks are installed on the opposite side also.

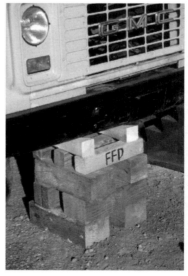

Figure 4.23 A typical box crib.

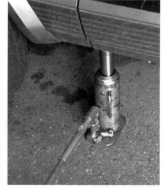

Figure 4.24 Hydraulic jacks can be used for stabilization.

to support the vehicle, in a four-point crib the support is placed aft of the front wheel well and at the equivalent point forward of the rear wheel well on both sides of the vehicle (Figure 4.25).

Six-Point Support. A six-point crib is most often needed to support a vehicle that is in danger of collapsing in the middle such as when the doors are opened or removed or when the roof is removed from a unibody vehicle. Cribbing should be installed under the middle of both sides of the vehicle (Figure 4.26). However, it is possible that additional support may also be needed under the front and rear of the vehicle (Figure 4.27).

On occasion, vehicles are found in positions other than upright such as on their side, upside down, or over an embankment. Under these circumstances, rescuers should use whatever means available to stabilize the vehicle. As always, the goal is to create as many points of contact between the vehicle and the ground as is reasonably possible given the resources available and the demands of the incident.

Vehicle on Side

When a vehicle has come to rest on its side, establishing fire protection is a high priority because gravity causes fuel, oil, and other fluids to flow into areas where they do not belong. These fluids may come into contact with hot exhaust system components or electrical

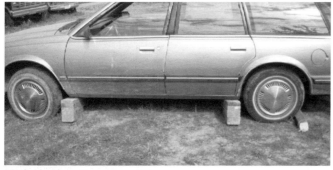

Figure 4.25 A typical four-point crib.

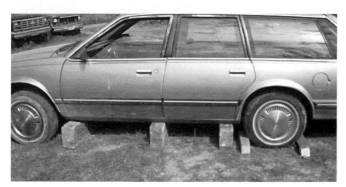

Figure 4.26 A typical six-point crib.

components that can serve as sources of ignition. At least one 1½-inch (38 mm) or larger hoseline should be charged and ready. If fuel has been spilled, Class B foam should be applied to suppress the production of flammable vapors.

The exposed doors on the top side and rear may or may not be operable. If they are, occupants can escape through the door/window openings. If the vehicle is not on fire and rescue personnel are going to assist occupants through these openings, they should first stabilize the vehicle. A four-point crib with step chocks and wedges may be sufficient. Again, depending upon the situation, rescue personnel should use the best means available to quickly and safely prevent the vehicle from moving in any direction. This may involve the use of cribbing and/or step chocks as previously described, but it may also involve the use of webbing and rope.

Webbing/Rope. Especially when a vehicle has come to rest on a sloping, sandy, or other unstable surface, webbing/rope may be needed to stabilize the vehicle. The webbing/rope may be used alone or in combination with shoring or step chocks. As described earlier in this chapter, webbing, ropes, and/or chains can be attached to the vehicle and to a secure anchor point. Rope and webbing should be protected from chafing and/or contact with chemicals (such as battery acid) that may reduce their strength and cause them to fail. The need for redundancy must be weighed against other factors in the situation when deciding whether to back up rope or webbing with a second system.

Vehicle Upside Down

When a vehicle has come to rest upside down, the same fire potential exists as with the vehicle on its side, so the same fire protection should be set up. The vehicle's roof posts may be supporting the chassis

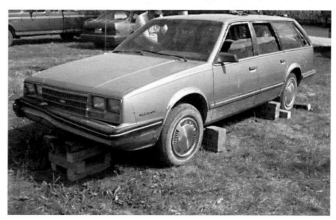

Figure 4.27 Another form of six-point crib.

more or less intact, or they may have collapsed. If the posts have collapsed, the normal window openings may have been reduced to narrow slits, too small to serve as access openings. If the A- and B-posts have collapsed but the vehicle has a rear door, it may still be operable and can be used to access the occupants, or the rear window can be removed. The occupants are likely to be hanging upside down, being held in place by their seat belts. They cannot survive long in this position, so they must be extricated as quickly as safely possible. After establishing fire protection, stabilizing the vehicle is critical.

Because the roofs of most vehicles are rounded above the door openings, and their surfaces have a smooth, painted finish, there is less purchase for cribbing or step chocks in contact with the roof surface than with other parts of the vehicle. Therefore, it is often faster and more effective to turn step chocks upside down and slide them under the vehicle's roof surface in at least two places on each side of the vehicle (Figure 4.28). Because of the rounded contours of vehicle roofs, it may also be necessary to support the vehicle front and rear with cribbing and/or hi-lift jacks (Figure 4.29).

Vehicles in Other Positions

Because of the ballistic movement and inertial forces involved in collisions, vehicles can come to rest in a variety of positions other than those already described. For example, a vehicle may be found at a steep angle resting against a tree or other solid object or partially atop another vehicle. Just as with spinal immobilization of an injured victim, the challenge in stabilizing a vehicle in an unusual position is to stabilize as it is found — without moving it. This may involve the use of box cribbing or wooden or pneumatic shores to span the distance between the vehicle and a stable surface (Figure 4.30). It may also involve the use of tow trucks.

Use of Tow Trucks

If a tow truck is already on the scene, it may be a very valuable resource for stabilizing vehicles. In some cases, depending upon the situation and the other resources available, it may be prudent to wait for a tow truck to arrive before attempting to stabilize a vehicle. For example, if the vehicle is teetering on the edge of a high cliff or a bridge and the rescue units on scene do not have the necessary equipment to secure the vehicle, it may be safer for both the trapped occupants and rescue personnel to wait for a tow truck that is already en route. Attaching the cable from a tow truck's winch to an unstabilized vehicle can provide the initial stability needed for rescue personnel to safely access the trapped victims (Figure 4.31).

Lifting

While the objective of vehicle stabilization is to secure it in place without moving it, there may be times when

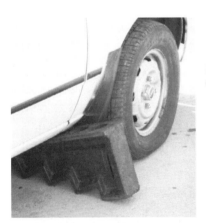

Figure 4.28 Step chocks can be used upside down.

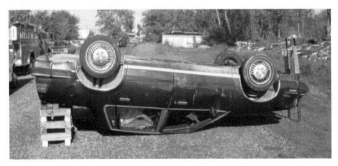

Figure 4.29 Hi-lift jacks can be used to temporarily stabilize an overturned vehicle.

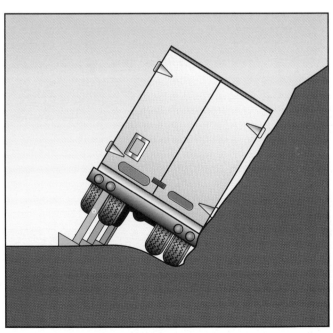

Figure 4.30 Shoring may be needed to stabilize a vehicle.

it is necessary to move something from the vehicle. For example, if the vehicle struck a tree, power pole, or a building, the struck object may have collapsed onto the vehicle, trapping the occupants inside. The challenge in these situations is for rescue personnel to be able to lift the collapsed object from the vehicle while limiting the amount of vehicle movement.

Depending upon the situation and the resources available on scene, lifting objects from crashed vehicles may involve the use of jacks, extension rams, pneumatic or hydraulic shoring devices, pneumatic lifting bags, or even booms or cranes (Figure 4.32). The most critical point in these operations is the security of the attachment of the lifting mechanism to the object being lifted. If the attachment should fail during the lift and allow the object to drop back onto the vehicle, the time and effort will have been wasted and it may have done more harm than good.

In some cases, the object resting on the vehicle may be too massive to be lifted intact. This may leave only one choice — dividing the object into pieces that can be lifted. If the object is a tree or wooden power pole, it can be cut into smaller, more manageable pieces with a chain saw. The point of the operation is to free the underlying vehicle while making as few cuts as possible. Also, to the extent possible, the crushed vehicle must be stabilized to reduce the amount of reaction movement when the overlying burden is lifted. The same is true if the overlying object is made of metal and will be cut with a power saw, oxyacetylene cutting torch, or other thermal cutting device. If the overlying object is a wood frame wall, it can be cut into sections with a chain saw or rotary saw. If it is a

masonry wall, it can be cut into smaller pieces with a rotary saw — or if necessary, broken apart using an electric concrete breaker (jack hammer).

In cases of this type where the IC is convinced that the operation is not a rescue but a body recovery, one other option remains — removing the vehicle from the object. This involves supporting the overlying object so that it will not settle any further and lowering the vehicle enough that it can be pulled from beneath the object. If the vehicle's tires are still inflated, the valve cores can be removed or the valve stems cut off to allow the tires to deflate. If this creates the necessary clearance, the vehicle can then be pulled out with a tow truck's winch. If deflating the tires does not create the needed clearance, it may be necessary to use shovels to dig out beneath the vehicle's wheels.

Glass Removal

One of the fastest and easiest ways of gaining access to the interior of a vehicle is by removing glass from the vehicle. Removing the glass may be necessary if the doors are inoperable, the doors are operable but locked, or the roof needs to be removed or flapped. There are two types of glass used in vehicles: laminated safety glass and tempered glass.

Laminated Safety Glass
Laminated safety glass consists of two sheets of glass bonded to a sheet of plastic sandwiched between them. This type of glass is most commonly used for windshields and some rear windows. Impact produces many long, pointed shards with sharp edges. The plastic laminate sheet holds most of these shards and fragments in place. When broken, the glass remains attached to the laminate and moves as a unit (Figure 4.33). This makes windshield removal easier. Some

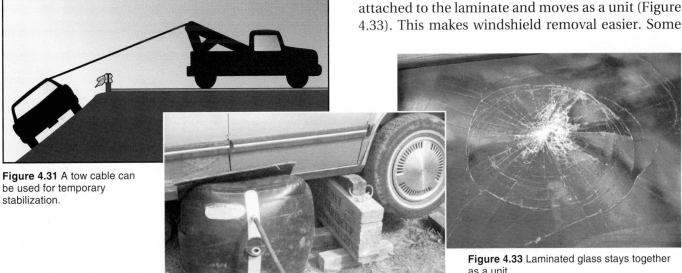

Figure 4.31 A tow cable can be used for temporary stabilization.

Figure 4.32 Low-pressure lifting bags may be needed.

Figure 4.33 Laminated glass stays together as a unit.

manufacturers have laminated an additional layer of plastic to the passenger side of the windshield for added protection. Some laminated glass side windows are more than ⅓-inch (9 mm) thick. Many laminated windshields and rear windows are now held in place with polyurethane glue. These windows can be identified by the black shading around the perimeter of the window, designed to protect the glue from sun damage (Figure 4.34).

Removing Laminated Glass

Removing windshields and laminated rear windows is somewhat more complicated and time-consuming than removing tempered side or rear windows. This is mainly because of the difference in glass types. Windshields and rear windows constructed of laminated safety glass do not disintegrate and fall out like tempered glass windows. Because more laminates are being added to windshields, it may not be as easy to chop through the windshields of newer vehicles. In this case, the best method of removing glass is with a saw. After providing a means of protecting vehicle occupants from glass dust and chips, the following common hand tools can be used to cut laminated glass:

• Bypass-type pruning shears (not anvil type)

• Axe (standard or aircraft crash axe)

• Reciprocating saw

• Hand saw with a coarse blade such as those used in commercially produced rescue tools

• Air chisel

If the roof is to be removed, total windshield removal is unnecessary. Instead, the windshield is cut across its full width near the bottom. Then, when the A-posts are cut, the cuts are made at the same level as the windshield cut (Figure 4.35). This allows the roof and the windshield to be moved as a unit.

WARNING!

Backboards or other rigid devices should not be used to shield vehicle occupants if there are undeployed air bags in the vehicle.

If the windshield or rear window must be removed, the glass may have to be cut on all four sides. There are a number of tools that can be used to cut the glass. However, both the tool operator and the vehicle occupants need to be protected from the glass dust and chips produced during the cutting operation.

If bypass-type pruning shears are used, the following procedure is suggested:

Step 1: Drive the point of the shears into the upper corner of one side of the windshield to create an access hole (Figure 4.36).

Step 2: Starting from the hole just created, cut across the top of the glass to the middle (Figure 4.37).

Step 3: Repeat Steps 1 and 2 from the other side (Figure 4.38).

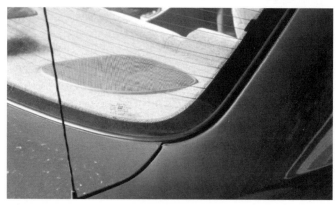
Figure 4.34 Black shading identifies this window as one that is glued in.

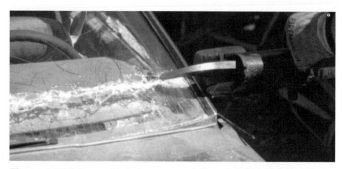
Figure 4.35 If the roof is to be removed, the windshield is cut across the bottom.

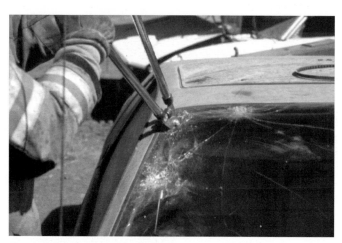
Figure 4.36 Create an access hole in an upper corner of the windshield.

Step 4: Cut from the top of the windshield to the bottom on both sides (Figure 4.39).

Step 5: With someone holding the top of the windshield at the other end, cut across the bottom of the windshield (Figure 4.40).

Step 6: Both rescuers lift the windshield up and out (Figure 4.41).

If bypass type shears are not available, a glass saw can be used. In that case, the following steps are recommended:

Step 1: With the point of the saw, cut an access hole in the middle of the windshield at the top (Figure 4.42).

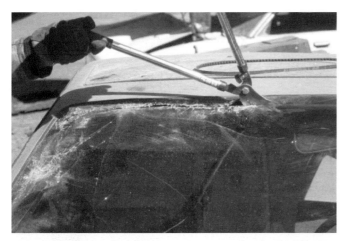
Figure 4.37 Cut across the top.

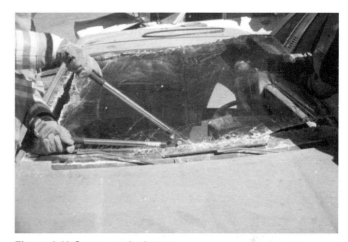
Figure 4.40 Cut across the bottom.

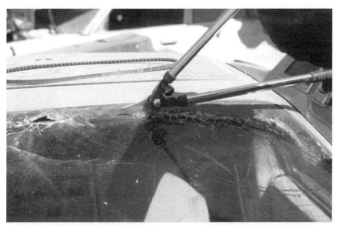
Figure 4.38 Repeat Steps 1 and 2 from the other side.

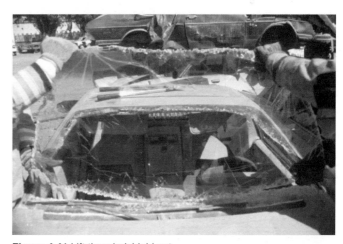
Figure 4.41 Lift the windshield out.

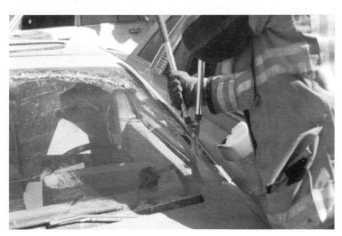
Figure 4.39 Cut from the top down both sides.

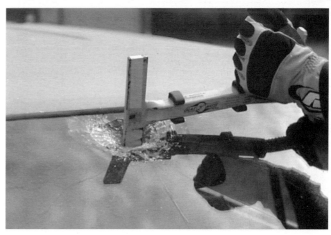
Figure 4.42 Create an access hole at the mid point of the top of the windshield.

Step 2: Insert the saw blade and cut from the middle to the near edge of the windshield (Figure 4.43).

Step 3: Repeat Step 2 from the other side of the vehicle (Figure 4.44).

Step 4: Cut from the top of the windshield to the bottom edge (Figure 4.45).

Step 5: With someone supporting the windshield at the top corner, repeat Step 4 on the other side of the windshield (Figure 4.46).

Step 6: Cut across the bottom of the windshield as described in Steps 2 and 3 (Figure 4.47). The windshield can now be removed and placed safely out of the way.

Older type windshields can be removed as follows:

Step 1: Create an access hole in an upper corner of the windshield. The hole must penetrate all layers of lamination (Figure 4.48).

Step 2: Insert the blade of the saw into the hole and cut to the bottom corner of the windshield (Figure 4.49).

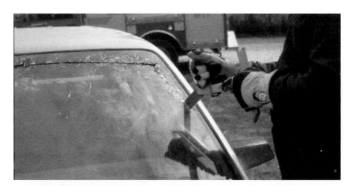

Figure 4.46 Repeat Step 4 from the other side.

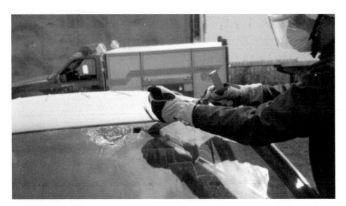

Figure 4.43 Cut from the middle to the near edge.

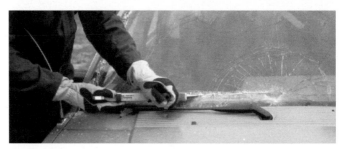

Figure 4.47 Cut across the bottom and remove the windshield.

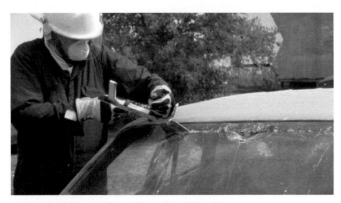

Figure 4.44 Repeat Step 2 from the other side.

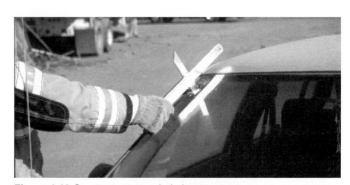

Figure 4.48 Create an access hole in an upper corner.

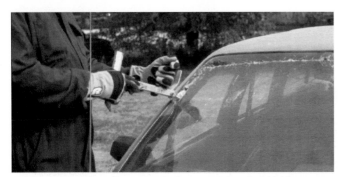

Figure 4.45 Cut from the top to the bottom of the windshield.

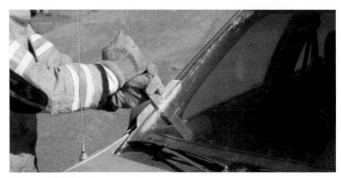

Figure 4.49 Cut from top to bottom.

Step 3: Repeat Steps 1 and 2 on the opposite side (Figure 4.50).

Step 4: Cut across the top edge of the windshield to connect with the side cuts (Figure 4.51).

Step 5: Gently pull the top of the windshield outward and downward, laying it forward over the hood of the vehicle (Figure 4.52). This will separate the windshield from the lower mount, and it can then be placed under the vehicle or in some other out-of-the-way location.

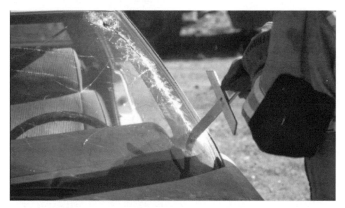

Figure 4.50 Repeat on the other side.

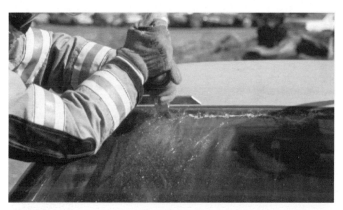

Figure 4.51 Cut across the top edge of the windshield from side cut to side cut.

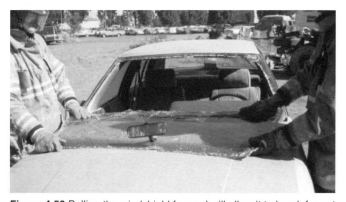

Figure 4.52 Pulling the windshield forward will allow it to break free at the bottom.

Tempered Glass

Tempered glass is most commonly used in side windows and some rear windows. Tempered glass is designed to spread small fracture lines throughout the plate when struck. This results in the glass separating into many small pieces, decreasing the hazards of long, pointed pieces of glass. However, new problems are created such as small nuisance lacerations to unprotected body parts and the possible contamination of open wounds and the eyes with tiny bits of glass.

Removing Tempered Glass

If it is necessary to break a window to access a victim, choose a window as far away from the victim as possible, and protect the victim from glass dust and chips. To protect themselves, rescue personnel should wear full PPE including eye protection.

Removing side and rear windows made of tempered glass is a relatively simple operation. These windows can easily be broken by being struck with a sharp, pointed object such as a glass hammer or even the end of a radio antenna or a windshield wiper arm (Figure 4.53). Or, they may be broken by a spring-loaded center punch being pressed against the glass. These tools are usually applied at a lower corner of the glass but they may work at any point on the glass surface. When using a spring-loaded center punch, the hand holding the tool should be braced with the other hand to increase control of the tool (Figure 4.54). Having

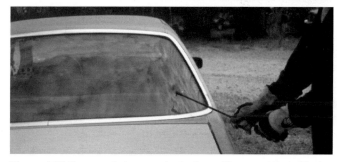

Figure 4.53 Tempered glass can be broken with any pointed object.

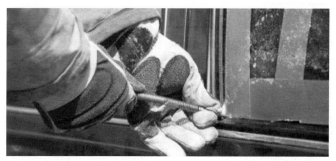

Figure 4.54 Both hands are used when operating a spring-loaded center punch.

control prevents the rescuer from sticking his hand into the glass when it breaks. It also prevents the center punch from being pushed through the window opening and possibly striking a vehicle occupant who may be near the window. A standard center punch or Phillips® screwdriver can also be used. Both of these tools must be driven into the glass with a hammer or other striking tool (Figure 4.55). The pick end of a pick-head axe or Halligan tool will also work if nothing else is available.

One method of controlling the glass fragments is to apply strips of duct tape to the surface of the glass. Enough tape can be applied to cover the entire window surface, or in a crosshatch pattern. The crosshatch pattern is faster to apply and is equally effective (Figure 4.56).

Another method of controlling broken glass is to spray the glass surface with an aerosol adhesive that forms a coating on the glass (Figure 4.57). This coating sets up in seconds and allows the glass to be broken and retained in a sheet. Then the glass can be removed in sheets instead of tiny pieces.

As mentioned earlier, some rear windows are tempered glass and some are laminated. If a window does not respond to removal techniques for tempered glass, it is probably laminated glass and must be removed in the same way as a windshield. If the glass resists all attempts to remove it, it is probably the newer 9 mm glass that is virtually unbreakable. This glass can be left intact while doors and other vehicle components are removed.

Door/Side Panel Removal

When removing the glass from a crashed vehicle does not allow sufficient access to those inside the vehicle, other means must be used. The most obvious means is by simply opening the vehicle's doors. If the doors will not open because they are locked, the interior door lock release can be reached through the window opening. If unlocking the doors does not allow them to open when both the inside and outside latches are used simultaneously, the doors must either be forced open or removed from the vehicle entirely. On two-door vehicles, it is sometimes advantageous to also remove the side panel between the door opening and the rear wheel well.

Door Opening/Removal

Depending upon the situation, it is sometimes sufficient to merely open a jammed vehicle door, at other times it is necessary to remove the door entirely from the vehicle. The following sections describe both of these techniques.

WARNING!

Frontal air bags, side-impact air bags, head protection systems, and seat belt pretensioners can be unintentionally deployed when doors are being forcibly opened or removed. Make sure that rescuers, victims, and loose objects (including seat belt buckles) are out of the deployment path of any of these devices.

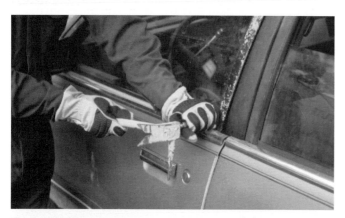

Figure 4.55 Other tools must be driven into the glass.

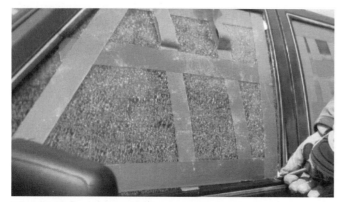

Figure 4.56 Duct tape will help control the broken glass.

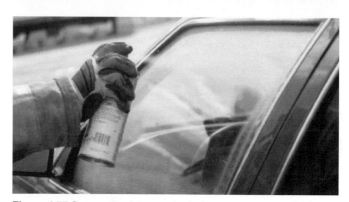

Figure 4.57 Spray adhesive can also help control broken glass.

Door Opening

Obviously, the first thing that should be tried is to simply open all doors in the usual way. If that fails, it may be because the doors are locked. If the collision did not remove the door windows, they should be broken and removed as described earlier. Once the windows have been removed, rescuers can reach inside and unlock the doors. If the doors still cannot be opened, they will have to be forced. Even if a door is ultimately removed from the vehicle, having the door open makes removal easier.

As is true of most evolutions in emergency rescue, there is more than one way to open a jammed door. The fastest and most commonly used method of forcing a jammed door is with a hydraulic spreader. After protecting those inside the vehicle, a safety strap is looped loosely around the B-post and the door frame. The tips of the spreader are inserted into the seam between the door and the B-post above the door handle. The spreader is then opened in a downward and outward direction (Figure 4.58). This allows the door latch to roll off the Nader pin and open the door.

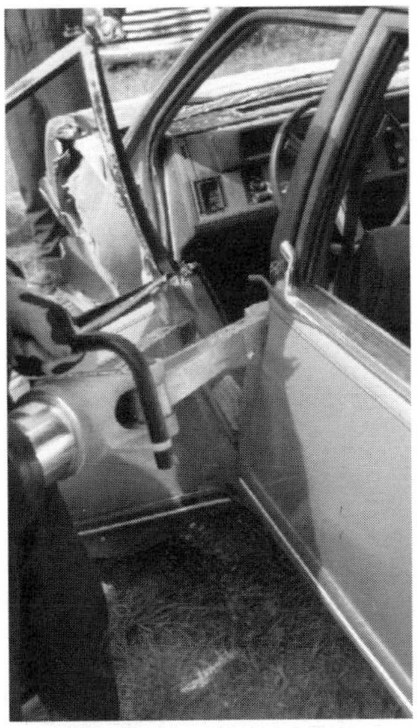

Another way is to cut around the door handle with an air chisel or similar tool so that the

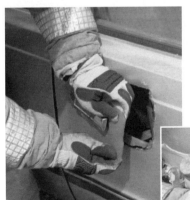

Figure 4.58 One way of opening a jammed door.

Figure 4.59 Cutting the skin of the door exposes the latch mechanism.

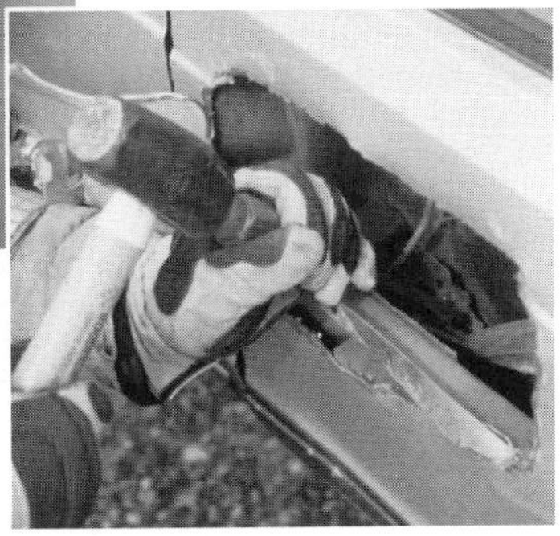

Figure 4.60 The latch can then be released.

skin of the door can be folded back to expose the door latch/lock mechanism (Figure 4.59). The latch/lock housing must be broken open to expose the latch cogs that engage the Nader pin. Once exposed, the cogs can be rotated with a striking tool to disengage the Nader pin (Figure 4.60). Once disengaged, the door should be free to open. If it still resists being opened, it can be pried open by inserting the end of a prying tool into the space between the door and the door post even with the handle.

Door Removal

To provide unencumbered access to victims inside a vehicle, it is often necessary to remove one or more of the vehicle's doors. However, if the vehicle door contains an air bag, a cable (possibly yellow) will be exposed between the door and the A-post when the door is removed.

> ## WARNING!
> DO NOT cut any cable unless you are sure that the battery has been disconnected and the reserve power has dissipated. Otherwise, cutting this cable will deploy the air bag.

If the wires between the door and the A-post *must* be cut, after the battery has been disconnected and the reserve power dissipated, the wires should be separated and cut one at a time with handheld cutters — *never* with power shears (Figure 4.61).

As with door opening techniques, there is more than one way to remove a door. One method is to use an air chisel or reciprocating saw to make three cuts in the skin of the front fender. The first cut is made vertically approximately 6-inches to 1-foot (150 mm to 300 mm) forward of the A-post, from the bottom of the fender to the top — or vice versa (Figure 4.62). A short horizontal cut is then made from the bottom of the first cut to the A-post, and a similar one is made at the top of the first cut (Figure 4.63). This allows the flap of metal to be folded back to expose the door hinges. The hinges can then be unbolted using an impact wrench or ratchet and a socket of the appropriate size (Figure 4.64). This is one good method of door removal on vehicles equipped with air bags in the doors.

Another method uses a power spreader. With the vehicle occupants protected and a safety strap looped around the B-post and the door frame, an access

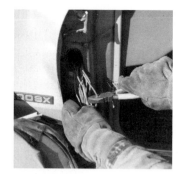
Figure 4.61 Air bag wires should be cut one at a time.

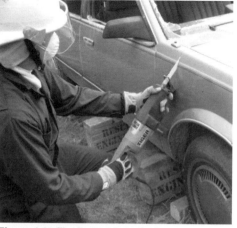
Figure 4.62 The first cut is vertical.

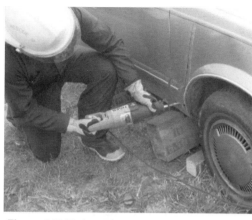
Figure 4.63 Horizontal cuts are made to the A-post.

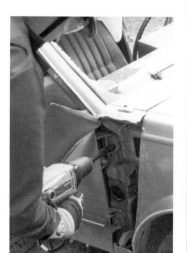
Figure 4.64 The hinges can then be unbolted.

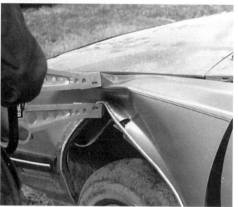
Figure 4.65 Pinch the fender above the wheel well.

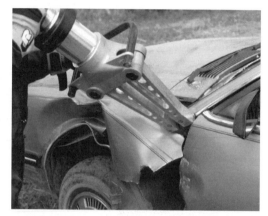
Figure 4.66 Insert the spreader tips near the top hinge.

opening is made in the seam between the A-post and the door by pinching the front fender with a spreader (Figure 4.65). Or, an opening can be made with a Halligan or any other prying tool with a blade narrow enough to fit into the seam. The spreader tips are then inserted very close above or below the top hinge (Figure 4.66). The door is then pried open in a downward and outward direction (Figure 4.67). This pulls the top hinge loose, and if the movement is continued, the bottom hinge breaks away also (Figure 4.68). It may be necessary to break the door loose from the latch mechanism as described earlier.

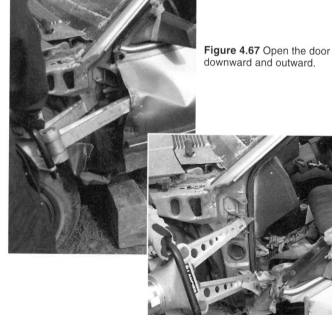
Figure 4.67 Open the door downward and outward.

Figure 4.68 The bottom hinge will break away also.

> ## WARNING!
> Do not lean against a door being forced open with a power spreader. Loop a nylon strap loosely around the front door frame and the B-post to suppress the door's movement when it releases.

An alternate method of removing a door with a power spreader is to place the spreader tips slightly

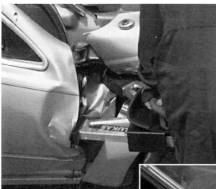

Figure 4.69 The spreader tips are inserted near the top hinge.

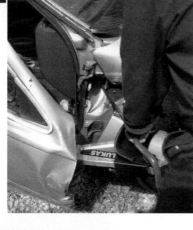

Figure 4.70 The spreader tips are inserted below the bottom hinge.

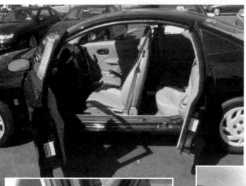

Figure 4.71 There is no B-post between the front door and the third/fourth door.

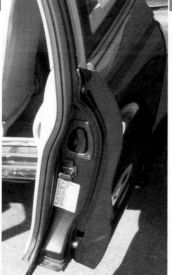

Figure 4.72 A typical door latch on a third door.

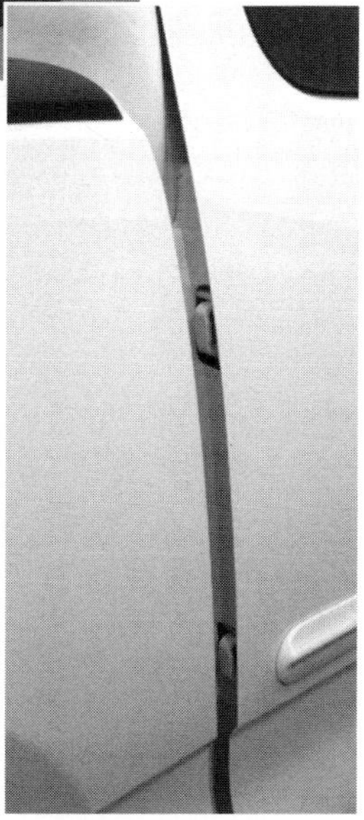

Figure 4.73 The third/fourth door hinges may be exposed.

above or below the top hinge to pull it away from the A-post (Figure 4.69). The spreader tips are then inserted slightly below the bottom hinge to pull it away from the A-post (Figure 4.70). The purpose of this procedure is to remove the door while avoiding the sensors that may deploy the side-impact air bags and to roll the door out and down away from the victim. This redirects the air bag deployment path away from the trapped victim. Otherwise, the procedure is exactly the same as the one previously described.

Factory Third/Fourth Doors

Some automobiles and light trucks are now available from the factory with a third door that is smaller than the regular door. On automobiles, the third door is located directly aft of the driver's door. On light trucks, the third door is located aft of the passenger door. Some light trucks now have this type of door on both sides of the vehicle. Regardless of how many of these doors a vehicle has, there is no B-post between the front door and the third/fourth door (Figure 4.71). Since there is no B-post, the front door latches to the leading edge of the third/fourth door (Figure 4.72). Therefore, the third/fourth doors cannot be opened unless the adjacent front doors are opened first.

Factory third/fourth doors latch at the top and bottom, and even though some of them have inside door handles, they can normally be opened only when the front door is open. On some light trucks (but not all), the third/fourth door hinges are slightly exposed behind the trailing edge of the door (Figure 4.73). This allows access to these hinges, and they can be cut from outside the vehicle with power shears. All factory third/fourth doors have a window with tempered glass. However, since the inside door handle (if so equipped) will not work with the front door closed, there is no advantage to breaking this window in an attempt to gain access into the vehicle.

Third Door Conversion

The term "third door conversion" refers to the technique that is sometimes used to create a wider door opening on two-door vehicles. Because rear seat passengers in two-door vehicles are virtually trapped as long as the front seats are intact and in place, it is sometimes necessary to move the wall of the vehicle to allow the passengers to escape or to allow rescuers to gain access to them for medical evaluation and stabilization.

Those in the rear seat must be protected as the rear window is removed. A third door conversion is much easier to accomplish if the roof is removed first. If the roof has not been removed, use power shears to cut through the B-post at the roof junction (Figure 4.74). Relief cuts must be made at the side panel/C-post junction and at the base of the B-post (Figure 4.75). When cutting the B-post, be careful not to cut into the seat belt pretensioner. Using an air chisel or reciprocating saw, the skin of the panel is then cut from the base of the B-post upward to the top of the panel, across the top of the panel to the C-post junction, and down to the rocker panel (Figure 4.76). This allows the outer skin of the panel to be pulled outward and toward the rear in a large flap (Figure 4.77). Any supporting structure within the panel area can then be cut and the inner wall of the panel folded out and back (Figure 4.78). Once the inner wall has been folded back, any sharp edges should be taped or otherwise covered (Figure 4.79).

A similar technique can be used on four-door automobiles. In this case, the B-post is cut completely through just below its junction with the roof and at its base. When cutting the base of the B-post, be careful not to cut into the rocker panel as the battery cable and/or fuel line may be inside it. Once the cuts are completed, the rear door and the B-post can be removed as a unit creating a clear operating space from the A-post to the C-post (Figure 4.80).

Kick Panel Roll-Up

When a vehicle driver's feet and legs are pinned by the brake and/or clutch pedal, it is often necessary to

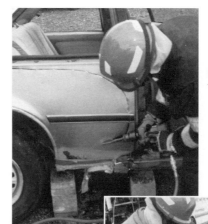

Figure 4.76 Cut the skin of the rear quarter panel.

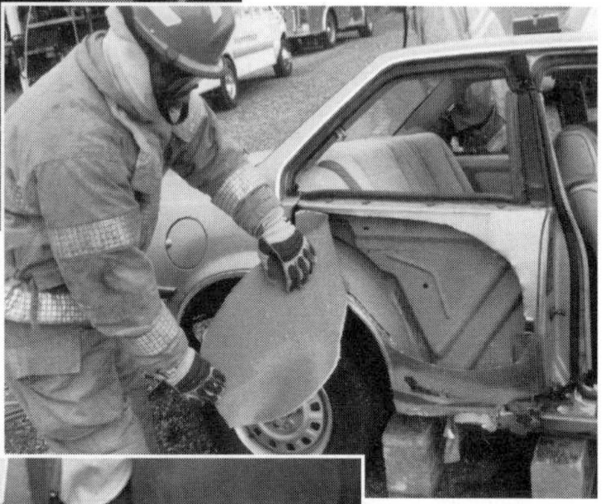

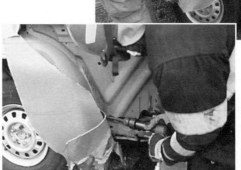

Figure 4.77 Flap the outer skin rearward.

Figure 4.78 Cut the internal support structure and fold the panel back.

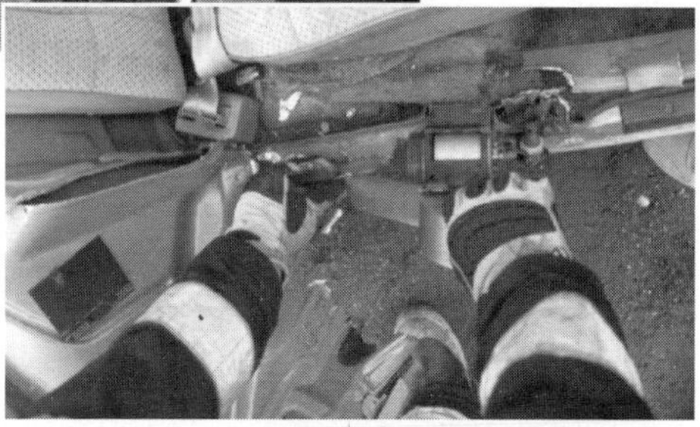

Figure 4.79 Tape the exposed sharp edges for safety.

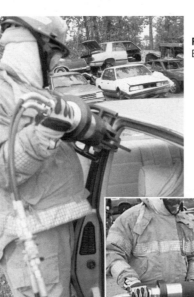

Figure 4.74 Cut through the B-post.

Figure 4.75 Make relief cuts at the bottom of the B- and C-posts.

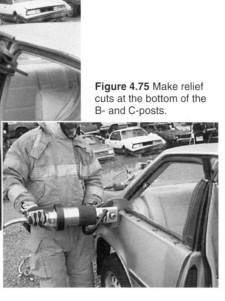

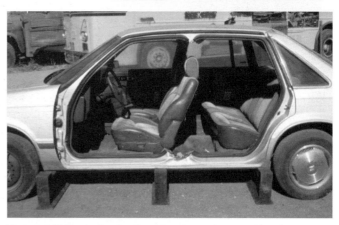

Figure 4.80 Removing the B-post and rear door creates a large opening.

move the kick panel out of the way to allow access to the victim's feet. One of several ways to create this access is to perform a kick panel roll-up. To make a kick panel roll-up, the door is removed as described earlier. The kick panel roll-up is easier to complete if the front fender is removed. In either case, shears are used to cut through the A-post at its base and make a relief cut in the A-post at the dashboard level (Figure 4.81). If the fender has not been removed, an air chisel or reciprocating saw is used to cut the skin of the kick panel from the base of the A-post forward to the wheel well and vertically to the level of the top door hinge (Figure 4.82). This should allow the skin of the kick panel to be pulled outward and upward to expose the substructure. After the substructure has been cut away with an air chisel or reciprocating saw, a spreader can be used to fold the kick panel upward exposing the foot well area (Figure 4.83).

The disentanglement procedures used on different collisions vary depending upon the circumstances. Gaining access to trapped victims by removing a vehicle's roof is a common and frequently performed evolution. Removing the roof also eliminates the possibility of SIPS or inflatable window curtains deploying. Before a vehicle's roof is removed, the doors should be removed.

The doors can be removed with a spreader as described earlier in this chapter. Because unibody vehicles are designed to function as a unit, removing the doors and roof can seriously compromise the vehicle's structural integrity. Therefore, a step chock or other support should be placed under the B-post of unibody vehicles before removing the roof (Figure 4.84).

The roof can then be removed by cutting all the door posts (being careful not to cut into the seat belt pretensioners) and lifting the entire roof off as a unit (Figure 4.85).

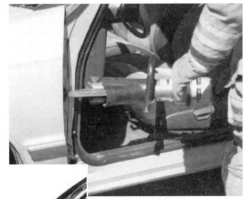

Figure 4.81
The A-post is cut at its base and at the dashboard level.

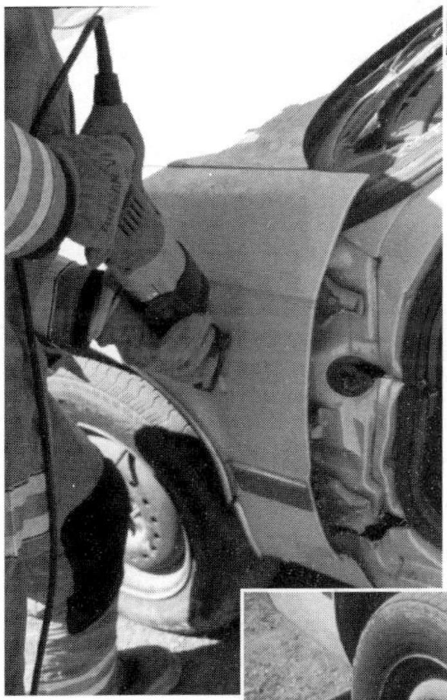

Figure 4.82 The external skin of the panel is cut away.

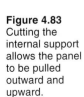

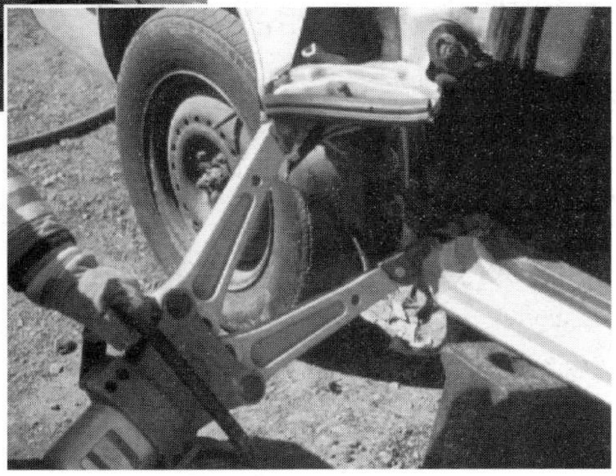

Figure 4.83
Cutting the internal support allows the panel to be pulled outward and upward.

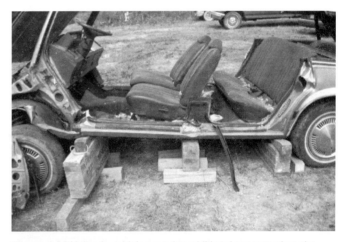

Figure 4.84 Unibody vehicles require additional support when the roof is removed.

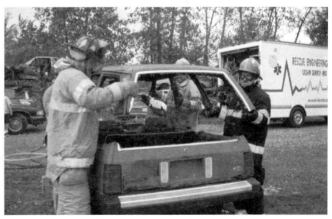

Figure 4.85 The roof can be lifted off as a unit.

Historically, it was SOP in some agencies not to remove the roof but merely to fold it back onto the trunk or forward onto the hood. These procedures were sometimes called "making a roof flap" or simply "flapping the roof." Flapping a roof forward did eliminate the need for removing the windshield. However, flapping a roof takes as long as removing it and may not serve as well. In addition, the materials used in the construction of some newer vehicles may prevent the roof from being folded, so removing the entire roof is the only option.

Dashboard Roll-Up

After a front-end collision, victims are often pinned under the steering wheel and/or wedged under the dashboard. Running a chain attached to a come-along or other device through the windshield opening and pulling the steering wheel up has been standard procedure in many departments for decades. However, in newer vehicles, pulling up the steering wheel up can cause the steering column to pivot at the dashboard and force the end of the column into the driver's torso. The steering wheel can also suddenly

break free and fly forward with tremendous velocity. Therefore, it is recommended that the entire dashboard be moved away from those in the front seat. (**CAUTION:** When applying the following techniques, rescuers must protect themselves and the entrapped victims from any undeployed front-impact or knee-bolster air bags.)

A dashboard roll-up can be accomplished in several ways. One way starts with removing the windshield and both front doors, cutting the roof posts, and removing the roof or folding it back. The other method leaves the windshield in place, the roof posts are cut, and the roof is folded forward onto the hood of the vehicle. Both of these methods involve the following steps:

Step 1: Make a relief cut in both A-posts just above the rocker panel or midway between the hinges (Figure 4.86).

Step 2: Place a ram support at the bottom of the B-post (Figure 4.87).

Step 3: Position extension ram in door opening (Figure 4.88).

Step 4: Extend the ram to push the dashboard up and away from the front seat area (Figure 4.89).

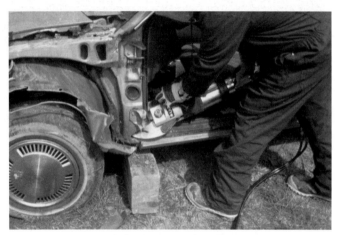

Figure 4.86 Relief cuts are made in the A-posts.

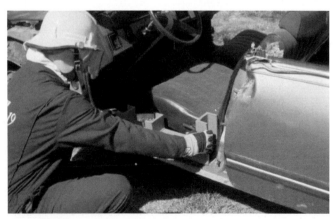

Figure 4.87 Ram support is placed at the bottom of the B-post.

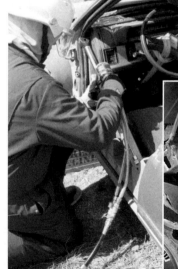

Figure 4.88 Extension ram is then put in place.

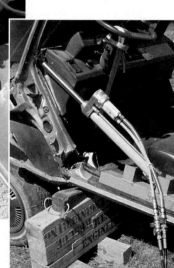

Figure 4.89 The ram is then extended to displace the dashboard.

Cribbing or other suitable spacers should be inserted under the base of the A-post on unibody vehicles, or between the frame and the body on full-frame vehicles, to prevent the dashboard from returning to its original position. The extension ram can be retracted and removed.

Seats

The seats of many newer automobiles contain side-impact air bags. In most vehicles so equipped, the air bags can be disabled by cutting the cable between the sensor and the air bag. This cable is usually in a corrugated black plastic sheath inside the outer edge of the seatback near the bottom (Figure 4.90).

The seatbacks on bucket seats in many vehicles can be reclined several degrees. On bucket seats that do not recline, it will be necessary to cut the seat frame on both sides in order to lower the seatback.

WARNING!

If there are SIPS in the seats, the seat frame *must not be cut*, as this can deploy the air bags. The only safe way to work around any undeployed air bag is to keep rescuers, victims, and any loose objects out of the air bag deployment path.

A vehicle's seats are designed to allow the occupants to sit in relative comfort for long periods of time. To accomplish this end, the driver's seat and front passenger's seat are usually adjustable to a greater or lesser extent. The range of adjustments vary from a simple mechanical system for moving the seat forward or backward or adjusting the angle of the seatback, to electrically operated systems with 8-way movement and adjustable lumbar support. The seats in some newer automobiles also contain the side-impact air bags. These features designed to increase passenger comfort and safety can sometimes cause injuries to passengers and rescuers alike.

To be adjustable forward and back, vehicle seats slide in tracks mounted on the floor of the vehicle. Small metal teeth hold the seats in the desired position in the tracks. However, the inertial forces generated by a high speed impact often break the teeth of these mechanisms allowing the seats to move rapidly forward carrying the seat occupants with them. If the vehicle is not equipped with front-impact and knee-bolster air bags, the driver may "submarine" under the dashboard — that is, become wedged under the dashboard and/or entangled in the steering wheel and brake pedal. In these cases, it may be necessary to move the seats to access the victims.

WARNING!

Be careful to not damage the electronic controls for the front-impact air bags. These controls are often located between the front seats, and damage can cause undeployed air bags to suddenly deploy.

Before a seat is moved, the occupant must be properly packaged as dictated by his injuries, and he must be closely monitored during the seat movement. If the occupant cannot be packaged without moving the seat, the seat must be left in position and the vehicle removed from the victim. In general, it is better to move the vehicle from around the victim by doing a dashboard roll-up than to move the seat. If the victim can be properly packaged and monitored, the seat can be moved to facilitate removing the victim from the vehicle.

To move the front seat rearward, the tips of a spreader are placed between the base of the A-post and the bottom front corner of the seat (Figure 4.91). The tip in contact with the seat must be positioned on the seat frame and not on the seat cushion. Then, with the seat occupant being carefully monitored, the tips of the spreader are slowly opened to force the seat back (Figure 4.92).

If it is necessary to lay the seat back down to a horizontal position, the seat frame must be cut at its base on both sides of the seat — but the caution mentioned earlier must be considered. To make this

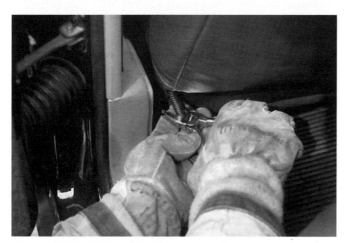

Figure 4.90 The SIPS can be disabled by cutting the cable in the seat.

cut easier and more controlled, the upholstery covering the seat frame should be stripped away.

It is sometimes necessary to remove a front seat entirely — such as to provide room to work on a rear seat passenger. In this case, the seat mounts at the point of attachment to the tracks can be cut with shears (Figure 4.93). Or, they can be broken away by inserting the tips of a spreader between the rocker panel and the bottom of the seat frame (Figure 4.94). Once the attachments on the door side are loose, the tool can be inserted between the seat and the transmission hump to separate it from the track on the inside (Figure 4.95).

Pedals

It is not uncommon for a vehicle driver's right foot to be pinned to the transmission housing or driveshaft tunnel by the brake pedal. If the vehicle has a standard transmission, the clutch pedal may also pin the other foot. In either case, the pedal must either be moved away from the victim's foot or removed entirely.

Once access to the pedal area has been accomplished — either through the door opening or after a kick panel roll-up — the pedals can either be cut or moved out of the way. If available, a hydraulic pedal cutter can be used to quickly cut the pedal arms and free the victim's feet (Figure 4.96). If not, the pedals can be moved by securely attaching a chain or length of webbing around the pedal arm near the foot pad and pulling laterally. The pull can be applied as simply as by a number of rescue personnel physically

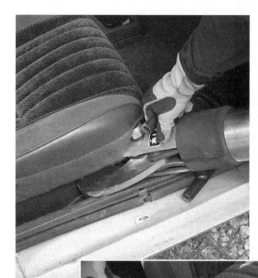

Figure 4.93 The seat mounts can be cut with shears.

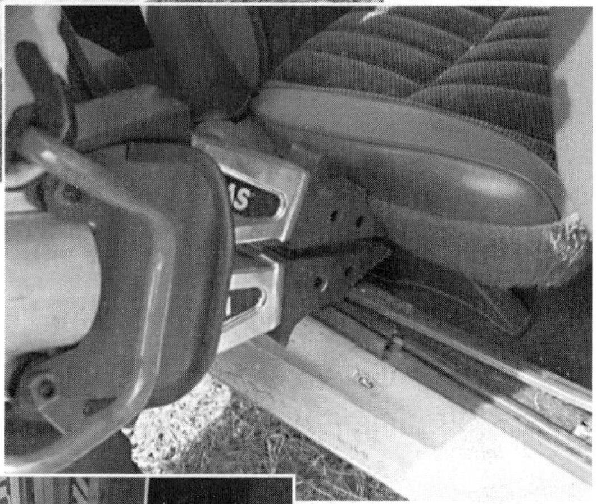

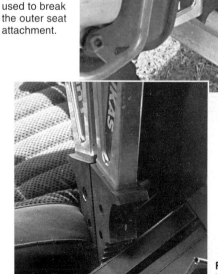

Figure 4.94 A spreader is used to break the outer seat attachment.

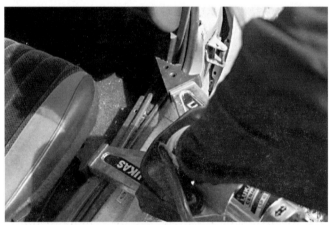

Figure 4.91 Place spreader tips between the A-post and the base of the seat.

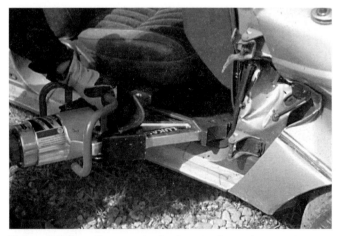

Figure 4.92 Open the spreader tips to move the seat.

Figure 4.95 The spreader is then used to break the inner attachment.

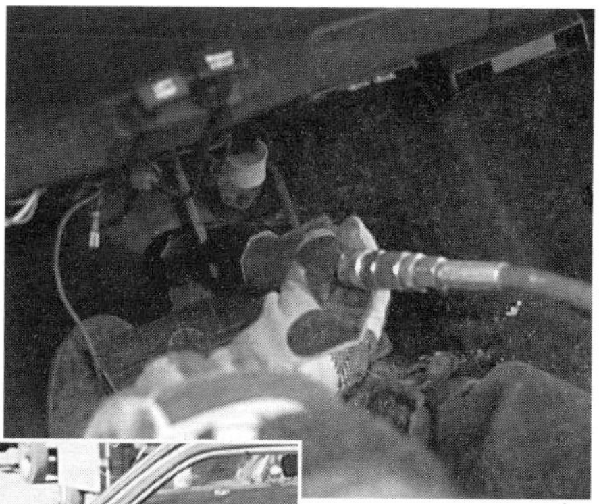

Figure 4.96 A pedal cutter can be used to remove the pedal.

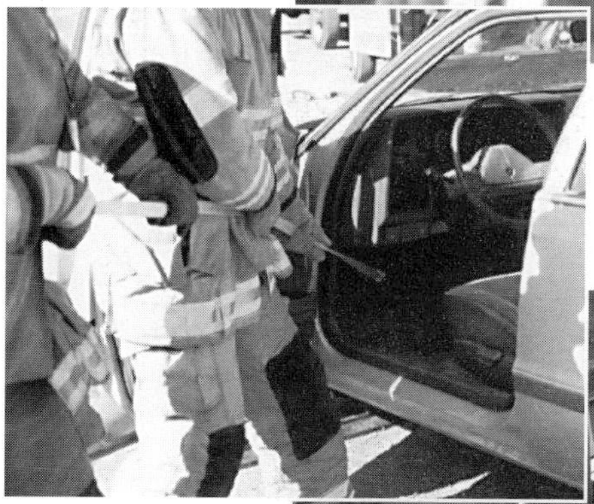

Figure 4.97 A pedal can be moved manually.

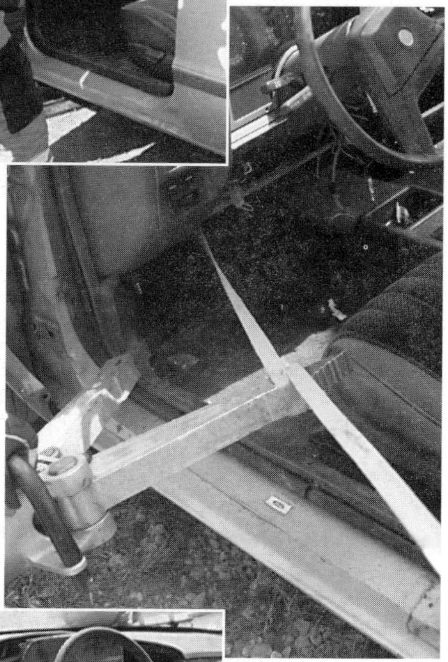

Figure 4.98 A spreader can be used to move a pedal.

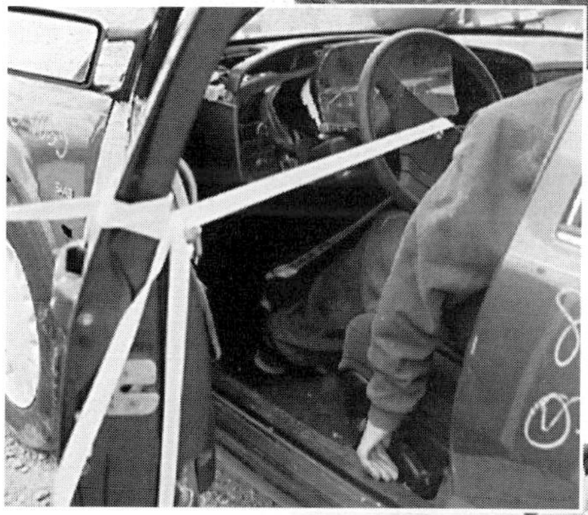

Figure 4.99 A pedal can be moved by opening a door.

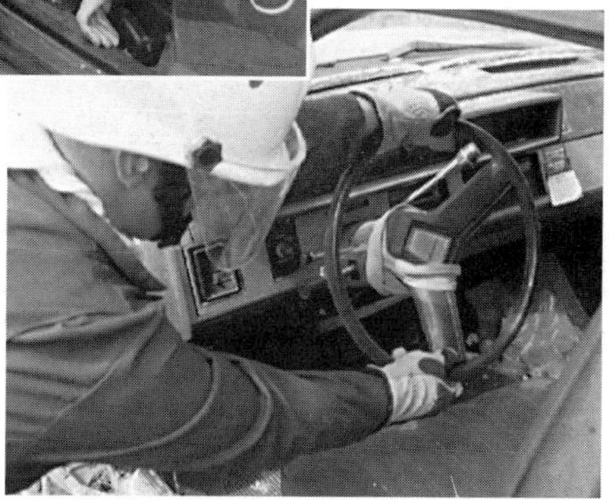

Figure 4.100 A pedal can be moved by turning the steering wheel.

pulling on the attachment (Figure 4.97). It can also be applied by forming the attachment into a short loop and slipping one end of the loop over a spreader tip. The other tip is placed against the rocker panel near the A-post. When the tips are spread apart, the attachment pulls the pedal clear of the victim's feet (Figure 4.98).

If the doors are still attached, the pedal can be moved by strapping it to the frame of a partially opened door. Opening the door fully will move the pedal (Figure 4.99). The pedal can also be bent upwards by strapping it to the steering wheel and then turning the wheel (Figure 4.100).

Entry Through the Floor

Gaining access through the floor of a vehicle may be necessary if the vehicle has come to rest upside down in a ditch and there is limited access to the windows — either because the roof has collapsed or because the vehicle is wedged between the sides of the ditch. In either case, entry through the sides of the vehicle is difficult if not impossible. A far easier technique is to enter the vehicle through the floor.

There are two ways to enter a vehicle through its floor. The choice of which way is best is determined by the type of vehicle, the number of trapped occupants, their locations within the vehicle, and their conditions. One way is to mark an area approximately 2 feet x 2 feet (0.6 m x 0.6 m) over the rear foot well area between the rocker panel on unibody vehicles (the inside of the frame on other types) and the centerline of the vehicle (Figure 4.101). If little is known about the occupants, cutting in this area is least likely to cause additional injury to those inside the vehicle. Using a reciprocating saw, three sides of the square are cut — one parallel to the rocker panel or frame and two more from the ends

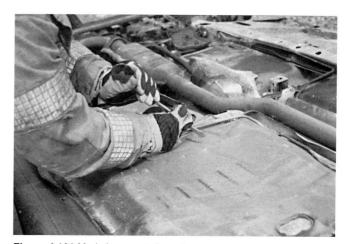

Figure 4.101 Mark the area to be cut.

of the first cut toward the centerline (Figure 4.102). The flap thus created can then be bent upward and toward the centerline (Figure 4.103). This will allow a rescuer to enter the vehicle to assess the condition of those inside.

The other way to gain access to the vehicle's interior through its floor can be used only on unibody vehicles *and* if the front passenger seat is unoccupied. Using a spreader, the bottom of the passenger door is pried away from the rocker panel at least far enough to allow the blade of an open shear to be inserted into the opening—farther if possible (Figure 4.104). The rocker panel is then cut through at a point near the base of the A-post and at a point near the B-post (Figure 4.105). A reciprocating or rotary saw can then be used to extend these cuts toward the centerline of the vehicle (Figure 4.106). The flap of floorboard, with the

passenger seat attached, can then be lifted and folded toward the centerline of the vehicle (Figure 4.107). It may be necessary to cut the seatback from the passenger seat as it is being rotated out of the vehicle.

Entry Through the Roof

Gaining access through the roof of a vehicle on its side can be very effective. Using an air chisel or reciprocating saw, a vertical cut is made in the roof panel about 6 inches (150 mm) away from the edge of windshield down to a point near the ground (Figure 4.108). A similar vertical cut is then made about 6 inches (150 mm) away from the edge of the rear window (Figure 4.109). A horizontal cut is then made connecting the top ends of the two vertical cuts (Figure 4.110). The roof panel can then be flapped down, exposing the headliner (Figure 4.111). The headliner

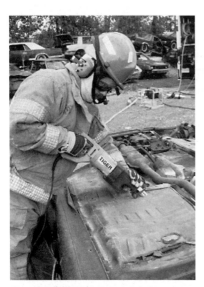

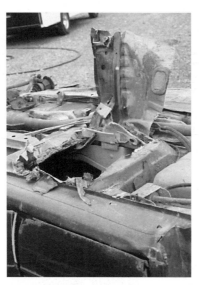

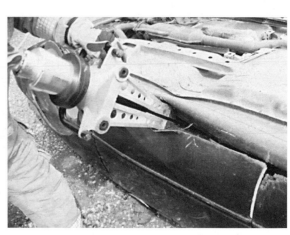

Figure 4.104 The bottom of the door is spread apart.

Figure 4.102 Three sides of the square are cut.

Figure 4.103 The floor panel is then flapped over.

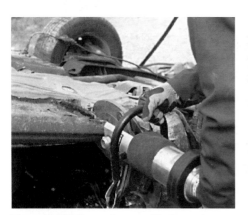

Figure 4.105 The rocker panel is then cut.

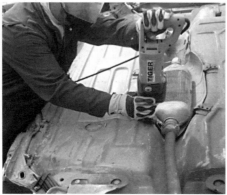

Figure 4.106 The cuts are extended to the center of the floor panel.

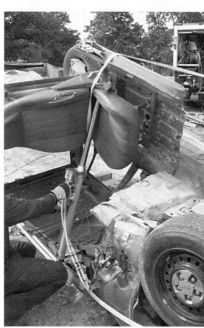

Figure 4.107 The floor panel and seat are then folded toward the middle.

support struts can be cut with shears or bolt cutters (Figure 4.112). If necessary, the headliner can be cut out with a knife in the same pattern as the roof panel.

Summary

Rescuers should choose the easiest route available to gain access into a vehicle. They should first try to open the doors normally, but if they are jammed, the windows would be the next logical choice. Once a suitable opening has been created, at least one medically qualified rescuer should be placed inside the vehicle to begin stabilizing the victim and to protect the victim while disentanglement procedures are in progress. Initial medical assessment and treatment must follow local EMS protocols.

Once the victim's injuries have been assessed, treatment and preparation for removal from the vehicle can be performed simultaneously. It is important to remember that in most cases the vehicle is removed from the victim and not the reverse. Various parts of the vehicle, such as the steering wheel, seat, pedals, and dashboard, may trap the occupant. Their own and the victim's safety should be foremost in the rescuers' minds when selecting and applying the method of extrication.

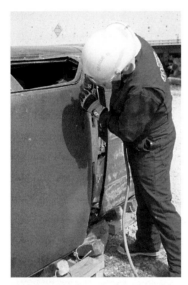

Figure 4.108 A vertical cut is made near the windshield.

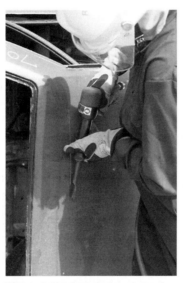

Figure 4.109 A vertical cut is made near the rear window.

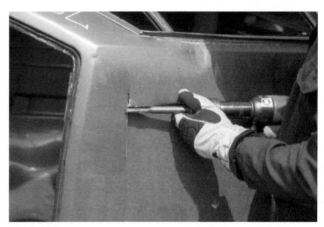

Figure 4.110 A horizontal cut connects the upper ends of two vertical cuts.

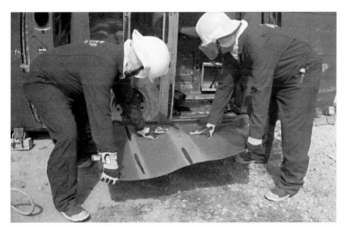

Figure 4.111 The roof panel is then flapped down.

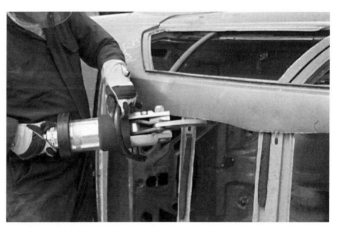

Figure 4.112 The headliner supports are cut.

Chapter 5

Passenger Vehicle Extrication

The majority of all vehicle extrication incidents involve one or more passenger vehicles. These vehicles may be any of several types—automobiles, station wagons, sport utility vehicles, pickup trucks, or minivans. Each vehicle may be occupied by the driver only or by as many as ten or more passengers. To successfully deal with incidents involving passenger vehicles, rescue personnel must know how each type of vehicle differs from other vehicles, how each behaves in a collision, how to stabilize the vehicles and the occupants, and how to extricate the occupants quickly and safely.

This chapter reviews the various types of passenger vehicles and their anatomy. Passenger vehicle safety features and concerns are discussed along with the mechanisms of injury typical of passenger vehicle collisions. Also discussed are the operational aspects of passenger vehicle extrication incidents—sizing up these incidents, stabilizing the vehicles, gaining access to the trapped occupants, and performing extrication on vehicles that have come to rest upright or in various other positions.

Types of Passenger Vehicles

The most common types of small passenger vehicles are automobiles and station wagons, sport utility vehicles, pickup trucks, and minivans—motor homes and other recreational vehicles are discussed in other chapters. Although passenger vehicles all are intended for one basic function — to transport their occupants from one point to another in relative comfort and safety — each is designed to perform that function in a slightly different manner. Automobiles are intended to provide their passengers with the maximum level of comfort. Sport utility vehicles are designed to offset a somewhat lower level of comfort with higher performance off-road and in snow and other

hazardous driving conditions. Pickup trucks sacrifice even more amenities for practicality. Minivans compromise on other features to maximize passenger load. Each of these different designs behaves differently in a collision, and each presents different challenges for extrication personnel.

Automobiles and Station Wagons

Automobiles and station wagons are available in an incredible variety of sizes, shapes, colors, and capabilities. They range from tiny economy models with few amenities and only those safety features that are required by law, to large luxury models with every amenity imaginable and a host of innovative safety features. It is an ongoing challenge for rescue personnel to stay current on the design and safety features unique to each make and model. In the U.S., the National Highway Transportation Safety Administration (NHTSA) classifies automobiles and station wagons according to wheelbase—the distance between the front and rear axles. The NHTSA passenger vehicle classes are subcompact, compact, intermediate, and full size.

Subcompact

NHTSA classifies passenger vehicles with a wheelbase of less than 100 inches (254 cm) as *subcompact*. In general, subcompact cars are primarily *economy* cars. As such, they are relatively tiny vehicles that typically have unibody construction, 4-cylinder engines, and standard transmissions. Because they often do not have a trunk, they have a third door (hatchback) in the rear. They have only those safety features required by law, and they do not fare well in collisions with larger and heavier vehicles or with solid objects. This combination often translates into serious injuries for the driver and other occupants when involved in a collision. However, because of their lightweight construction, subcompact cars are relatively easy to dismantle during extrication operations.

An anomaly in this size class is the sports car. Unlike the rest of the ultrasmall vehicles, these are not economy cars, and they are neither underpowered nor lacking in safety features. Instead, they may have 12-cylinder engines that produce hundreds of horsepower, and they may be equipped with roll bars, racing suspension, disk brakes, and other features that make them very responsive, highly maneuverable, and generally much safer to drive than other vehicles of this size. As a weight-saving measure, sports cars may have large amounts of aluminum and magnesium in their construction, and some may have plastic body components. However, despite there superior engineering and construction, they are still quite small and are therefore vulnerable in a collision. Many of these cars are involved in very high speed collisions, perhaps rolling over numerous times before coming to rest.

Compact

Compact cars, according to NHTSA, are those with a wheelbase between 100 and 104 inches (254 cm and 265 cm). They are typically slightly larger versions of those in the subcompact class, with only the required safety features and few amenities. The majority of compact cars also have unibody construction, 4-cylinder engines, and standard transmissions. Unlike the subcompacts, some compact cars have four doors and a trunk.

There are also compact station wagons. Most have 4-cylinder engines and standard transmissions. Even though their lightweight construction and relatively few safety features make them vulnerable in collisions, their rear door can sometimes make extrication easier.

Intermediate

According to NHTSA, *intermediate* class vehicles are those with a wheelbase of 105 to 109 inches (265 cm to 278 cm). They are somewhat larger than compacts and may have 4- or 6-cylinder engines with either standard or automatic transmissions. Many have unibody construction and are front-wheel drive. Because they are larger than the compacts, they tend to fare better in collisions with other vehicles — but not as well as full-size automobiles or other types of vehicles.

This size class also includes station wagons. Midsize station wagons usually have 6- or 8-cylinder engines

and may have automatic transmissions. Midsize station wagons may have either three or five doors and may or may not have a rigid frame. They are heavier than the compact station wagons, so they tend to fare better in collisions than do the compact versions.

Also included in this size class are sport coupes. These cars are not large enough to be classified as full size, but they usually have 6- or 8-cylinder engines, automatic transmissions, and many luxury features. Some of these vehicles are front-wheel drive, but many are not. While these vehicles are called "sport" coupes, they are more like small luxury cars than true sports cars. They tend to have electrically adjustable seats, high quality sound systems, and luxury car suspension and brakes.

Full Size

While still not the largest or heaviest automobiles and station wagons — full-size passenger vehicles have a wheel base of 110 to 114 inches (278 cm to 291 cm). This class includes what some call *luxury* automobiles. Depending upon the make and model, they typically have 8-cylinder engines, automatic transmissions, plush interiors, soft suspension, and the latest in safety features. These vehicles are relatively heavy, but they may incorporate some aluminum and/or magnesium components to reduce weight. Many are built on rigid frames, others have space frame or unibody construction. Because they are larger and heavier vehicles, they tend to fare better than the other automobiles in collisions.

Also in this size category are the larger and heavier station wagons. Like their smaller counterparts in the midsize category, full-size station wagons usually have five doors and rooftop luggage racks. Because they are full-size vehicles, they tend to have 8-cylinder engines and automatic transmissions. In general, they are more luxuriously appointed than the smaller versions. Their heavy construction can make extrication operations more difficult and time consuming.

The largest automobiles are those with a wheelbase of more than 114 inches (291 cm). This category includes those that have been manufactured as or converted into *limousines*. They are all heavy vehicles built on rigid frames but are still vulnerable in side-impact (T-bone) collisions. Limousine passengers may not wear seat belts, so they can be seriously injured by being thrown about inside the vehicle in the event of a collision. Also, these vehicles almost always have darkly tinted windows, so it can be very difficult for rescue personnel to see into the vehicle without removing the windows.

Sport Utility Vehicles

Sport utility vehicles have replaced the family station wagon in many North American households. While some sport utility vehicles have 4-cylinder engines, most have either 6- or 8-cylinder engines. Most, but not all, have 4-wheel drive capability. Sport utility vehicles are generally larger and heavier than many automobiles, so they tend to fare better in collisions. However, because of their off-road capability, sport utility vehicles are involved in a greater number of nonhighway incidents than any other class of vehicle. The off-road environment can add considerably to the challenges for rescue personnel in these incidents.

Minivans

In many North American households, minivans perform the same functions as both station wagons and sport utility vehicles. Of course, their primary function is to transport people — often an entire family or a children's sports team. While most minivans do not have 4-wheel drive, when the rear seats are removed, they can accommodate cargo that is larger and bulkier than can most other family vehicles. While some minivans have a sliding door on the left side of the vehicle, aft of the driver's door, most do not. While there are exceptions, most minivans have only a driver's door on the left side, and a passenger's door and a conventional or sliding door on the right side. They have either a single or double door in the rear of the vehicle. From a safety standpoint, their large profile makes them vulnerable to crosswinds, and their relatively high center of gravity makes them vulnerable to rollovers.

Pickup Trucks

Pickup trucks are available in a wide range of sizes and styles. Their carrying capacity ranges from ½ to 1 ton, and many have 4-wheel drive capability. This makes them ideal as agricultural or construction vehicles, as well as for hunting, fishing, and other recreational uses. While some pickup trucks are as plush and comfortable as many automobiles — their owners would not think of putting anything more than groceries in the bed of their trucks — pickups are designed to be capable of hauling a load if the owner so chooses. Therefore, these vehicles — whether tiny imports or leviathans made in North America — are all made on rigid frames. This feature alone makes them less vulnerable in collisions than vehicles with unibody construction.

Safety Features and Concerns

As discussed in Chapter 4, Extrication Techniques, a variety of safety features and systems have been incorporated into modern passenger vehicles. They include air bags and other restraint systems, roll bars, and energy-absorbing bumpers. While each of these items is intended to enhance the safety of the vehicle occupants, they can also represent a safety hazard to the occupants and to rescue personnel after a collision. Also of concern from a safety standpoint are vehicles with alternative fuel systems such as LPG, CNG, LNG, or hydrogen.

Air Bags

Since their inception, many falsehoods, myths, and half-truths have developed about vehicle air bags. Understandably, these systems have been the source of endless discussions among rescue personnel. Based on test data from controlled crashes, and the investigative results from actual collisions, the information in the following sections is the most reliable available regarding air bags.

Deployed Air Bags

Air bags that deploy during a collision represent little threat to either rescuers or trapped vehicle occupants. Hopefully, the air bags will have minimized the trauma suffered by those in the vehicle during the crash. The interior of the vehicle and all those inside may be covered with a dusting of fine white powder. This powder is the residue from the sodium azide used to inflate the bag and talcum powder used to lubricate the bag during deployment. In the chemical reaction that deploys an air bag, the sodium azide converts to sodium hydroxide, a highly alkaline powder that becomes ordinary lye when wet. Obviously, the eyes and any open wounds should be protected from contamination by this residue or any other foreign material.

Undeployed Air Bags

Any air bags in a crashed vehicle that did not deploy during the collision are a serious potential safety threat. As mentioned in an earlier chapter, front-impact air bags deploy at speeds in excess of 200 mph (322 k/mh) — side-impact air bags deploy at even higher rates — in fact, *twice* as fast. The reason that side-impact air bags are designed to deploy faster than front-impact bags relates to the differences in the volume of structural material between the passenger compartment and the exterior of the vehicle. The rate at which front-impact air bags deploy takes into account that there is considerable mass — the engine, radiator, front fenders, and front bumper — between the exterior of the vehicle and the passenger compartment. However, the mass between the passenger compartment and the exterior of the door is minimal; therefore, the amount of time needed for the energy of a side-impact collision to be transmitted through the door is measurably less than for the energy of a front-impact collision to reach the passenger compartment. Consequently, side-impact air bags must deploy in a much shorter amount of time than front-impact bags if they are to be effective in protecting the occupants.

Electrically activated air bags continue to be armed as long as the vehicle's battery is connected — and even after it has been disconnected until the reserve power has drained down. The amount of time needed for the reserve power to drain down varies from 1 second to 30 minutes depending upon the make and model of vehicle involved (Table 5.1). All rescue vehicles should carry a laminated sheet showing the latest information from vehicle manufacturers regarding air bag deactivation times for various vehicles.

When the driver's side front-impact air bag did not deploy during a collision, the driver and rescue personnel must be protected from that air bag. Attempting to shield the occupants with a backboard, or by wrapping the air bag housing with duct tape, will have little likelihood of success, and can be extremely dangerous. The best way to protect the occupants is by using a steering wheel cover manufactured specifically for that purpose (Figure 5.1).

Mechanically activated air bags respond to shock or pressure. Therefore, if rescue personnel strike the sensor unit or put too much pressure on it during extrication operations, the bag can suddenly and unexpectedly deploy. Some side-impact air bags are mechanically activated and the sensor units are located inside the front seat cushions on the door side (Figure 5.2). Enough pressure to activate the air bag can be produced if some object is between the sensor unit and the inside of the door as the door is closed. Each air bag operates independently, so accidentally activating one of them does not activate both.

Some passenger vehicles are also equipped with air bags called *knee bolsters* (Figure 5.3). They are designed to inflate beneath the dashboard in a front-impact collision and prevent the driver from sliding forward ("submarining") and becoming wedged under the dashboard. The same precautions must be used with knee bolsters as with other front-impact air bags.

Some passenger vehicles have *head protection systems* — another form of side-impact air bags. These air bags are stored between the headliner and the roof of the vehicle above the side doors. In a side-impact collision, these bags instantly activate. At the time of this manual's publication, there were two types of head protection systems — inflatable tubes and window curtains.

Inflatable Tubes. When inflatable tubes are activated, they instantly inflate. This shortens them and snaps them down into place across the side window (Figure 5.4). Unlike other air bags, inflatable tubes remain inflated after deployment. They are easily deflated by being punctured with a sharp tool or being cut with a knife.

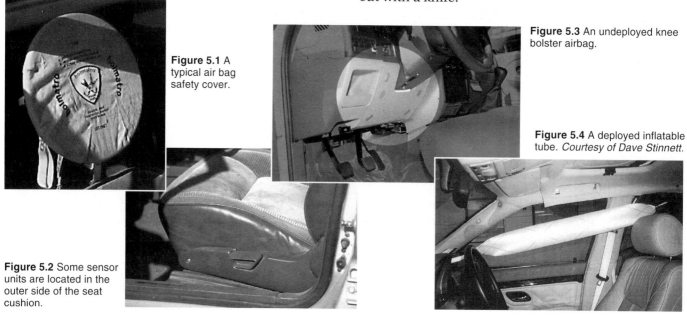

Figure 5.1 A typical air bag safety cover.

Figure 5.3 An undeployed knee bolster airbag.

Figure 5.4 A deployed inflatable tube. *Courtesy of Dave Stinnett.*

Figure 5.2 Some sensor units are located in the outer side of the seat cushion.

Table 5.1
Air Bag Deactivation Times

Acura

Integra	(MY 87-94) – 1.5 min. (MY 95-97) – 3 min.
Legend	(MY 87-88) – 15 sec. (MY 89-92) – 30 sec. (MY 93-94) – 2 min. (MY 95-97) – 3 min.
Legend Coupe LS	(MY 91) – 2 min. (MY 92) – 30 sec. (MY 93-94) – 2 min. (MY 95-06) – 3 min.
Sedan STD	(MY 94) – 2 min. (MY 95-97) – 3 min.
NSX	(MY 91-92) – 30 sec. (MY 93-94) – 90 sec. (MY 95-97) – 3 min.
Vigor LS	(MY 92-94) – 30 sec. (MY 95-97) – 3 min.
Vigor GS	(MY 93-94) – 90 sec. (MY 95-97) – 3 min.
SLX	(MY 96-97) – 15 sec.

Audi

	(MY 89-95) – 10 sec. (MY 96-97) – 3 sec.

Bentley and Rolls Royse

	(MY 90-93) – 30 min. (MY 94-97) – 6 min.

BMW

	(MY 86-93 and MY 94 for the "7-Carline") – 20 min. (MY 94 Vehicles made after 9/93) – 1 sec.

Chrysler

LHS and Concorde	(MY 89-94) – 2 min. (MY 95-97) – 90 sec.
LeBaron Convertible	(MY 89-94) – 2 min. (MY 95) – 90 sec. (MY 96-97) – NA
Town & Country	(MY 89-94) – 2 min. (MY 95-97) – 15 sec.
Sebring Convertible and Sebring Coupe	(MY 89-94) – 2 min. (MY 95) – NA (MY 96-97) – 15 sec.

Dodge

Caravan, Ram Van, and Stratus	(MY 89-94) – 2 min. (MY 95-97) – 15 sec.
Dakota and Neon	(MY 89-94) – 2 min. (MY 95-96) – 90 sec. (MY 97) – 15 sec.
Intrepid and Ram Pickup	(MY 89-94) – 2 min. (MY 95-97) – 90 sec.
Spirit	(MY 89-94) – 2 min. (MY 95) – 9 sec. (MY 96-97) – NA
Viper	(MY 89-94) – 2 min. (MY 95-96) – NA (MY 97) – 15 sec.

Ferrari

456 GT	(MY 1995, Vehicles made up to 12/95) – 30 sec. (MY 1996, Vehicles made after 7/96) – 1 sec.
456 GTA	(MY 1996-1997, Vehicles made beginning 7/96) – 1 sec.
F355	(MY 1995, Vehicles made up to 3/96) – 30 sec. (MY 1996-1997, Vehicles made after 3/96) – 1 sec.

Ford

	(MY 85-89) – 0 sec. (MY 90) – 15 sec. (MY 91-97) – 1 min.

GM and Saturn

	(MY 87-97) – 10 min.

Geo

	(MY 94-97) – 60 sec.

Honda

Accord Wagon	(MY 91-93) – 45 sec. (MY 94) – 2 min. (MY 95-97) – 3 min.
Accord Coupe/ Coupe SE	(MY 92-93) – 45 sec. (MY 94) – 2 min. (MY 95-97) – 3 min.
Accord Sedan	(MY 92-93) – 45 sec. (MY 95-97) – 3 min.
Civic 3D and 4D	(MY 94) – 90 Sec. (MY 95-97) – 3 min.
Civic del Sol, Sedan, Coupe DX and EX, and Hatchback	(MY 89-93) – 30 sec. (MY 94) – 90 sec. (MY 95-97) – 3 min.
Honda Passport	(MY 89-94) – 90 sec. (MY 95-97) – 15 sec.
Honda Prelude S and Si	(MY 92-93) – 30 sec. (MY 94) – 90 sec. (MY 95-97) – 3 min.
Other Preludes	(MY 92-94) – 90 sec. (MY 95-97) – 3 min.

Hyundai

	(MY 94-97) – 30 sec.

Isuzu

Impulse and Stylus	(MY 89-94) – 10 min.
Rodeo	(MY 89-97) – 15 sec.
Trooper	(MY 89-95) – 2 min. (MY 96-97) – 15 sec.

Jaguar

XJS	(Up to MY 96) – Mechanical air bags (MY 97) – 60 sec.
Sedan Models X100	(MY 89-97) – 60 sec. (MY 95-97) – 60 sec.

Jeep and Eagle

Grand Cherokee (Laredo)	(MY 89-94) – 2 min. (MY 95-96) – 90 sec. (MY 97) – 15 sec.
Cherokee and Wrangler	(MY 89-94) – 2 min. (MY 95-96) – NA (MY 97) – 15 sec.
Vision	(MY 89-94) – 2 min. (MY 95-97) – 90 sec.

Land Rover

	(MY 94-97) – 10 min.

Lincoln

	(MY 1985-89) – 0 sec. (MY 90) – 15 sec. (MY 91-97) – 1 min.

Mazda

MX-5 All others	(MY 95-97) – 10 min. (MY 89-94) – 10 min. (MY 95-97) – 1 min.

Mercedes Benz

Side air bags	(MY 89-97) – 1 sec. (MY 95-97) – 1 sec.

Mercury

Villager	(MY 85-89) – 0 sec. (MY 90) – 15 sec. (MY 91-93) – 60 sec. (MY 94-96) – 10 min. (MY 97) – 3 min.
Others	(MY 85-89) – 0 sec. (MY 90) – 15 sec. (MY 91-97) – 1 min.

Mitsubishi

	(MY 89-97) – 1 min.

Nissan and Infinity

	(MY 89-94) – 2 min. (MY 95-97) – 3 min.

Plymouth

Breeze	(MY 89-94) – 2 min. (MY 95) – NA (MY 96) – 90 sec. (MY 97) – 15 sec.
Voyager	(MY 89-94) – 2 min. (MY 95-97) – 15 sec.
Acclaim	(MY 89-94) – 2 min. (MY 95) – 90 sec. (MY 96-97) – NA
All other models	(MY 89-94) – 2 min. (MY 96-97) – 15 sec.

Porsche

944	(MY 90-94) – 20 min. (MY 95-97) – 1 sec.
968 and 928	(MY 90-94) – 20 min. (MY 95-97) – 1 sec.
911	(MY 90-94) – 5 min. (MY 95-97) – 1 sec.

Saab

900	(MY 90-93) – 20 min. (MY 94) – 0 sec. (MY 95-97) – 20 sec.
9000	(MY 90-93) – 20 min. (MY 94) – 0 sec. (MY 95-97) – 20 sec.

Subaru

	(MY 89-97) – 80 sec.

Suzuki

Esteem	(MY 95) – 15 sec. (MY 96) – 15 sec. (MY 97) – 90 sec.
Swift	(MY 95) – 10 sec. (MY 96) – 15 sec. (MY 97) – 90 sec.
Sidekick-2 door, Sidekick-4 door, Sidekick Sport, & X-90	(MY 95-96) – 15 sec. (MY 97) – 90 sec.

Toyota and Lexus

	(MY 90-91) – 20 sec. (MY 92-97) – 90 sec.

Volvo

	(MY 89-97) – 10 sec.

Volkswagon

Cabriolet All other models	(MY 90-93) – 20 min. (MY 94-97) – 1 sec.

Window Curtains. When window curtains are activated, they instantly inflate also (Figure 5.5). However, unlike inflatable tubes, window curtain head protection devices quickly deflate automatically.

Restraint Systems

All newer passenger vehicles are equipped with passive restraint systems — seat belts. These systems consist of a belt that attaches across the wearer's lap and extends across the upper torso. They are intended to restrain the wearer in his seat and keep him from bolting forward in a front-impact collision. More importantly, they are designed to keep the wearer inside the vehicle if the doors come open. Following a collision, these restraints can easily be removed by releasing the buckle or by cutting the belt.

Both testing and experience have made it clear that seat belts are most effective when they are pulled tightly across the wearer's body. But because this can be rather uncomfortable, few vehicle occupants tighten their belts as snugly as they should. Therefore, some manufacturers have added seat belt pretensioners to their vehicles (Figure 5.6). These devices are activated when the front-impact air bags

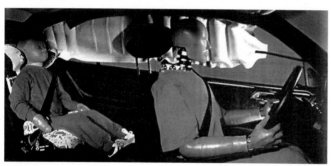

Figure 5.5 A deployed window curtain. *Courtesy of Insurance Institute for Highway Safety.*

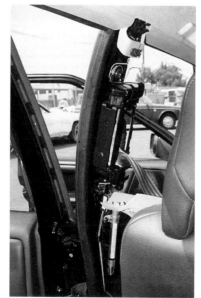

Figure 5.6 Some vehicles are equipped with seat belt pretensioners. *Courtesy of Holmatro Rescue Equipment.*

activate, and they instantly tighten (pretension) the seat belts so that the wearer receives maximum benefit of the belts when the crash energy reaches him. Since these devices are hidden inside the B-posts or the center console, rescuers cannot easily access them to deactivate them. Therefore, the best thing to do is unbuckle and retract the seat belts, and avoid cutting into these units during extrication operations.

Energy Absorbing Bumpers

As discussed in Chapter 4, Extrication Techniques, all vehicles manufactured in North America since 1974 are equipped with some form of energy absorbing bumper system. Therefore, if an automobile or other small passenger vehicle is involved in fire, rescue personnel should avoid the area directly in front of or behind the vehicle, and a distance from the vehicle's front or rear corners equal to the length of the bumper (see Figure 4.15). Also, if the vehicle is equipped with a crushable bumper system, the involved bumper should be flushed with large quantities of water after the fire is out, and personnel should avoid skin contact with any clear liquid that may form on the surface of the bumper as it cools. For a more detailed discussion of these systems and the appropriate safety precautions, see Chapter 4.

Roll Bars

Many convertible automobiles are equipped with roll bars (Figure 5.7). Usually made of hardened tubular steel stock, these roll bars are intended to protect the vehicle occupants in rollover crashes. All other passenger vehicles are now required to have roof supports (commonly called roll cages) that will withstand a force equal to 1.5 times the weight of the vehicle without the roof collapsing in a rollover crash (Figure 5.8). Even though roll bars and cages are designed to withstand significant impact without

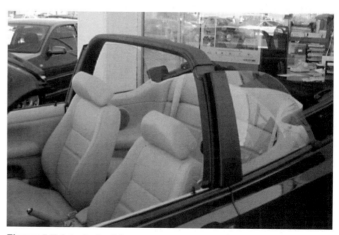

Figure 5.7 A typical roll bar.

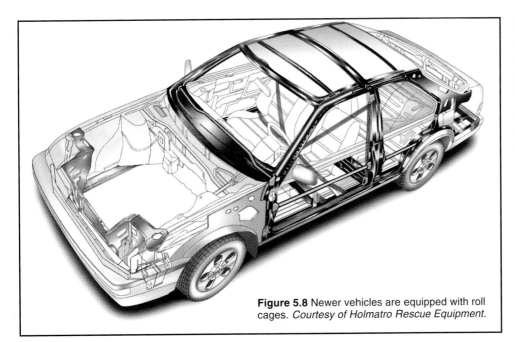

Figure 5.8 Newer vehicles are equipped with roll cages. *Courtesy of Holmatro Rescue Equipment.*

Front-Impact Collisions

Some of the worst injuries to vehicle occupants are produced by front-impact collisions. Inertia forces the driver and any passengers forward as the vehicle is recoiling rearward in the split second following impact. Depending upon the speed of impact, as the front of the vehicle collapses, the dashboard and steering column may be displaced rearward into the passenger compartment.

As the vehicle recoils, if the occupants are unrestrained, the driver's chest and face collide violently with the steering wheel and steering column, causing severe facial, cranial, spinal, and thoracic trauma. The driver's hands fly forward and strike the dashboard, and if the driver's legs were stiffened in the moment before impact, they are likely to be broken. An unrestrained front seat passenger will violently collide with the dashboard, perhaps breaking both arms and suffering massive facial, cranial, spinal, and thoracic trauma. He will either be propelled over the dashboard and into the windshield (and perhaps through it), or under the dashboard to become wedged there. One or both legs may be broken in the process. As the front of the vehicle collapses further, the kick panels may collapse and enfold the feet, legs, and any other body parts wedged under the dashboard. One or both front doors may fly open allowing those inside to be thrown out — or the doors may crumple and jam.

Unrestrained rear seat passengers will also be at the mercy of inertia. They may be propelled forward into the backs of the front seats, perhaps slipping between the front seats and colliding violently with the dashboard. The G-forces generated by their weight impacting the backs of the front seats will be added to the already tremendous forces acting on those in the front seats.

However, if the vehicle were equipped with air bags, and the occupants were wearing their seat belts, the results could be dramatically different. Depending upon the speed of impact, a properly belted driver may survive the crash virtually unscathed or with only minor injuries. If one of the driver's hands were in the

collapsing, they are not indestructible and can collapse onto the occupants, pinning them in their seats. Obviously, roll bars and cages can add to the challenge for rescuers in extrication situations.

Fuel Systems

Passenger vehicle engines can run on any of a variety of fuels currently available — and some on a combination of fuels. The most common passenger vehicle fuel is still gasoline, but diesel and other fuels are gaining in popularity. Some passenger vehicles are equipped with a fuel selector that allows the engine to run on either gasoline, propane or other liquified petroleum gas (LPG), or compressed natural gas (CNG). Because the fuel cylinder is most likely to be installed in the trunk of an automobile or the bed of a pickup truck, checking these areas should always be part of the vehicle size-up process. Obviously, adding highly flammable gaseous products to a vehicle crash increases the potential danger for everyone involved.

Kinematics of Injury

The types of injuries suffered by vehicle occupants vary with the types of collisions. The point, direction, and speed of impact will dictate what injuries are most likely to be produced by any given collision. Knowing what types of injuries are produced by front-impact, rear-impact, and side-impact collisions, as well as rollovers, can help rescuers function more effectively at these incidents.

12 o'clock position at the top of the steering wheel when the air bag deployed, the force of the inflation could push that hand back into the driver's face. This may result in a broken nose, and perhaps facial lacerations if the driver were wearing glasses. If a knee bolster air bag protects the driver's lower legs as the front of the vehicle collapses, there may be little if any injury. Quite a different result when compared to the preceding scenario.

Front seat passengers could expect similar protection if they were buckled up in a vehicle equipped with passenger air bags. Their extremities may flail about until the vehicle comes to rest, but any resulting injuries are likely to be relatively minor. Rear seat passengers may also flail about some, but any resulting injuries are also likely to be relatively minor.

Rear-Impact Collisions
Again, depending upon the speed of impact, rear-impact collisions can create their own unique problems for vehicle occupants and rescuers alike. In relatively low speed impacts, the rear-end structure of large sedans and station wagons can act as a crumple zone softening the impact on those inside. In higher speed impacts, those inside are susceptible to whiplash trauma resulting in spinal injuries. Unrestrained occupants can also be thrown upward making violent contact with the roof of the vehicle. Also, since the rear of most passenger vehicles is lighter than the front end, a rear-end collision can raise the rear of the vehicle off the ground while the vehicle is being pushed forward. This can result in the rear-ended vehicle rolling over. When this happens, the physical effects of being thrown about inside the passenger compartment are added to any other rear-impact injuries.

Side-Impact Collisions
Side-impact collisions can also produce some very serious injuries to the vehicle occupants. Whether the impact is the result of a so-called T-bone collision by another vehicle, or if the vehicle slid sideways into a tree or other solid object, the results are often the same. T-bone collisions can also result in the struck vehicle rolling over. Regardless of how the collision occurs, a vehicle that is struck in the side tends to fold itself around the point of impact. If the speed of impact is high enough, side-impacted vehicles sometimes tear completely apart leaving them in two separate pieces. Obviously, this does not bode well for anyone inside the vehicle.

While side-impact injuries can be prevented or reduced by side-impact air bags and head protection systems, many passenger vehicles still do not have these safety features. The result is that vehicle occupants on the side that is impacted suffer cranial, spinal, and thoracic injuries when they are thrown into the doors and windows by the force of the collision. They can also suffer injuries to the arm and leg on the impact side.

Rollovers
This very common type of incident can also produce a variety of serious injuries to those inside vehicles that roll over one or more times. The most common type of rollover involves a vehicle rolling sideways — that is, rolling onto its side and perhaps continuing to roll onto its roof, its other side, and back onto its wheels. Depending upon the speed at which the vehicle was traveling, the terrain and other variables, a vehicle may roll from one to several times before coming to rest. If the vehicle occupants are properly restrained by their seat belts, they may survive a sideways rollover with relatively minor injuries — provided that the roof does not collapse. If the occupants were not wearing their seat belts and/or the roof of the vehicle collapses on them, the injuries are likely to be much more serious, perhaps fatal. In addition to being tumbled over and over inside the vehicle, unrestrained occupants can be thrown out of the vehicle if the doors come open — and they often do.

Less common, although not rare, are incidents involving a vehicle rolling end-over-end. In most cases, vehicles traveling at normal highway speeds may flip forward onto their roofs and remain in that position. To generate the force necessary to cause a vehicle to flip end-over-end repeatedly, it must be traveling at a very high rate of speed. However, the environment in which the rollover occurs can be a major contributor to this type of incident. For example, if a vehicle traveling at normal highway speed plunges down a steep slope and strikes a boulder or other solid object, inertia may cause it to flip once and the effects of gravity and the angle of the slope may cause it to continue to flip until it reaches the bottom of the slope. Because the roof of a vehicle involved in this type of incident is very likely to collapse, the occupants may suffer cranial and spinal injuries even if they were properly restrained. However, unlike similar crashes staged in the movies, vehicles involved in this sort of crash rarely explode, although they may subsequently catch fire.

Passenger Vehicle Size-Up

Sizing up a passenger vehicle extrication incident follows the same process described in earlier chapters. It is an ongoing process that continues throughout the incident, and the steps involved are: scene assessment, vehicle assessment, victim assessment, and extrication assessment. Depending upon the number of rescue personnel initially at the scene and their capabilities, the steps in the size-up process may have to be done sequentially or they may be done simultaneously.

Scene Assessment

At a passenger vehicle extrication incident, scene assessment involves observing a variety of variables and factoring them into the initial decision-making process. These variables include, but may not be limited to, the weather; day of the week; time of day; emergency and nonemergency vehicular traffic approaching and at the scene; pedestrians in and around the scene; the number of vehicles apparently involved; and any hazards that may be apparent. All these variables must be considered by the first-arriving officer when he is attempting to see the "big picture" — to make a general assessment of the situation and to decide whether more resources will be needed.

Weather

Inclement weather may or may not have contributed to the incident occurring. The important things to be considered are if and how the weather may affect emergency response to the incident, how it might affect those trapped in the vehicles, and the effect it may have on the extrication operations. Inclement weather can slow the response of emergency vehicles. It can obscure the vision of other motorists approaching the scene and may make it more difficult for them to stop short of the scene or to drive around it. Cold weather can make trapped victims more susceptible to hypothermia, and extremely hot weather can put them at risk of suffering heat-related conditions and dehydration. These temperature extremes can also affect rescue personnel who must perform all of the functions necessary for a safe and efficient extrication.

Day of the Week

An incident that occurs on a weekday may be very different from one occurring on a weekend. Pedestrian and vehicular traffic patterns can vary significantly depending upon the day of the week. For example, during the week, many people are either at work or at school during the day, and relatively few are engaged in leisure and recreational activities. However, on the weekends, the reverse may be true. These variables can seriously affect the volume of traffic to be expected in the vicinity of a particular crash scene.

Time of Day

The time of day can also have a significant effect on an extrication incident. Incidents occurring during the morning or afternoon commute can be very difficult for emergency units to reach. Those occurring at night have the added problems associated with darkness and limited visibility. At certain hours of the day, large numbers of school children might be expected to be walking to and from school. Likewise, heavy pedestrian traffic might be expected around shopping areas, theaters, and sports arenas at particular times of the day or night.

Vehicular Traffic

The volume and speed of both emergency and nonemergency vehicular traffic approaching and already at the scene must also be considered as part of scene assessment. While it is important for emergency vehicles to reach the scene as quickly as safely possible, excessive speed and/or overly aggressive driving by emergency vehicle operators can cause additional collisions. Regardless of how well emergency vehicle operators drive, the greater the volume of traffic, the slower the response is likely to be. These possible delays must be factored into the initial size-up.

Pedestrians

Pedestrians at the scene of a vehicle crash may be curious spectators drawn to the scene by the sound of the crash, by others running toward the scene, or by the red lights and sirens of emergency vehicles. They may be witnesses who saw the crash and can contribute valuable information during the extrication operations and/or during the subsequent investigation. They may also be occupants of the involved vehicles who were able to free themselves from the wreckage. In any case, they need to be protected, and their presence needs to be factored into the initial scene assessment.

Vehicles Involved

While a detailed assessment of each involved vehicle is part of a subsequent step in the size-up process, observing the number of vehicles involved is a part of scene assessment. This, too, is part of the process of seeing the "big picture." Obviously, the initial assessment will be very different if the incident involves a single automobile or one that involves multiple vehicles and/or multiple victims.

Hazards

There are a number of possible hazards that could place those at the scene in some danger. Traffic control and crowd control/protection require the response of law enforcement personnel. Obviously, fire crews are required immediately if any vehicles are on fire or are in danger of catching fire. However, leaking fuels and/ or other flammable or combustible liquids also indicate a need for foam-making or other fire protection capabilities. Downed power lines represent a potentially lethal hazard if not isolated until the power is shut off, and they require the response of emergency personnel from the utility provider. Broken power poles also require the response of utility personnel even if there are no downed wires. Hazardous materials spilled at the scene must be isolated, and a hazardous materials response team may be required.

Vehicle Assessment

The second step in the initial size-up of vehicle extrication incidents involves a more detailed assessment of the vehicles involved than was done as part of scene assessment. Each vehicle involved in the collision must be assessed in terms of its position, stability, and condition.

Position

Is the vehicle upright, on its side, or upside down? Is it in some other position, such as partially over or under another vehicle or object? The vehicle's position relates directly to the next consideration — its stability.

Stability

This part of vehicle assessment seeks to determine if the vehicle is or is not stable, and if not, what will be required to stabilize it. Is the vehicle on a stable surface and just needs to be chocked or cribbed, or is it teetering on the brink of a cliff or other precipice? Will jacks, cribbing, step chocks, and/or shoring suffice, or will ropes, chains, or webbing be required to secure it? Will it require a four- or six-point crib, or will the cable from a tow truck's winch be needed? The answers to all these questions can be affected by the next consideration — the vehicle's condition.

Condition

Depending upon the size and type of passenger vehicle involved, the speed of impact and other variables, the vehicle may look significantly different than it did a moment before the collision. As described earlier in this chapter, a front-impact collision may "accordion" the engine compartment and the rest of the front end straight back or to one side or the other, making it difficult to locate and disconnect the battery. It may also displace the dashboard and steering column rearward into the passenger compartment, along with one or both kick panels. The doors may be jammed shut. The windshield and other windows may or may not be intact. Fuel, coolant, and hydraulic fluid may be leaking from the engine compartment.

In a rear-end collision, the rear fenders and trunk may be crumpled, and there may be heavy fuel leaks if the tank has been punctured. The valves and piping associated with an LPG tank may have been damaged and are allowing flammable gas to leak.

In a side-impact collision, the chassis may or may not be in one piece. The chassis may be wrapped around whatever it came into contact with. The doors on the impact side may be seriously damaged and virtually inaccessible, while the doors on the opposite side may be fully functional.

In a rollover incident, depending upon whether the vehicle rolled sideways or end-over-end and how many times it rolled, the damage may be relatively minor or nearly total. The main questions are whether the roof has collapsed or whether the roof posts continue to support it in or near its original configuration, and whether the doors came open or remained shut during the rollover. How the doors behaved as the vehicle rolled over has a serious and direct effect on the next consideration — victim assessment.

Victim Assessment

The third step in the initial assessment of a passenger vehicle extrication incident involves a more detailed assessment of the trapped victims than was done during vehicle assessment. Hopefully, there will be a sufficient number of rescue personnel on scene initially to allow this process to be started simultaneously with vehicle assessment.

Depending upon the dynamics of the collision, there may be one or more victims outside of the involved vehicles. They may have been pedestrians struck by one of the vehicles, or vehicle occupants who were ejected from one of the vehicles. In any case, they must be located and assessed as soon as possible.

The initial assessment of those trapped inside a vehicle must be performed from outside the vehicle until it is stabilized. This precaution is necessary to prevent sudden and unexpected movement of the vehicle as a result of rescue personnel entering and moving around inside the vehicle. To the extent possible under these circumstances, rescue personnel must attempt to determine how many victims are trapped in each vehicle and the apparent condition of each victim (Figure 5.9).

Based on the kinematics of injury discussed earlier in this chapter, what do the victims' major injuries appear to be? Are they wedged under the dashboard and/or entangled in the foot pedals? Are they conscious or unconscious? Can they communicate, or are they dazed and disoriented? Are they bleeding, and if so, how profusely? Are they breathing, and if so, is it nearly normal or very labored? Are their limbs in a normal position, or are they contorted? Are a sufficient number of ambulances on scene or en route, or are additional ones needed? The answers to these questions have a direct bearing on the final consideration in sizing up a passenger vehicle incident — extrication assessment.

Extrication Assessment

The final step in the process of sizing up a passenger vehicle extrication incident involves an assessment of what will be needed to safely and quickly extricate the trapped victims. This step will provide the incident commander (IC) with the final bit of information needed to make the critical decisions regarding operational priorities and how available resources can be used to best advantage.

The vehicle assessment step in the size-up process attempts to determine what actions will be needed to extricate those trapped in the vehicle. Are flammable or toxic materials leaking or spilled? Do the vehicle's windshield and/or windows need to be removed? Do the vehicle's doors need to be forced open or removed? Does the roof need to be flapped forward or backward or removed all together? Is a kick panel roll-up or roll-down needed? Is a third-door conversion needed? Is a steering column and/or dashboard roll-up needed?

An assessment of the equipment and other resources that are available to take these actions is the other half of the equation that the IC must solve. Given all the information supplied by all the steps in the size-up process, the IC must determine what personnel and equipment resources are needed to provide fire protection and/or hazard mitigation, victim care and management, and the needed extrication operations. If those resources are not already at the scene or en route, they must be requested *immediately* (Figure 5.10).

Passenger Vehicle Stabilization

As mentioned earlier in this chapter, before rescue personnel can enter a crashed vehicle to conduct a more thorough assessment of the victims inside and to properly package them for extrication, it is imperative that the vehicle be stabilized first. The essence of vehicle stabilization is to prevent sudden and unexpected movement of the vehicle by creating a sufficient number of points of contact between the vehicle and a stable surface — the ground or the

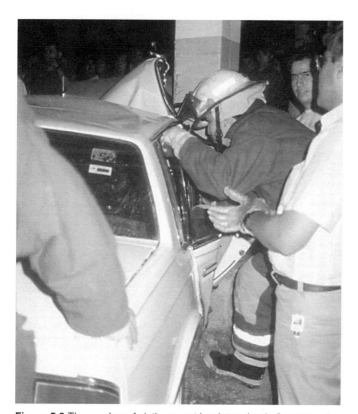

Figure 5.9 The number of victims must be determined. *Courtesy of Steve Taylor.*

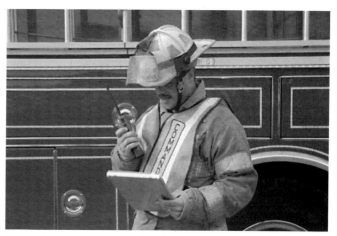

Figure 5.10 The sooner additional resources are called, the better.

pavement — to prevent it from moving in any direction. While the equipment used remains the same, the techniques employed to stabilize a passenger vehicle will vary depending upon the position in which the vehicle is found. The following sections discuss the stabilization techniques used for a passenger vehicle that is upright, on its side, on its roof, and in other positions.

Upright

The majority of vehicles involved in collisions will be found upright. However, because a vehicle is resting on its wheels does not mean that it is stable. The inflated tires allow a certain amount of movement, especially laterally. Also, the vehicle's suspension system is designed to allow the vehicle's chassis to move in various directions. Even these small amounts of bounce and sway are enough to aggravate a trapped victim's injuries. Therefore, the vehicle must be stabilized as quickly as reasonably possible.

In many cases, chocking the wheels and doing a four-point crib by installing one step chock aft of the front wheel well (forward of the door) and one forward of the rear wheel well on both sides of the vehicle will suffice (Figure 5.11). Once the chocks are shimmed into a tight fit, the vehicle should be stable enough to start the next phase of the operation.

On Side

A passenger vehicle on its side can sometimes be a challenge to stabilize. This is because the contours of the side of the vehicle are usually more rounded and offer fewer positive purchase points than a vehicle that is upright. The sheet metal or plastic fenders and side panels are not as strong as other structural members, and they tend to simply bend when supports are wedged under them, so chocks or other supports should be installed at the door posts. Because of the roundness of the roof edge, it may be advisable to invert the step chocks before sliding them under the vehicle (Figure 5.12). Depending upon how stable the vehicle is after cribbing is installed as just described, it may be advisable to shore the floor pan of the vehicle to prevent any possibility of the vehicle rolling back onto its wheels. This can be done by using hi-lift jacks, manufactured metal shores, or pieces of 4-x 4-inch (100 mm x 100 mm) shoring secured with webbing (Figure 5.13). Securing the vehicle with rope, chain, or webbing in addition to the shoring is also recommended.

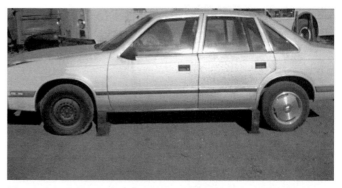

Figure 5.11 A four-point crib may be all that is necessary.

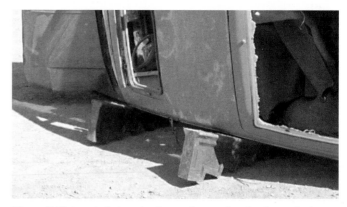

Figure 5.12 Inverted step chocks can be used under the roof edge.

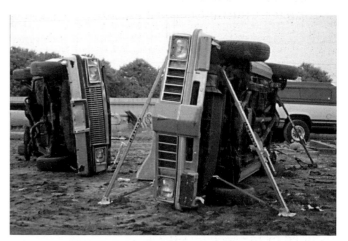

Figure 5.13 Shoring devices should be secured with webbing. *Courtesy of Steve Bourne.*

On Roof

A passenger vehicle on its roof can be even more of a challenge to stabilize than one on its side. The roofs of most passenger vehicles are rounded and offer few if any positive purchase points. Initially, a four- or six-point crib with inverted step chocks installed at the door/roof posts will prevent most movement (Figure 5.14). To prevent the vehicle from rocking fore and aft, and to prevent further roof collapse, the front and rear of the vehicle should be supported with cribbing or hi-lift jacks (Figure 5.15).

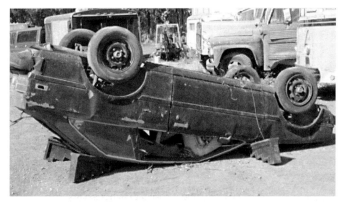

Figure 5.14 Inverted step chocks may prevent the vehicles from rocking.

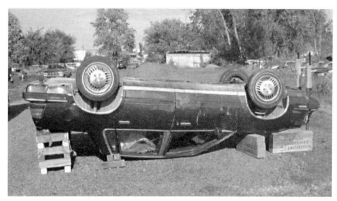

Figure 5.15 The front and rear of the vehicle should be supported.

Other Positions

Stabilizing vehicles found in positions other than those already described will test the ingenuity of rescue personnel assigned to perform this task. However, regardless of what technique is used to stabilize a vehicle, the emphasis must be on safety. While speed and efficiency are highly desirable, the security and effectiveness of the stabilization measures are far more important. A rapidly installed crib that fails is far worse than one that takes longer to install but does the job.

When deciding how to stabilize a vehicle that has come to rest in an unusual position, rescue personnel should remember the discussions in Chapter 4 regarding center of gravity, mass, and vehicle integrity. These basic physical principles will dictate how a vehicle is likely to move when its components are manipulated or removed during extrication operations. If a vehicle is on a steep slope or hanging over the edge of a bridge or cliff, shoring and/or rigging can be used to offset the forces of gravity and secure the vehicle in place. If the vehicle is wedged under another vehicle or other object, the goal is to limit if not eliminate the vehicle's reaction when the overlying object is removed. Exactly how this is done will be dictated by the specific situation.

Gaining Access

Once a crashed passenger vehicle has been stabilized, the next step is to gain access to the interior of the vehicle. As mentioned earlier, this may be as simple as opening the doors in the normal way — as in all forcible entry, *try before you pry* (Figure 5.16). However, in many cases, the doors are either locked or jammed, or both.

Windows

If the doors are either locked or jammed, removing the side windows to allow access to the door locks/

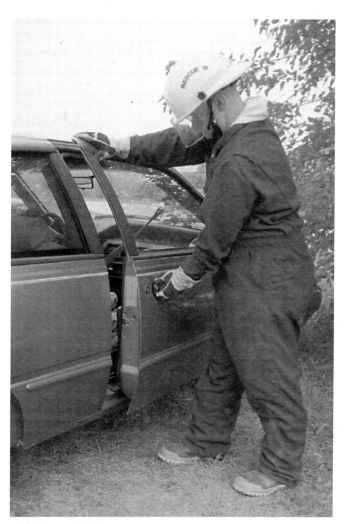

Figure 5.16 Try before you pry.

handles is often necessary. The windows can be removed using the tools and techniques described in Chapter 4. Once the windows have been removed, the door lock/handle can be reached through the window opening. Depending upon the specific situation, it may or may not be necessary to remove the vehicle's windshield. If it is, it should be done using the tools and techniques described in Chapter 4.

Doors

When the door has been unlocked, the door handle should be tried. If that allows the door to be opened, the door handle can be held in the open position by inserting a short piece of angle-iron — cut specifically for this purpose — between the handle and the door handle recess (Figure 5.17). Holding the door handle in the open position prevents the door from latching again if it closes when released.

If the doors are jammed, they must be forced open using the tools and techniques described in Chapter 4. Whether the doors need to be removed or merely opened will be dictated by the specific situation. In two-door passenger vehicles, even opening or removing the doors may still not provide sufficient working room for safe and efficient extrication operations. In these cases, a third-door conversion may be needed.

Third-Door Conversion

As described in Chapter 4, this technique involves using shears and either a reciprocating saw or air chisel to flap back the side panel between the B-post and the rear fender well. This creates an unobstructed opening from the A-post back to the rear fender well (Figure 5.18).

Roof Removal

When victims are trapped inside a vehicle that has come to rest on its side, one of the fastest and most efficient ways of gaining access to them is by opening the doors that are on the top side of the vehicle. However, this is usually not the best route to use for extricating the victims. This is more often done by removing all or part of the vehicle's roof.

Again, as described in Chapter 4, shears or other suitable cutters can be used to cut through the door/roof posts that are accessible, depending upon how the vehicle is lying. If the vehicle is lying on its side doors, but the door/roof posts are accessible, all the posts can be cut and the entire roof removed (Figure 5.19). If the vehicle is lying on the door/roof posts on one side of the vehicle, the other posts can be cut and the roof flapped down to the ground. Or, as described in Chapter 4, using an air chisel to cut around the edge of the roof and removing the sheet metal and any cross members will create a relatively large opening through which victims can be extricated. However, compared to roof removal, cutting through the roof will probably take longer (Figure 5.20). (**CAUTION:** Flapping or removing the roof of a passenger vehicle on its side may compromise the vehicle's stability.)

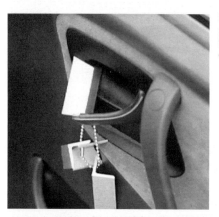

Figure 5.17 A short piece of angle-iron will hold the door latch open.

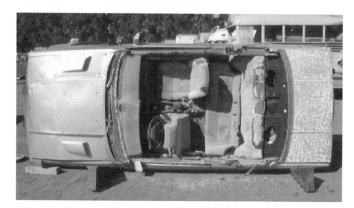

Figure 5.19 If all posts are accessible, the roof can be removed.

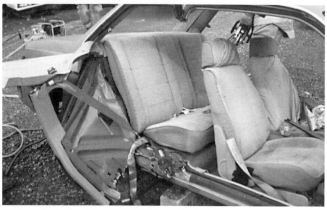

Figure 5.18 A third-door conversion may be needed.

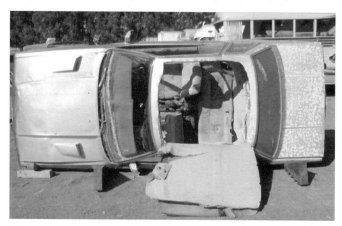

Figure 5.20 Cutting through the roof may be the best option.

Extrication Process

Once the vehicle has been stabilized and access to its interior has been gained, all that remains of the extrication phase of the operation is the sometimes challenging process of disentangling the trapped victims and removing them from the vehicle. As mentioned earlier, the techniques and procedures involved in medically stabilizing and properly packaging an injured victim for extrication are beyond the scope of this manual. Therefore, in the extrication techniques that follow, it is assumed that medical stabilization and packaging have been or are being done. As with the other phases of the process, the extrication techniques used will vary depending upon the position of the vehicle — upright, on its side, on its roof, or in other positions.

Upright

Regardless of where the trapped victims are located within the vehicle, rescuers must focus their efforts on disentangling the victims — that is, removing the vehicle from the victims. And, they must do so in a way that will not aggravate the victims' injuries. This means that the extrication team must closely coordinate their efforts with those who are stabilizing and packaging the victims.

Disentanglement may involve cutting the brake and/or clutch pedals or bending them out of the way to free the driver's feet. It may involve removing the front seat backs or the entire seats. Or, it may involve removing or flapping the roof or doing a third-door conversion and/or a dashboard roll-up. These operations, too, can be performed using the tools and techniques described in Chapter 4.

Once the vehicle has been removed from the victims, and they have been properly packaged, the extrication team should work with the medical team to secure each victim to the appropriate size backboard. Then, working together, the team members carefully lift each victim and remove them from the wreckage. Once clear of the wreckage, the victims can be transferred to those responsible for transporting them to a medical facility.

On Side

Disentangling and extricating victims from a vehicle on its side can sometimes be very challenging. However, because the victims may still be belted into their seats or piled on top of each other at the bottom of the wreckage, the greatest challenge may be for the medical team responsible for stabilizing and packaging the trapped victims. As described in the preceding section on gaining access, roof removal is probably the best option for creating a clear opening through which the victims can be extricated — provided that it can be done without compromising the vehicle's stability. Given a well-trained and equipped extrication team, the roof of a passenger vehicle can be flapped down or removed in less than a minute.

On Roof

When a vehicle has come to rest on its roof, the occupants may be in dire need of extrication — and as quickly as safely possible. Unconscious victims hanging upside down from their seat belts will not survive very long, even if their injuries are not otherwise life-threatening. In addition, the possibility of the vehicle catching fire is greater than when in other positions because of the fuel and other hazardous fluids that are almost surely to be leaking from the vehicle. Therefore, time is of the essence. However, the safety of rescue personnel and victims should not be compromised to expedite the extrication.

Depending upon the structural condition of the vehicle, members of the extrication team may be available to assist the medical team in freeing victims hanging from their seat belts and with packaging them for extrication. As in all extrication operations, all rescue personnel must work together cooperatively for the good of those in need of their help.

Disentanglement and extrication from a vehicle on its roof may be complicated by the fact that removing door posts or other components may weaken the vehicle's structural integrity. This could cause the vehicle to suddenly and unexpectedly move in some way, perhaps aggravating the victim's injuries. Therefore, rescue personnel must anticipate the consequences of each of their actions before it is taken. If removing a structural component will weaken or destabilize the vehicle, steps must be taken to counteract those effects or another option must be considered. Otherwise, disentangling and extricating victims from a vehicle on its roof are no different than from vehicles in the other positions already discussed.

In those cases where the roof posts have collapsed to form what is known as a *pancake roof collapse*, one proven method of gaining access through the door opening is as follows:

Step 1: Using a power spreader, pinch the rocker panel midway between the A- and B-posts to create an access opening (Figure 5.21).

Step 2: Insert the spreader tips into the access opening and slowly spread the center of the door outward (Figure 5.22).

NOTE: If it becomes necessary to reposition the spreader tips during this operation, insert cribbing into the opening before removing the spreader tips to prevent the opening from closing or the metal from recoiling and possibly striking a victim.

Step 3: When the upper edge of the door has been pulled away from the chassis, use the opening thus created to look inside the vehicle to determine the victims' locations and assess their conditions. As the vehicle's interior will be quite dark, use a flashlight to illuminate the interior (Figure 5.23). If available, a search camera can be used (Figure 5.24)

To gain access into the vehicle, use the tools and techniques described in Chapter 4 (see Figures 4.101 through 4.107).

Other Positions

When a vehicle has come to rest in a position other than those already discussed, rescue personnel may have to use all of their ingenuity and skill to safely and efficiently disentangle and extricate the victims trapped inside. For example, if the victims are trapped inside a vehicle that is wedged under a collapsed bridge or other structure, the working room inside the vehicle may be extremely limited. The space limitation may render the most reliable extrication techniques impractical, if not impossible to perform. Members of the medical and extrication teams may have to work in either the prone or supine position inside of the vehicle. They may also have to take turns working inside the vehicle. However, regardless of how innovative the situation forces rescuers to be, they must never forget that the techniques employed must be safe for them to apply and as safe as possible for the victims. While the goal of extricating all victims without doing further injury still applies, these unusual situations may not allow that to happen. In some extremely rare instances, it may be medically necessary to sacrifice a limb to save a life. Such a decision must be made according to local protocols and through consultation between the IC and a physician at the scene.

Incident Termination

After the last victim has been extricated from the wreckage, the emergency phase has ended and all that remains is to terminate the incident. There are

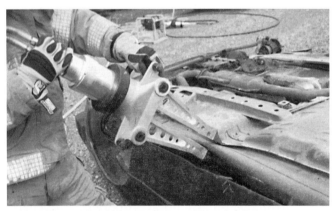

Figure 5.21 Pinch the rocker panel to create an access opening.

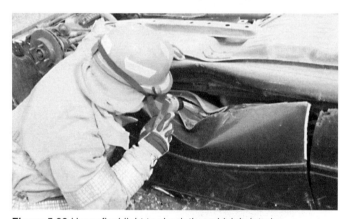

Figure 5.23 Use a flashlight to check the vehicle's interior.

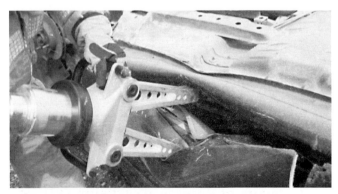

Figure 5.22 Insert the spreader tips and enlarge the opening.

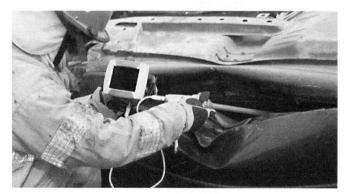

Figure 5.24 A fiber optic search camera can also be used.

three important goals to be accomplished during the termination phase:

- Restoring the scene
- Restoring traffic flow
- Restoring operational readiness

Restoring the Scene

Local protocols vary regarding who is responsible for restoring a vehicle collision scene to as nearly normal as possible. In some jurisdictions, the emergency response agency is responsible, in others it is the responsibility of the tow truck driver. However, regardless of whose responsibility it is, scene restoration must be delayed until law enforcement personnel have finished taking measurements and photographing the scene (Figure 5.25). Once the law enforcement officer in charge gives permission, scene restoration can begin.

Some response agencies prefer to retain responsibility for scene restoration so that they can be sure that any hazardous materials spills are adequately cleaned up and the materials properly disposed of. They also want to ensure that downed power lines or other damaged utilities are properly isolated from the public until they can be repaired.

Regardless of who restores the scene, the point is to make sure that the area is safe for the public to use after emergency units have departed. This will obviously require that all broken glass and other vehicle parts be picked up. Such debris is often swept up and deposited in one of the wrecked vehicles. Of course, the wrecked vehicles themselves must be removed from the scene. Any fluids that were spilled during the incident must also be properly cleaned up and contained. Any hazards, such as downed power lines, broken power poles, or damaged guardrails, that were not repaired during the incident must be isolated using barricades, brightly colored caution tape, and appropriate signage to alert the public to avoid these areas.

Restoring Traffic Flow

The traffic pattern that was established early in the incident must be maintained until the crash scene has been restored. This is necessary to protect those who are engaged in scene restoration activities. However, once all the previously mentioned tasks have been completed, law enforcement can be given permission to restore normal traffic flow.

Restoring Operational Readiness

As soon as the last victim has been extricated and transferred to EMS for treatment and release or transport to a medical facility, rescue and fire fighting units involved in the incident should start preparing for the next call. This process can be started while the scene is being restored — even if some rescue personnel are involved in scene restoration. Power units must be refueled and made ready for service. All tools and equipment used in the incident must be retrieved, inspected, and replaced on the apparatus. This process is simplified if each item is clearly marked with the unit designator. When emergency response units have returned to quarters, the tools, equipment, and PPE used in the incident should be inspected more carefully than was done at the scene, and they should be thoroughly cleaned. Damaged items should be removed from service until they can be repaired or replaced.

When the hardware and rolling stock have been restored to operational readiness, the personnel involved in the incident should also be considered. It may be prudent to relieve them early if they are physically, psychologically, and/or emotionally spent. The wisdom of sending thoroughly exhausted

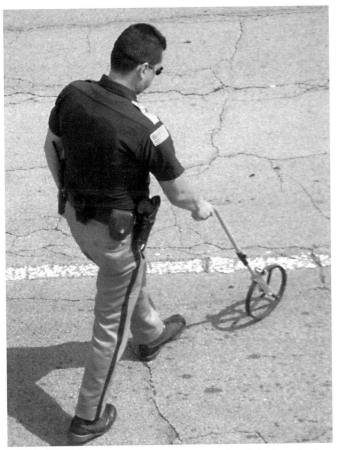

Figure 5.25 Scene restoration must be delayed until the investigation is complete.

personnel out on subsequent calls — perhaps having to make critical, even life-and-death decisions — must be weighed against the trouble and extra expense of relieving them before the end of their scheduled work shift. Those who were directly involved with seriously injured — perhaps even dismembered — victims almost certainly need to attend a critical incident stress debriefing (CISD). To assess these needs, the officer in charge of each unit should conduct an informal debriefing, sometimes called "defusing," with his crew as soon as the apparatus and equipment have been restored to readiness.

The debriefing can be a casual review of the incident over a cup of coffee with the crew. Knowing the members of his crew should allow the officer to detect signs of uncharacteristic behavior such as unusual silence, moodiness, withdrawal — or at the other end of the spectrum — excessive and inappropriate joviality. Any or all of these uncharacteristic emotional displays can indicate a need for CISD.

Because some firefighters and other emergency responders may have an unhealthy "macho" attitude and may believe that it is a sign of weakness to need psychological counseling after a particularly gruesome incident, many jurisdictions make attendance at professionally conducted CISD sessions mandatory within 72 hours of the incident. While attendance is mandatory, *participation* is not. However, any crew member who clearly exhibits uncharacteristic behavior following such an incident, but refuses to participate in the CISD, should be referred for individual counseling.

Once all personnel and equipment are operationally ready, it is critically important that the incident be documented. The officer in charge of each unit involved in the incident should submit a detailed written report describing his unit's actions. The IC should combine all of these individual reports into a single comprehensive report on the entire incident. Because these reports may someday be used as evidence in court, perhaps years after the incident, the reports need to be as accurate and clearly written as possible.

Once the documentation has been completed, it is valuable to conduct a formal review, sometimes called a critique, of the incident. All emergency response personnel who participated in the incident should attend. The review should be conducted in an objective and low-key manner, with the goal being to learn from the experience, not to find fault. The incident should be reviewed chronologically from start to finish to see what went according to SOP and what did not. Any deviations from SOP should be discussed to see if the plans need to be changed or if there is a need for more training and/or better equipment. However, because all incident reports are public records, and because of potential liability litigation, many agencies choose to conduct their incident critiques orally only. This eliminates any written record of actions or inactions by agency personnel who deviated from agency SOP and therefore might be considered mistakes or deficiencies for which the agency and/or the individual could be held liable.

Summary

Rescue personnel should be well trained and adequately equipped to safely and efficiently handle extrication incidents involving passenger vehicles of all types. This means that rescue personnel must be familiar with the types of passenger vehicles, their anatomy, and their individual safety features and concerns. They must also be familiar with how and why vehicle occupants are injured in collisions. When sizing up a passenger vehicle incident, the IC must assign a priority to each vehicle involved in the collision based on the potential for saving lives. In general, this potential relates to the condition of the trapped victims and the time that will be required to extricate them. Rescue personnel must then be capable of stabilizing the involved vehicles, gaining access to the trapped victims, and extricating them as quickly as possible. Finally, an orderly process for terminating these incidents must be used.

Chapter 6

Bus Extrication

With the exception of railroad passenger cars, buses are the largest passenger vehicles with which rescue personnel may have to contend. Like other passenger vehicles, buses are manufactured in a variety of shapes and sizes. They range from 10-passenger commuter vans, to transit and commercial buses capable of carrying more than 40 passengers, to school buses capable of carrying in excess of 90 passengers, to a variety of specialty buses. From the smallest commuter van to the largest passenger coach designed for transcontinental travel, buses are all designed for the same purpose — to convey a relatively large number of passengers from one point to another in relative safety and comfort. However, the fact that a large number of vehicle occupants may be trapped in a bus collision sets this type of extrication problem apart from those involving automobiles and trucks. Therefore, if emergency response organizations are to function safely and effectively during bus extrication incidents, pre-incident planning and realistic training exercises involving mass casualty scenarios are imperative.

This chapter reviews how the various types of buses are classified, along with bus anatomy and how each type is constructed. How bus extrication incidents should be sized up is discussed. Also discussed are bus stabilization, gaining access, and the extrication process as applied to buses.

Bus Classifications

There are four main classifications of buses: school buses, transit buses, commercial buses, and specialty buses. Each type has certain characteristics in common with the other types and other characteristics that are unique. The level of familiarity that rescue personnel have with the anatomy of any particular type of bus will dictate how effectively they can handle

extrication problems in that type of vehicle. Therefore, it is important that rescue personnel learn as much as possible about the common and unique features of each type of bus.

School Buses

Federal Motor Vehicle Safety Standards define a school bus as "a passenger motor vehicle designed to carry more than 10 passengers in addition to the driver, and which the Secretary of Transportation determines is to be used to transport preschool, primary, and secondary school students to or from such schools or school-related events." While this definition limits this type of vehicle to school functions, these and similar vehicles are used by church groups, civic groups, and others. The rescue procedures for these vehicles are the same regardless of who is using the vehicle.

Transit Buses

Transit buses are designed to move a large number of people over relatively short distances. They are most commonly found in urban or metropolitan areas that operate mass transit systems. In some cases, these systems may have bus routes that extend far into the suburbs that surround the core coverage area. Similar types of buses are often used as parking shuttles at airports, large amusement or entertainment facilities, or as employee shuttles within large business or industrial complexes. Because transit buses generally operate in heavy traffic, the potential for involvement in accidents is very high. The potential for a large number of casualties is also present because of the high passenger load and the fact that people may be sitting in an irregular and unrestrained manner or may even be standing. Transit buses have capacities for more than 60 seated passengers — plus a number of standees.

Also included in this classification are articulated transit buses. In some areas, budget limitations have forced transit systems to reduce the frequency of bus service. To offset this reduction, some now use larger buses that can transport more passengers per trip. Because it is impractical to design a single chassis vehicle longer than about 40 feet (12 m), some transit authorities have switched to articulated buses. The advantages in maneuverability offered by these buses are similar to those that the tractor-tiller aerial apparatus offers to the fire service. The vehicle's ability to flex in the middle makes it able to maneuver extremely well in areas that single-chassis vehicles of comparable size could not.

The articulated transit bus consists of a tractor section and a trailer section. The two are connected by a pivoting joint that is enclosed by a large, bellowslike seal. The tractor section is nearly the size of a standard transit bus. The trailer section is considerably shorter. These vehicles are unique in that they have two separate engines. The vehicle is powered by a six- or eight-cylinder engine located in the middle of the tractor section. A separate four-cylinder engine is located in the rear of the trailer section. This rear engine is used solely to power the air-conditioning system. Aside from these specifically mentioned features, articulated buses are constructed in the same manner as conventional transit buses.

Commercial Buses
Commercial buses (also called motor coaches, charter buses, and touring buses) are primarily designed to transport large numbers of people over relatively long distances. These buses may travel regularly scheduled routes or may be chartered by groups to travel to a specific location. Because charter buses travel through almost every region and area, every organization responsible for extrication must be prepared to deal with this type of vehicle. Typically, these buses carry up to about 50 passengers.

Specialty Buses
Some specialty buses are similar to Type A and B school buses (see next section on Bus Anatomy) but have been converted into vehicles for transporting those with disabilities. Others are commercial buses that have been converted into mobile living quarters, offices, and recreational vehicles.

Transporters of those with disabilities may have fewer passengers than school buses of the same size but the occupants may be less able to help themselves in an emergency. Commercial bus conversions present the same extrication problems and challenges as any other commercial bus, but usually with fewer passengers.

Bus Anatomy

Even though all buses are intended for the same purpose — transporting a relatively large number of passengers from one point to another safely — there are significant differences in how the various types of buses are constructed. The following sections discuss the differences and similarities between each type.

School Buses
While school buses vary in size and configuration, all have at least one entry/exit door and at least one additional emergency exit, usually at the rear of the vehicle, that may or may not be an exit door. According to the National Standards for School Buses and School Bus Operations, school buses are divided into four types: A, B, C, and D.

Type A
Essentially large passenger vans, there are two classifications of Type A buses. Type A-I has a gross vehicle weight rating (GVWR) of more that 10,000 pounds (4 540 kg), and Type A-II has a GVWR of less than 10,000 pounds. The entry/exit door is aft of the front wheel well, there is a driver-side door, and the engine is either below the windshield or between the front seats (Figure 6.1).

Type B
These minibus-type vehicles have a GVWR in excess of 10,000 pounds (4 540 kg). The entry/exit door is aft of the front wheel, and there is typically no driver-side door. The engine is usually forward of the windshield (Figure 6.2).

Type C
These full-size conventional-type vehicles are perhaps the closest to a "typical" North American school bus of all the various types. They have a GVWR of greater than 10,000 pounds (4 540 kg), and the engine is forward of the windshield. The entry/exit door is aft of the front fender and there is no driver-side door (Figure 6.3).

Type D
These full-size vehicles are easily distinguished by their rather boxy appearance (Figure 6.4). There is no driver-side door, and unlike all the previously described types, the main entry/exit door is forward of

the front wheels. The engine may be in the front, midship, or rear of the vehicle.

Although most of the full-size school buses have an authorized carrying capacity of up to 66 passengers, changes in the technology of school bus construction have resulted in school buses with larger carrying capacities. All U.S. school bus manufacturers now offer a "super" school bus, 8 x 40 feet long (2.4 m x 12.2 m) (Figure 6.5). The engine in a super bus is located inside, at the front or rear of the bus. The front engine position is similar to the engine location in a typical van-type vehicle.

In the typical super bus, the interior of the bus has been extended forward to the front bumper. By lengthening the body of the vehicle, the flat-nosed bus now has a legal seating capacity of 90 passengers plus the bus driver. A legally permissible overflow of standees equal to 20 percent of the seating capacity is also permitted in some states, increasing the capacity by 16 persons. In addition to the usual door exits, roof hatches may also be provided, one toward the front of the bus and a second toward the rear (Figure 6.6).

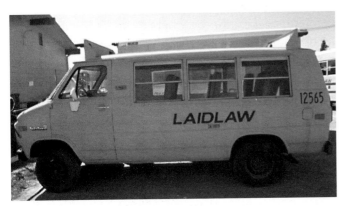

Figure 6.1 One form of Type A school bus.

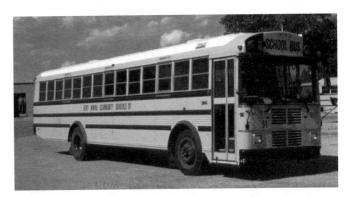

Figure 6.4 A typical Type D school bus.

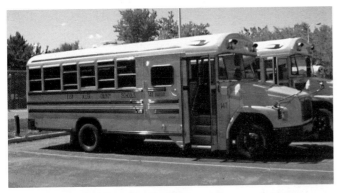

Figure 6.2 A typical Type B school bus.

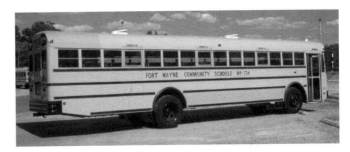

Figure 6.5 A typical "super" school bus.

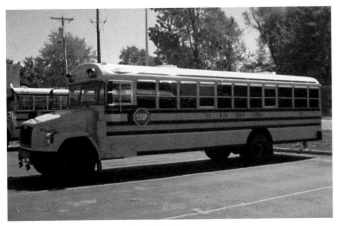

Figure 6.3 A typical Type C school bus.

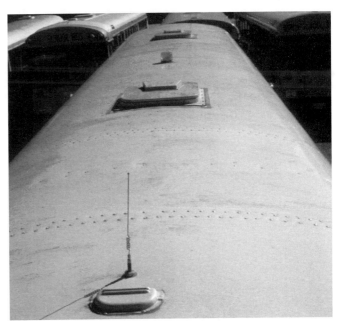

Figure 6.6 Super school buses have two roof hatches.

School Bus Construction

There are two basic construction methods used by major school bus manufacturers: integral construction and body-on-chassis.

Integral Construction. In this method, the body and chassis are formed as a unit. The manufacturer assembles the vehicle starting with the frame and chassis assembly and proceeds item by item to the finished vehicle.

Body-on-Chassis. The body and chassis are manufactured as separate units and joined by the bus manufacturer. As mentioned earlier, each construction method has similarities, and each method has its own unique features. The following sections highlight some of the common elements found on most school buses manufactured in North America.

School Bus Skeletal System. All school bus body units are comprised of a roof, a floor, two sidewalls, and front and rear assemblies. The finish and trim components of each area of the body are supported by a skeletal system beneath. This skeletal system forms the basic structure of the entire bus (Figure 6.7). It dictates how the vehicle will respond during a collision and forms the basis of the protective envelope designed to provide occupant safety and survival.

Sidewalls are comprised of vertical load-bearing frame members and in some models, the roof bows extend down to form the support members. These vertical members serve as partitions between window openings. Running horizontally along the base of each sidewall is a framing element referred to as a *collision beam.* This heavy-gauge steel member is strategically located to limit penetration of an object into the passenger compartment.

Finish panels of 20-gauge steel are typically mounted on the exterior and 22-gauge on the interior of the sidewall frame members. To meet requirements for interior noise attenuation and temperature control, insulation materials may be sandwiched between the interior and exterior panels.

Additional impact resistance is added to the exterior sidewall. Formed rub rails (4¾-inch [120 mm] wide) of 16-gauge steel run the full length of the sidewalls (Figure 6.8). They are intended to minimize penetration during collision and can also be used for identifying occupant location from the exterior. One rub rail will indicate the seat cushion level; if a second rail is present, it will identify the floor level. Some

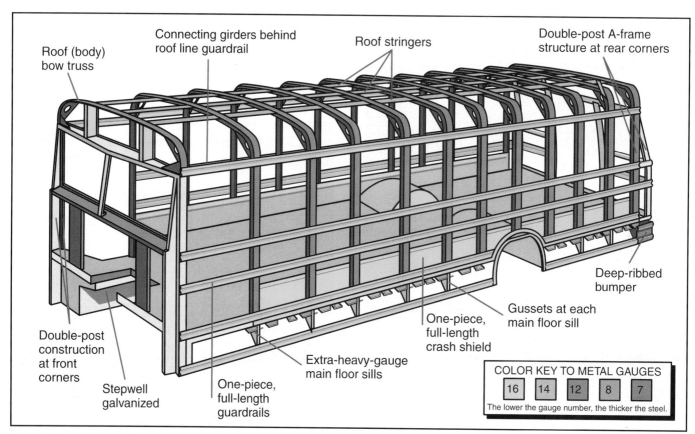

Figure 6.7 Typical school bus skeletal system. *Courtesy of The Wayne Corporation.*

school buses have as many as four rub rails from the bottom of the windows down to the bottom of the skirts.

The rear skeletal system is similar to the sidewall, with additional reinforcement installed to provide protection from rear-end collisions. The additional reinforcement may be a double-post A-frame structural member built into the rear corners of the bus.

The skeletal framework of the school bus roof commonly consists of 11- to 14-gauge steel frame members called *roof bows*. These members span the roof structure from side to side. Within this frame are 14- to 16-gauge girders (known as stringers) running from front to rear, strengthening and spacing the bows. There may be as many as three of these longitudinal members in the roof skeleton.

Insulation material and electrical wiring are located within the framework of the roof. The outside and inside of the framing members are generally covered with sheet metal panels. If breaching the roof structure becomes necessary, the location of the roof bows and stringers can be determined by the rows of rivets used to secure the roof panels.

Emergency escape hatches may also be located in the roof structure. These hatches are made of fiberglass or other lightweight materials, and they open by the activation of a release mechanism from inside or outside (Figure 6.9). If necessary, they may be forced open using conventional prying techniques. These hatches open fully to provide a clear opening of at least 11 x 14 inches (275 mm by 350 mm). Some buses may have larger hatches, especially if they are used to transport physically disabled passengers.

School Bus Floor and Undercarriage. The floor of a school bus consists of several components. In most of the full-size buses, a heavy-duty vinyl or rubber floor covering is typically applied over plywood decking and 14-gauge metal flooring panels. The smaller conversion-type vehicles may have ½- or ⅝-inch (13 mm or 16 mm) plywood sheets placed on top of the existing vehicle floor. Structural members, acting as floor joists, are spaced as close as every 9 inches (225 mm) along the underside of the floor.

> Because of the amount of time needed to breach the floor, **DO NOT** consider that as a primary entry point.

The undercarriage of a typical school bus is substantially reinforced with 8-gauge angle bar, 12-gauge channel stock, and 14-gauge sheet metal. There are guard loops around the entire length of the driveshaft to prevent the driveshaft from falling to the ground if it breaks or becomes disconnected (Figure 6.10). As mentioned earlier, forcible entry through the floor is difficult and time consuming — any other available entry route should be used.

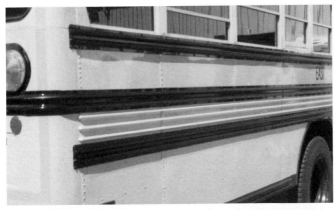
Figure 6.8 School buses have from one to four rub rails.

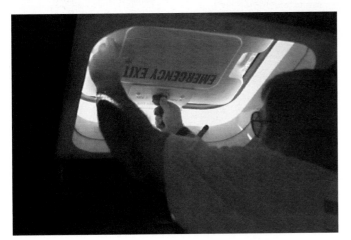
Figure 6.9 Escape hatches in the roof can be opened from the inside or outside.

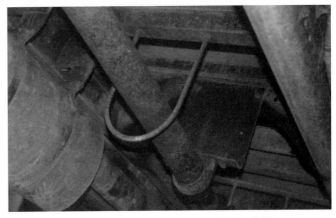
Figure 6.10 Guard loops prevent the driveshaft from falling.

School Bus Doors. There are various types of entry and exit doors on school buses, each serving a specific function. The doors are strategically located to maximize exit paths during an emergency.

Entry doors on some Type A and Type B buses are stock versions provided by the original manufacturer. The latch and lock mechanism is the Nader safety lock found on most motor vehicles since 1973.

The passenger side front door may be drastically altered to suit the needs of the school bus owner/operator. The passenger door may have the same general design as a standard passenger vehicle door, but the window glass is typically permanently fixed in a closed position. The door handles, armrests, and window cranks may be removed. Usually, the only means of opening or closing the front passenger exit door is a manual control arm operated by the driver (Figure 6.11). Some of these buses may also be equipped with the same type of split, folding doors that are typically found on larger buses (Figure 6.12). School buses of all types used to transport

handicapped passengers may be equipped with electric lifts at the side doors (Figure 6.13).

The passenger side front doors on the full-size Type C and D school buses open in a variety of ways. Some are two-part, split-type doors that open inwardly or outwardly, with outward being most common. When operated, these doors split in the middle, with each half of the door swinging to its respective side (Figure 6.14).

Another common type of door is a center-hinged type door that opens by folding forward or rearward (Figure 6.15). Regardless of the type of door, the most common way to open it or secure it in the closed position is with the manual control arm mechanism. When open, school bus front doors typically have a horizontal opening of between 22 and 24 inches (550 mm and 600 mm) and a minimum vertical opening of approximately 68 to 72 inches (1 700 mm to 1 800 mm).

Some school buses use air-operated mechanisms to control the front door. The main switch is usually located to the left of the driver on the instrument console. There will also be a backup emergency release mechanism in the exit stairwell inside the vehicle. The readily identifiable release button or switch causes the air lock device to release the door (Figure 6.16). Rescue personnel can then manually move the door through its normal path of travel. There may not be an

Figure 6.11 A typical manual control arm.

Figure 6.15 Center-hinged doors are common on school buses.

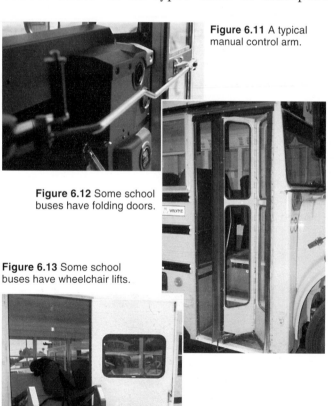

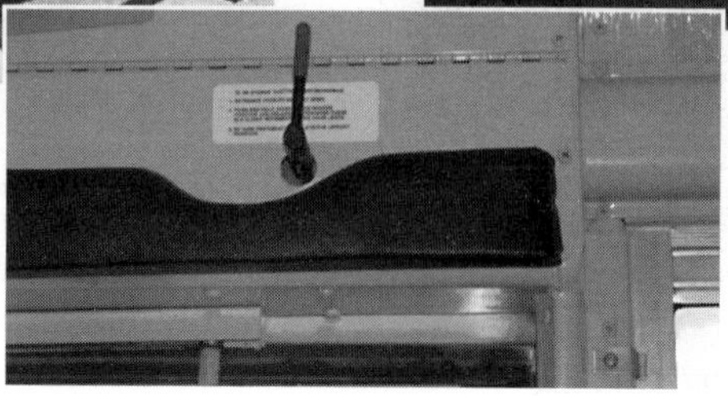

Figure 6.12 Some school buses have folding doors.

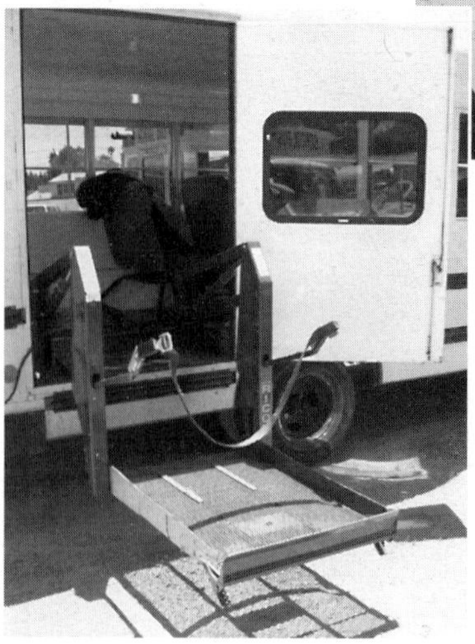

Figure 6.13 Some school buses have wheelchair lifts.

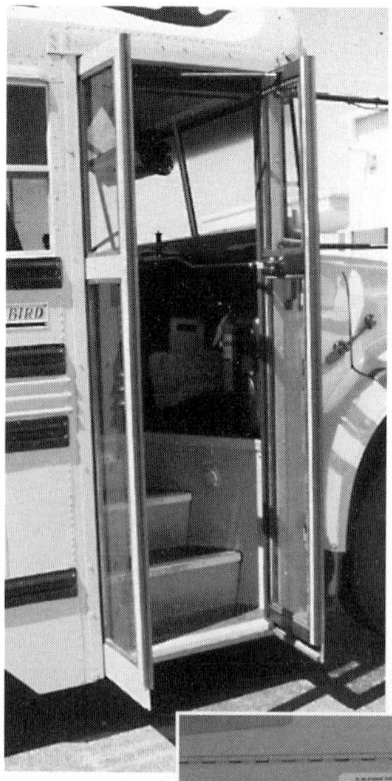

Figure 6.14 Some Type C and D school buses have dual-leaf swinging doors.

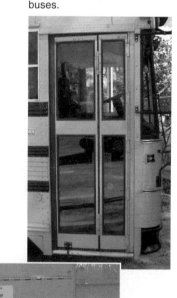

Figure 6.16 An emergency door release switch.

air override release mechanism if there are two similar doors located along the same side of the bus.

The rear exit door is designed to give occupants inside the vehicle a way to exit if the front door does not function or is blocked. On Type A school buses, there may be either one or two rear exit doors (Figure 6.17). On Type B and C, and some D school buses, there is usually one large rear exit door (Figure 6.18). There is no locking device on these rear doors, and they open outwardly by manipulation of a lever to release a latch mechanism. These doors may be opened from the exterior as well as from the interior.

The rear exit door is secured by a one-point or three-point latch system. The main latch is at the edge of the door near the control handle and the other two latches, if present, are found at the top and bottom of the door, engaging the bus body and the floor assembly. **NOTE:** Rear-engine Type D buses do not have a rear exit door but are required by U.S. Motor Vehicle Safety Standards to have a rear emergency window exit.

In some states, buses with larger capacities are required to have an additional exit door along the driver's side of the vehicle (Figure 6.19). This door, known as the "third door" or the "left-hand door," provides an opening of 24 x 48 inches (600 mm by 1 200 mm) and is secured with the same one- or three-point latch mechanism as the rear door. Access is easier from the exterior, since the interior access to the latch mechanism may be obstructed by the passenger seats.

School Bus Windows. The openings for the side and rear windows are defined by the vertical frame members, the roof edge, and the top of the sidewall.

The vertical posts between the windows are either extensions of the roof bows or are hollow tubular structures consisting of several layers of sheet metal. These posts can be removed with power shears or reciprocating saws (Figure 6.20).

The windows may be laminated or tempered safety glass framed in extruded aluminum. The windows are of the split-sash design and are affixed to the rough openings with screws, rivets, or similar fasteners. Typical school bus windows open from the top down, providing an opening of approximately 9 x 22 inches (225 mm by 550 mm), or one-half the total size of the window area (Figure 6.21).

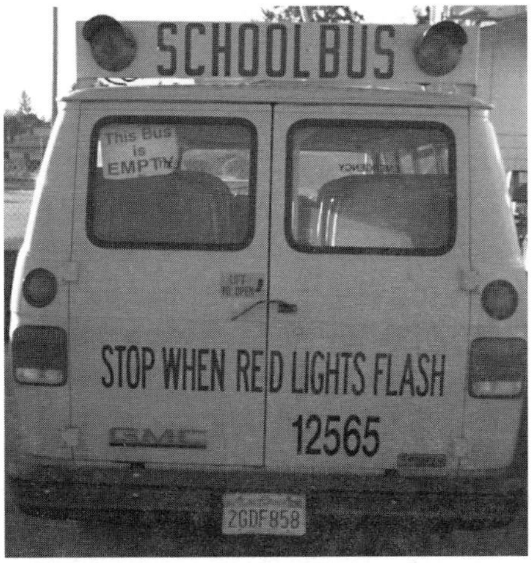

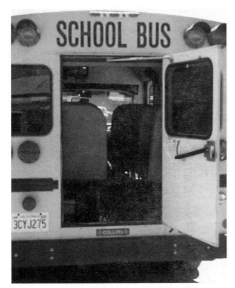

Figure 6.17 Type A school buses have either one or two rear exit doors.

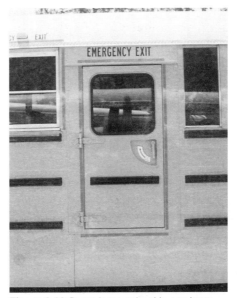

Figure 6.19 Some large school buses have an exit door on the driver's side.

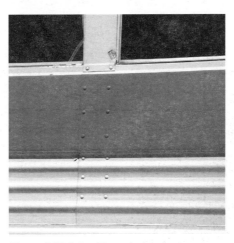

Figure 6.18 Type B, C, and D buses have large rear exit doors.

Figure 6.20 School bus window posts are extensions of the roof bows.

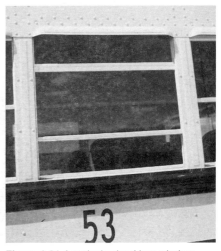

Figure 6.21 A typical school bus window.

To provide a larger opening, some states have regulations requiring that certain side windows be designed as emergency exits and labeled as such inside the vehicle (Figure 6.22). From the exterior, rescuers can identify these exits by the hinges located along the top side of the window frames. Once opened, these windows provide a larger opening through the side of the vehicle than do standard windows.

On the smaller conversion-type school buses, the stock one-piece laminated safety glass windshields are set into the vehicle body with a multipiece rubber mounting gasket. Windshields on full-size buses consist of two or more sheets of laminated safety glass. These sheets are also secured into the vehicle body with a multipiece rubber mounting gasket.

Rear windows are flat sheets of laminated safety glass and are also mounted with removable rubber gaskets. The mounting components for both the windshield and the rear windows are similar to those described in the preceding chapter on passenger vehicle extrication.

School Bus Seats. The two types of seats found in school buses are driver's seats and passenger seats. The driver's seat is an adjustable bucket-type seat with a floor-mounted seat belt and/or shoulder

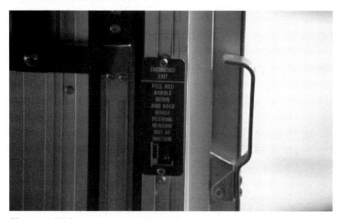

Figure 6.22 An emergency exit window.

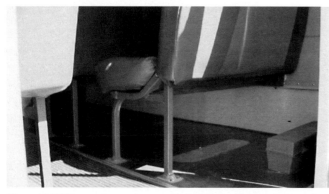

Figure 6.23 Passenger seats are attached to the floor and sidewall.

harness assembly. Passenger seats are framed with 1-inch (25 mm) tubular steel. The seats are bolted into the bus floor and into the sidewall area (Figure 6.23). Detachable foam rubber seat cushions and seat backs are covered with a vinyl upholstery material. Since 1977, school bus seat backs have been required to be of the high-back style, 24 inches (600 mm) high.

School bus passenger seats may be equipped with lap-style seatbelts if mandated by local ordinance or state law, but all Type A buses under 10,000 pounds (4 450 kg) GVWR must have lap belts. In buses used to transport physically or mentally handicapped persons, positive body restraint harnesses may be found in specially designated seats.

School Bus Aisles. The position of the seats inside the school bus dictates the width of the vehicle's center aisle. The aisle of suburban-type buses can be as narrow as 10 inches (250 mm). Aisle space in van-conversion buses increases to approximately 12 inches (300 mm). Full-size school buses may have aisle widths between 12 and 15 inches (300 mm and 375 mm) (Figure 6.24). Since the width of a typical backboard is 18 inches (450 mm), a narrow center aisle can make the process of removing victims more difficult. Wheelchair-equipped vehicles generally have a 30-inch (750 mm) wide aisle in the area where the chair will be maneuvered; however, the aisle may not be that wide throughout the entire vehicle.

School Bus Batteries. On Type A and some Type B buses, the batteries are usually located in the engine compartment. On most Type B, C, and D buses, the batteries are typically located in a separate compartment on the driver's side of the vehicle (Figure 6.25). If the bus is equipped as a handicapped

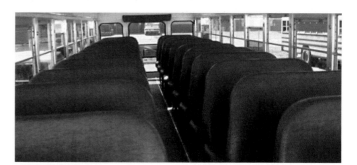

Figure 6.24 A typical full-size school bus aisle.

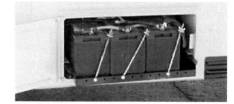

Figure 6.25 Larger school buses have a battery compartment on the driver's side.

transport with an electric lift, a separate battery may be provided for the lift. This battery is usually located in a separate compartment on the driver's side of the vehicle. Disconnecting this battery will not interrupt power to the engine.

Transit Buses

As mentioned earlier in this chapter, transit buses run on city streets, rural roads, and major highways. Therefore, rescue personnel in virtually every jurisdiction should be familiar with how these vehicles are constructed.

Transit Bus Construction

In general, transit buses are of integral body construction. This method combines the chassis framing and the body understructure into one integral module. The main undercarriage structure consists of longitudinal beams that support horizontal and vertical beams, all made of carbon steel. All other structural components are made of either galvanized or stainless steel or aluminum. These include tubular support members, cross bracing, inner or outer panels, plates, and any other formed members.

Formed tubular members are used to support the upper body portion of the bus. This upper body structure is welded to the vertical carline supports located near the floor of the bus. *Carline supports* are gussets that strengthen the side wall of a bus at the level most likely to be struck by a car. The roof is constructed of inner and outer panels that sandwich insulation and electrical wiring and fixtures between them. The most common material used for transit bus floor decking is ¾-inch (19 mm) plywood. The decking may be covered with any of a variety of floor coverings, most of them rubber or linoleum type.

Transit Bus Doors.

Nearly all transit bus doors are of the two-piece, center-opening type. While most swing toward the outside, some slide laterally (Figure 6.26). The opening mechanism may be pneumatic, hydraulic, or electric, depending upon the manufacturer. The operating control is usually located at the driver's left side. Most transit buses are constructed with two passenger side doors. One is at the very front of the vehicle, directly opposite the driver; the other midship, or slightly aft of midship (Figure 6.27). Both doors are intended for normal entry and exit by passengers. Normally, these doors will open and close simultaneously. Unlike school buses, transit buses generally do not have a specific emergency exit door. The two standard doors are considered to be sufficient for most emergencies. All

buses are equipped with window exits in addition to the regular exits (Figure 6.28).

Some transit buses are designed to accommodate disabled passengers. These buses may be equipped with one or a combination of features that allow easier

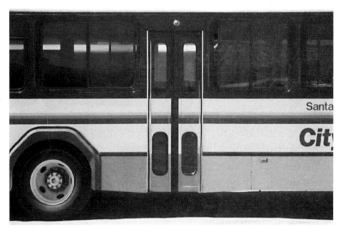

Figure 6.26 Transit bus doors may swing open or slide laterally.

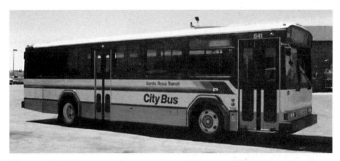

Figure 6.27 The second door is toward the rear of the bus.

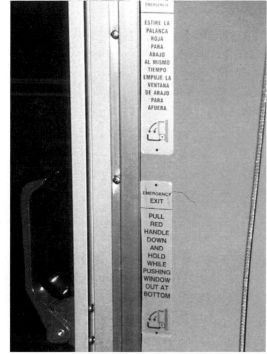

Figure 6.28 A typical transit bus emergency exit window.

access for passengers with limited mobility or those confined to wheelchairs. One such feature is a hydraulic lift designed to raise passengers in wheelchairs from curb height to assist them onto the bus and to lower them back to curb height when they wish to exit (Figure 6.29). The lift is often located in the midship door, but not always. By operating a control next to the door, the bus driver is able to convert the stairway into a lift. When the control is operated, the stairs fold out into a lift platform. From that position, the platform may be lowered or raised.

Another feature allows the front end of the bus to be lowered to curb level so that a passenger is not required to step up to get into the bus (Figure 6.30). By controlling the air in the suspension system bellows, the driver can lower the level of the step from its normal height of about 12 inches (300 mm) down to about 6 inches (150 mm). This feature demonstrates how important it is that rescuers stay clear of an unsupported bus with an air suspension system. If the air suspension system fails, anyone underneath would be crushed.

WARNING!

Never put any part of your body beneath an unsupported bus with an air suspension system. If the system fails suddenly, severe injuries or death may result. Be sure that the bus is properly supported by jacks and cribbing.

Figure 6.29 Some transit buses have wheelchair lifts.

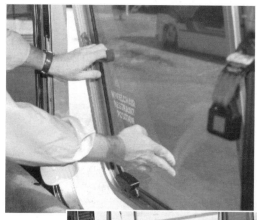

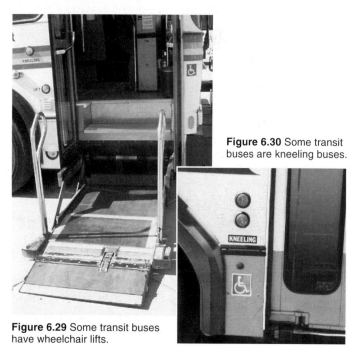

Figure 6.30 Some transit buses are kneeling buses.

Transit Bus Windows. Laminated safety glass is the most common type of glass used in transit bus windows, but some transit buses have side windows of tempered glass, Plexiglas®, or other synthetic material. Transit bus windshields and rear windows are similar to those in school buses or other large vehicles. The large windshields are typically of two-piece design. Transit bus windshields are held in place by a simple locking rubber filler strip.

The type of transit bus side windows varies greatly, depending on the age of the bus and the manufacturer. Older buses — those without air conditioning — may have windows that can only be opened by sliding the window to one side or the other. The glass is set into an aluminum or other lightweight metal frame designed to slide open a distance equal to one-half the width of the entire window unit. Transit buses are now commonly equipped with windows that are hinged at the top and are designed to tilt out when the latch on the lower side is released (Figure 6.31). Some transit buses have windows that are designed to slide open during normal operation; however, they still tilt out to provide an emergency exit. These windows will not stay open by themselves and have to be propped open.

Transit Bus Seats. Nearly all passenger seats found on transit buses are molded from some type of plastic (Figure 6.32). They may be further covered by a vinyl or plastic covering or cushions. The seats are supported

Figure 6.31 Some transit buses have awning type windows.

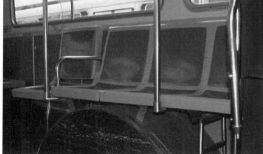

Figure 6.32 Many transit bus seats are molded.

by a metal framework that is bolted to the floor and the sides of the bus. In some cases, the supporting framework of the seats is combined with handrail systems that are also bolted to the ceiling of the bus.

A major difference between transit bus seating and that in other types of buses is the layout of the seats. Most transit buses do not have the standard, uniform front-facing seat arrangement. The seats in a transit bus may be arranged so that some seats face forward, and others face the center aisle. The layouts will vary depending on the owner/operator's specifications. They may even vary within the same transit fleet, depending on the age of individual buses and prevailing trends at the time the vehicles were purchased. The driver's seat in a transit bus is similar to those described in the school bus section of this chapter.

Transit Bus Aisles. In most transit buses, the width of the center aisle is considerably wider than those in typical school buses. This is because transit buses are designed for adults who may be carrying packages, briefcases, etc. The wider aisle also results from different seating arrangements. Depending on seat layout, transit bus aisles vary in width from about 20 inches (500 mm) to about 5 feet (1.5 m). This makes transit buses somewhat easier than school buses for rescue and EMS personnel to work and maneuver in.

Transit Bus Batteries. The battery banks on nearly all transit buses are located on the driver's side of the vehicle, just forward of the rear wheels. For ease of access, the batteries are grouped together on a tray that can be pulled out when the compartment door is open. However, sliding out the tray is usually unnecessary because most transit buses are equipped with a battery shutoff switch located in the battery compartment (Figure 6.33). Power from the batteries can be interrupted by simply moving this switch to the "off" position.

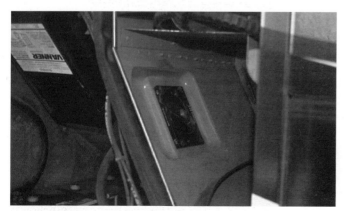

Figure 6.33 The battery shutoff switch.

Commercial Buses

Commercial buses travel local roads and city streets as well as major highways. Just as with transit buses, rescue personnel should be familiar with the construction of commercial buses that travel through their jurisdictions.

Commercial Bus Construction

Most manufacturers of commercial buses construct the entire frame of the vehicle as one integral unit. This method of construction is sometimes referred to as bird cage construction, since the assembled frame resembles a large bird cage. The majority of the frame is constructed of low carbon, square steel tubing 1 to 2 inches (40 mm to 50 mm) in diameter. The frame is covered with either aluminum or stainless steel sheeting. On some buses, the panels covering the front and rear modules are made of fiberglass.

Framing members that support the roof are generally separated by about 24 to 26 inches (600 mm to 650 mm) on center. Wiring and insulation are sandwiched between the outer (roof) and inner (ceiling) panels. A major difference in roof construction between commercial buses (sometimes called motor coaches) and other types of buses is that the panels in a commercial bus may not be riveted to every structural member. Some manufacturers rivet the panels to every other roof rafter; therefore, there is a structural member about halfway between each row of rivets. If the rows of rivets are more than about 2 feet (0.7 m) apart, expect to find a rafter between the two riveted members.

Commercial bus floors are constructed in a manner similar to those on transit buses. Most are ½- or ¾-inch (13 mm or 19 mm) plywood covered with a composite rubber or other synthetic covering.

Commercial Bus Doors. All commercial buses have a single door at the front, opposite the driver's position. This door is usually a one-piece, single-hinged door with hinges located on the forward edge of the door. A few models have a two-piece center-opening door, similar to those on a transit bus, or a folding door. The folding door is not a center opening door like those found on school or transit buses; rather, it has a hinge along one edge and in the center allowing it to fold to one side. The door folds toward the front of the bus instead of swinging open like a one-piece door.

Many commercial bus manufacturers use air-operated opening mechanisms on their doors. When the driver operates a dash-mounted control device, compressed air pressure moves the door. In the event of air compressor failure, or any other emergency, the driver can open these doors by operating an emergency release that dumps the air pressure from the system and allows the door to be manually operated. Emergency releases are located inside the bus near the top of the door (Figure 6.34). Exterior releases are usually located either in the right front wheel well, under or to the left of the door itself on the outside of the vehicle, or directly below the center of the windshield. Some motor coaches have mechanical pivot arm openers similar to those used on school buses. The emergency release for doors with a mechanical arm is a knob or latch located directly under the center of the windshield on the front of the bus (Figure 6.35).

Most commercial buses do not have emergency exit doors, although a few import models do. Most rely on window exits for emergencies. Window exits are covered in more detail in the next section.

Commercial Bus Windows. Because most commercial buses are air conditioned, there is little or no need for windows that open. Because of this, all modern motor coaches are designed with single-piece side windows, some of which can be opened in emergencies. These exit windows are set in metal frames that are hinged at the top (Figure 6.36). Typically, these windows are opened by lifting a horizontal bar located across the bottom of the window frame. When the mechanism is released, the bottom of the window can be pushed out to provide an exit path. These emergency exit window openings are at least 20 x 48 inches (500 mm by 1 200 mm), with many being considerably larger. These window exits will not stay open by themselves, so if it is necessary to keep them open, they will have to be propped. Pike poles are well suited for this purpose.

Commercial bus windshields and rear windows are set in a rubber molding, and they can be removed as described earlier. Windshields and rear windows are usually constructed of laminated automotive safety glass. Side windows may be laminated glass, tempered safety glass, Lexan®, or other synthetic material.

Commercial Bus Seats. Commercial buses are generally equipped with individual bucket-type seats for each occupant, similar to those on commercial airliners (Figure 6.37). These seats have high backs, can be inclined, and may or may not have armrests between the seats. They are usually mounted four to a

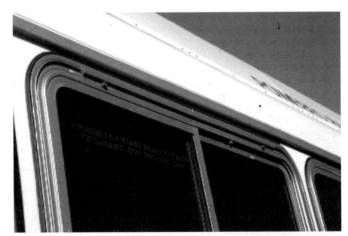
Figure 6.36 Emergency exit windows are hinged at the top.

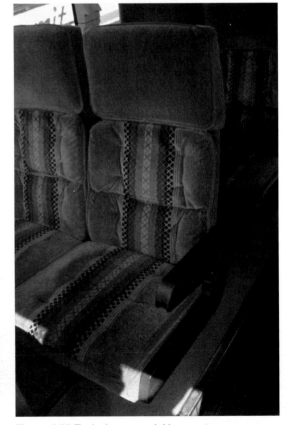
Figure 6.37 Typical commercial bus seats.

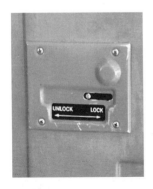
Figure 6.34 The emergency door release.

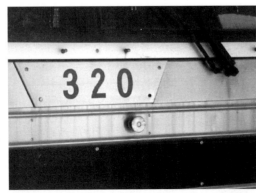
Figure 6.35 The external emergency door release.

row, two on each side of the center aisle. How the seats are mounted varies from manufacturer to manufacturer. Some seats are connected and mounted like the bench seats in a school bus. The legs on the aisle side are bolted to the floor, and the window side of the seat is bolted to the floor and/or the sidewall. Other seats may be mounted on an individual pedestal that is bolted to the floor. Most drivers' seats are pedestal mounted. Some motor coaches have a bench at the rear of the bus; this is usually molded into the rear frame design and removing anything other than the cushions is extremely difficult.

Commercial Bus Aisles. Most commercial buses have a uniform aisle width for most of the length of the seating area; however, there may be some variation in aisle width toward the rear of the bus near the restroom. The center aisle is usually between 13 and 18 inches (325 mm and 450 mm) wide. This narrow width creates problems for rescuers trying to remove victims on backboards, scoop stretchers, or other litters. The ceiling height in most motor coach aisles is generally 75 to 78 inches (1 875 mm to 1 950 mm). Because of the high seat backs and low overhead luggage racks, it may be difficult to carry the litters over the seat tops. In some cases, seats may have to be removed to make passage possible.

Commercial Bus Luggage Compartments. Most commercial buses are equipped with overhead storage compartments located directly above the seats. These compartments are designed for passengers to stow small articles of carry-on luggage. The compartments may be either open shelves or enclosed cabinets similar to those on commercial airliners. These storage areas reduce the ceiling height directly above the seats and may present some working space difficulties for rescuers.

Commercial buses also have large luggage compartments located below the seating area of the bus that open from the outside (Figure 6.38). While these compartments are primarily designed to carry large pieces of luggage, in many cases motor coaches also haul common freight. No matter what is hauled, there is a heavy fuel loading near these storage compartments and any ignition in this area could result in a serious fire. Because these lower compartments extend completely through to the other side of the bus. Firefighters may need to open the doors on both sides of the bus when attacking a fire in this area.

Once the fire has been knocked down, pike poles can be used to either pull or push the cargo out of the storage area and onto the ground. This will lessen the overall damage to the bus and make extinguishment and overhaul much quicker and easier. As with any other vehicle fire, firefighters should wear self-contained breathing apparatus.

Commercial Bus Batteries. The location of the batteries on commercial motor coaches varies depending on the manufacturer of the bus. Many are found just aft of the front wheel on the passenger side of the bus. Table 6.1 lists the locations of batteries for various manufacturers' buses.

Regardless of the location of the batteries, all manufacturers place an electrical disconnect switch in the battery compartment. This switch will either be directly above or below the batteries. Electrical service

Table 6.1 Motor Coach Battery Bank Locations	
Bus Model	**Battey Location**
MCI Model 7 and 8	Passenger side front of baggage compartment
MCI Model 9	Passenger side front of baggage compartment
GMC	Behind left rear wheel or behind right front wheel
Eagle Model 05	Driver and passenger side behind rearmost axle
Eagle Model 10	Passenger side behind rearmost axle

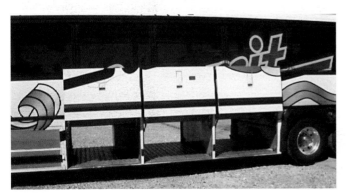

Figure 6.38 Typical commercial bus luggage compartment.

to the bus's 24-volt systems (power plant, air-conditioning systems, etc.) can be interrupted by operating this switch. In some cases, interior emergency lights will still have power even though the battery switch is off. To de-energize these systems, it will be necessary to disconnect or cut the battery cables. Follow the battery cable cutting precautions described in Chapter 5 of this manual.

Specialty Bus Construction

As mentioned earlier in this chapter, converted buses have the same general construction features as the conventional vehicles from which the conversions were made — with a few exceptions. The following sections discuss some of the exceptional features of bus conversions.

Type A/B School Bus Conversions

Many Type A/B school buses have been converted into transports for those with disabilities. These conversions are different from the conventional Type A/B units in several ways. First, they are usually designed to carry fewer total passengers because of the space requirements for wheelchairs and other devices (Figure 6.39). Secondly, the center aisles in these buses are significantly wider than those in conventional buses so there is more room for EMS personnel to maneuver inside the vehicle. Finally, many of these units are equipped with double entry/exit doors located midship on the passenger side. The entry/exit stairs also convert to an electrically operated wheelchair lift. When equipped with a wheelchair lift, a separate battery box for supplying power to the lift is usually located on the driver's side of the vehicle. Disconnecting this battery will not interrupt power to the engine.

Commercial Bus Conversions

Commercial buses have been converted for a variety of purposes. Some have been converted into transports

for prisoners. Others have been converted into large mobile field hospitals and ambulances. Some have been converted into mobile command posts and communications vehicles by fire departments and other public safety agencies (Figure 6.40). Others have been converted into mobile living quarters for entertainers and offices for others whose jobs require them to relocate with relative frequency.

In most cases, since these are conversions of conventional buses, the basic construction will remain the same as other conventional buses of that type. The major differences will be in how the interiors of the converted buses are configured. Those converted as prisoner transports may have more-or-less conventional seating but the windows may be covered with bars, heavy gauge wire screens, or even metal plates with louvers to allow for air circulation (Figure 6.41). Those converted for use as mobile offices may

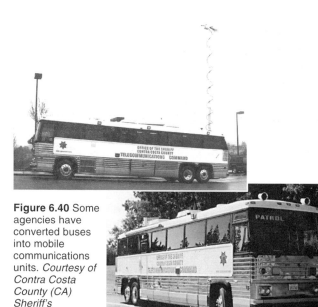

Figure 6.40 Some agencies have converted buses into mobile communications units. *Courtesy of Contra Costa County (CA) Sheriff's Department.*

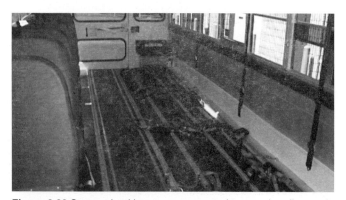

Figure 6.39 Some school buses are converted to carry handicapped passengers.

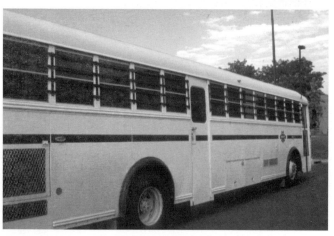

Figure 6.41 A typical prisoner transport bus.

have most of the original seating removed and replaced with typical office furniture. There may or may not be separate sleeping quarters. Those that have been converted into mobile living quarters may be more like motor homes than buses, but their basic structure is still that of a commercial bus, and rescue personnel should follow the protocols and procedures recommended for that type of bus. These conversions can often be identified by their blacked-out windows and the sometimes garish cosmetics on the vehicle's exterior.

Bus Fuels

Most school bus fuel systems use either gasoline or diesel fuel. Nearly all transit and commercial buses are powered by diesel fuel, although some are powered by a mixture of diesel fuel and kerosene. Depending upon their size and weight, motor homes may use any of these fuels. Fuel tanks on Type A and B buses are commonly in the rear of the vehicle. The fuel tank(s) on school buses, transit buses, and commercial buses may be as large as 180 gallons (720 L). In Type C and D school buses, as well as most transit and commercial buses, the fuel tank is located in the midship portion of the bus or slightly ahead of midship, just behind the front wheels. The fuel filler is usually located on the passenger side, just behind the front wheels, although some commercial buses may be equipped with fillers on both sides of the vehicle.

Alternative Bus Fuels

Many transit buses and motor homes are powered by engines using alternative fuels — those other than gasoline or diesel. Some are powered by compressed natural gas (CNG), and others liquefied petroleum gas (LPG). The presence of an alternative fuel system may be evident because of decals or other signs on the exterior of the vehicle indicating the type of fuel in use (Figure 6.42). Otherwise, the presence of a fuel filler and main supply valve at some point on the lower half of the vehicle body may be the only indication. In any case, the fuel filler and main supply valve will be located at the same point, and this point should be relatively easy to access because it is where the filler hose connects.

As will be explained in greater detail in the section on size-up, alternative fuels behave differently when released into the atmosphere because of their differing vapor densities. At this point, it is sufficient to remember that CNG is lighter than air, so it will rise when released, perhaps filling the passenger compartment. LPG is heavier than air, so it will fall when released and will collect in depressions and other low areas. In both cases, at the point of optimum fuel/air mixture, these are both highly flammable gases and represent significant safety hazards.

Some local transit buses do not have liquid or gaseous fuel because they are powered by electricity supplied from overhead wires through a rooftop apparatus called a pantograph (Figure 6.43). As discussed in greater detail in Chapter 8, Rail Car Extrication, rescue personnel should avoid working on the roof of any vehicle powered in this way — even if the pantograph is disconnected from the overhead wires.

Other buses are powered by alternative fuels such as hydrogen. These fuels and fuel systems are considered experimental, and their use is still limited to a very small number of vehicles. When buses using these or any other alternative fuels are introduced into an area, the rescue personnel in that jurisdiction should familiarize themselves with the fuels and their characteristics.

Bus Brakes

Buses generally have the same types of brakes as trucks of similar size and weight. For more information

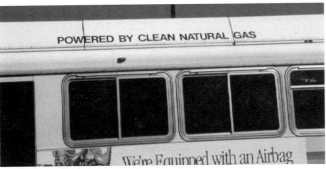

Figure 6.42 A sign identifies the alternative fuel.

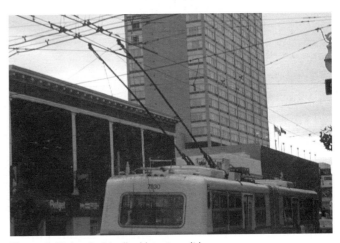

Figure 6.43 An electrically driven transit bus.

about bus brakes and brake systems, see Chapter 7, Medium and Heavy Truck Extrication.

Bus Extrication Size-Up

Given the possible number of trapped victims, and the potential for loss of life in a serious collision involving a fully loaded bus, the importance of performing a rapid but thorough size-up cannot be overstated. There may well be dozens of victims trapped inside a crashed bus — many of them needing immediate medical intervention to save their lives — so the first-arriving resources at this type of incident can easily be overwhelmed. Therefore, it is critical that the IC develop an incident action plan and order any other needed resources as soon as possible.

As in other types of vehicle extrication incidents, the initial size-up of a bus incident involves making a number of quick assessments. In general, the size-up focuses on scene assessment, vehicle assessment, victim assessment, and extrication assessment.

Scene Assessment

As in other types of extrication incidents, the scene assessment in a bus crash begins with the initial dispatch. Any incident involving an occupied bus may trigger an agency SOP that would increase the number of resources included in the initial response. Regardless of whether this occurs, as discussed in earlier chapters, those responding should consider such variables as the day/date/time, the weather, and the volume of traffic encountered during the response.

Approaching the scene, the officer in charge of the first-arriving unit should look for the following:

• Smoke and/or steam that would indicate a need for fire protection

• Sparks or the blue-white arc from downed power lines that would indicate a need for utility crews

• Cloud of vapor that would indicate a release of LP gas or other hazardous material

• Vehicular traffic in and around the scene to assess the need for traffic control

• Pedestrians in and around the scene to assess the need for crowd control

• Anything that might indicate a danger to rescue personnel and/or others at the scene

Once on scene, the officer in charge should attempt to confirm his initial observations and factor in any additional information obtained through closer observation and/or from questioning those at the scene. The scene should be surveyed immediately to ascertain if there are any injured victims outside of the crashed vehicles. Any additional resources that may be needed should be requested *immediately*. The sooner they are requested, the sooner they will arrive on scene where they are needed.

On-scene personnel should be assigned to perform those tasks that relate to protecting everyone at the scene — themselves, pedestrians, and trapped victims. The highest priority may initially be traffic control to prevent oncoming vehicles from crashing into spectators, rescue personnel, or the vehicles already involved in the incident. Or, the highest priority may be to mitigate hazards such as downed power lines, fuel leaks, or incipient fires. Finally, the highest priority may be to gain control of the scene by cordoning off the area into control zones as described in Chapter 2.

During the scene assessment phase, rescue personnel should attempt to determine the following:

• Any safety hazards at the scene

• What will be needed to mitigate the hazards

• The resources needed

• Any additional resources (law enforcement, fire protection, haz mat, utilities, lighting units, etc.) that may be needed

Vehicle Assessment

After the overall scene has been assessed and deemed safe for rescue personnel, they should turn their attention to assessing the vehicles involved in the incident. As a minimum, rescue personnel should attempt to determine the following:

• Number of vehicles involved

• Size/type of vehicles involved

• Condition of each vehicle

Victim Assessment

Simultaneous with the vehicle assessment, or as soon as possible thereafter, an assessment must be made of the victims trapped in the vehicles. This is the initial medical triage. As a minimum, rescue personnel should attempt to determine the following:

• Number of victims inside of the vehicles

• If victims are injured or merely trapped

• Each victim's individual medical priority

• Any additional resources (additional ambulances, medevac helicopter, etc.) that may be needed

Extrication Assessment

Once the number of vehicles involved and the number of victims and their conditions are known, rescue personnel will need to assess what will be needed to extricate those trapped inside the vehicles. As a minimum, rescue personnel should attempt to determine the following:

- How to stabilize the involved vehicles
- How to gain access to the trapped victims
- How to free the trapped victims
- Any additional resources (cutting tools/equipment, cranes, booms, air supply, lighting equipment, etc.) that may be needed

Bus Stabilization

In every vehicle extrication incident, one of the first tasks is to stabilize the vehicle. Stabilization must precede gaining entry to evaluate or extricate victims trapped inside the vehicle. Just as in Chapter 5, stabilizing vehicles upright and in various other positions is discussed in the following sections.

Bus Upright

If a bus is upright, the task is to prevent it from moving in the most likely directions — horizontally and vertically. Any bus, regardless of type or size, can usually be prevented from moving forward or backward by chocking the wheels. Whenever possible, wheel chocks — and not pieces of cribbing — should be used (Figure 6.44). Manufactured wheel chocks are usually more effective, and it saves the cribbing for use in stabilizing the vehicle. However, if the bus is on a slope — especially if it is in danger of rolling sideways down the slope — it may be necessary to supplement the wheel chocks with a chain, cable, or webbing attached to the bus and a "bombproof" anchor point.

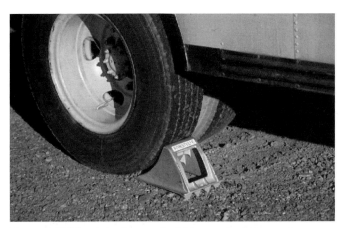

Figure 6.44 Wheel chocks — not cribbing — should be used.

The term *bombproof* is taken from rope rescue and it means any object that absolutely, positively cannot be moved by the weight of whatever is attached to it. To horizontally stabilize a bus may require a heavy-duty tow truck, a huge boulder, or a large, fully mature tree as an anchor point (Figure 6.45).

In general, vertically stabilizing a school bus is no different from vertically stabilizing any other bus. Most school buses built by either integral construction or the body-on-chassis method all have conventional heavy-duty suspension — that is, leaf and/or coil springs. Most transit, commercial, and some newer school buses are equipped with air suspension systems. In these systems, the conventional metal springs are replaced with compact rubber air bags that are similar to a bellows. At each wheel, there are two air suspension bags — one on each side of the axle (Figure 6.46). An on-board compressor maintains the air pressure within the bags as high as 120 psi (840 kPa). Depending upon the load of the vehicle and the condition of the road, the pressure within each bag is automatically increased or decreased to maintain the bus in a level state.

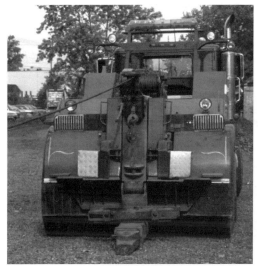

Figure 6.45 A heavy vehicle can serve as a secure anchor point for effective rigging.

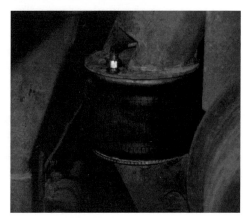

Figure 6.46 Typical bus air suspension bags.

If the pressure in an air suspension bag is lost because of damage to the bag or its associated piping, the chassis of the bus can suddenly drop without warning to within 3 to 3½ inches (76 mm to 89 mm) of the roadway surface.

WARNING!

No one should be allowed to place their head or extremities under any part of a bus until it has been positively stabilized.

Some transit and commercial buses are equipped with an emergency air inlet valve on the front end. This valve allows the bus to be hooked to an air compressor or cascade system to reinflate a collapsed suspension system. However, reinflating the suspension system should not be considered an alternative to proper cribbing techniques. Even though a small percentage of transit and commercial buses are equipped with a standard mechanical suspension system (similar to that of a school bus), unless rescuers are positive that the bus being worked on has a mechanical suspension system, the bus should be treated as one that has an air suspension system.

Because most transit and commercial buses do not have a rigid frame, they are equipped with specially designed jack plates for use as contact points for cribbing or jacks. On transit buses, these plates are located slightly behind each axle, near each wheel. On commercial buses, the jack plates are located under the body between the two rear axles and in back of the front axle. Again, cribbing may be used on these points, although they are designed more for use with hydraulic jacks. All four jack plates should be supported to completely stabilize the vehicle. If rescuers are unsure of the location of jack plates on a particular bus, the vehicle can be stabilized by cribbing the body at any solid frame member. If possible, the middle axle (also known as the bogie or tag axle) should also be cribbed.

When cribbing is used to stabilize a bus, it is important that the cribbing be large enough to hold the weight of the bus. Generally, 6- x 6-inch (150 mm by 150 mm) wooden cribbing is the minimum size that should be used. If hydraulic jacks are being used to stabilize or lift the bus, they should be of at least 8-ton (7 250 kg) capacity. On many buses, each axle is equipped with a piece of tubing welded on the axle near each wheel. This tubing is designed to accept the shaft of a jack to prevent the jack from slipping.

In some cases, the engine supports can be used as jack points. However, this should be done only if there is no other alternative *and* if it is possible for rescuers to access these supports without having to place themselves beneath the unsupported bus. Because of their location beneath the bus, using these engine supports as jack points can be dangerous.

As mentioned earlier, rescuers should *never* place any part of themselves under any portion of an unsupported vehicle. Cribbing or jacks should be pushed into position using another piece of cribbing, a pike pole, or some similar device. Jacks should be equipped with handles that allow them to be operated from outside the perimeter of the vehicle.

To stabilize a bus, cribbing and wedges or shims should be installed at a sufficient number of points to prevent the bus from settling any further. If jacks are used, they should be extended only to the point where they would begin to lift the bus. If the objective is to lift the bus, the jacks should be extended slowly and evenly. As the bus is raised, cribbing should be added to minimize the distance the bus will fall should the jack(s) fail. Remember — *raise an inch, crib an inch.* The bus should be raised only as much as necessary to stabilize it — and no more.

Hazard Control

Another very important part of stabilizing a bus in any position is controlling and mitigating the other hazards that may be present. Among these other hazards are the vehicle's engine, its electrical power supply, leaking fuel or other hazardous substances, and downed power lines.

Power Shutoffs. As in the crash of any type of motor vehicle, one of the most important functions rescuers must perform as part of stabilizing a bus is to disconnect the vehicle's batteries (Figure 6.47). This eliminates a possible ignition source for flammable vapors and also de-energizes any power equipment that may still be functioning.

Before shutting off or disconnecting the batteries, rescuers should first shut off the engine, if it is still running. A running engine causes vibration that may further injure victims, may add noise that can upset victims and hinder communications, and it could cause the bus to move. Rescuers should first attempt to turn the ignition key or push the ignition system switch to the "off" position. This will minimize the chance of an electrical system malfunction and will shut off the vehicle's engine. On buses equipped with an alternate fuel system, such as LPG or propane, shutting off the fuel system main supply valve will also stop the engine (Figure 6.48).

Transit and commercial buses have engine stop switches located on the driver's console, usually to the left of the driver's seat (Figure 6.49). In addition, a stop switch is located in the rear engine compartment. It should be clearly marked and is usually found in the top left or right corner of the compartment (Figure 6.50). The stop button may have either an on/off position or it may be a push button that has to be held down until the engine comes to a complete stop.

> **WARNING!**
>
> Use extreme care when opening the engine compartment door(s). There are no safety guards around the fans and their speed of rotation makes them difficult to see. Contact with a moving fan may result in serious injury.

If these methods do not stop a running engine, CO_2 can be discharged into the air intake located at the rear corner of the vehicle. Air intakes may be located on either or both sides of the vehicle. Rescuers should discharge the CO_2 into the air intake screen area, aiming the main stream of it inward and toward the front of the vehicle. Because this method is dangerous, it is to be used ONLY if all other attempts to stop the engine have failed.

> **WARNING!**
>
> Use ONLY CO_2 to try to stop an engine. Using other extinguishing agents may cause the engine to break apart and injure personnel with flying shrapnel.

Batteries on Type A and B school buses are usually located in the engine compartment. If the bus is equipped as a handicapped transport with an electric lift, a separate battery may be provided for the lift. This battery is usually located in a separate compartment on the driver's side of the vehicle. However, disconnecting this battery will not interrupt power to the engine.

On Type C and D school buses, the batteries will be located either under the hood or in a separate compartment on the driver's side of the bus. In some buses, a hex key or Allen wrench must be used to unlatch the compartment door. The required key is usually located inside the school bus near the driver's area. In the absence of a key device, battery compartment doors may have to be forced open.

Just as with school buses, the batteries of transit buses and commercial buses should be disconnected to interrupt the flow of electrical power to the rest of the bus. The batteries should not be disconnected

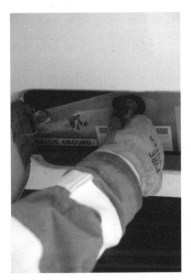

Figure 6.47 Disconnecting the batteries is an important part of vehicle stabilization.

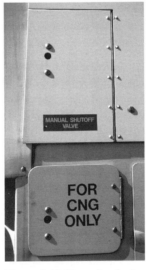

Figure 6.48 Alternative fuel supply valve should be closed.

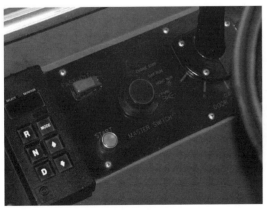

Figure 6.49 The driver's engine shutoff switch.

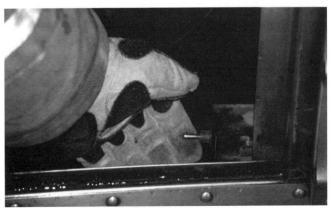

Figure 6.50 An engine shutoff switch in the engine compartment.

while the engine is running. This is dangerous, and the engine will continue to run after the batteries have been disconnected. Rescuers can interrupt the electrical power supply by operating the battery shutoff switch located in the battery compartment, disconnecting the battery cables, or cutting the cables. Whenever working with or around batteries, full PPE (including eye protection) should be worn.

Fuel Leaks. Many Type A, B, and C school buses, and other buses of similar size, have gasoline-powered engines. Other buses of all sizes operate on alternative fuels such as LPG or LNG. Because of the volatility and flammability of these fuels, it is critically important that any leaks be controlled and any spilled fuel be covered with Class B foam. As mentioned earlier, shutting off the main fuel supply valve on those buses operating on alternative fuels will interrupt the flow of fuel. Because of the possibility of LPG or LNG becoming trapped in and around a crashed bus, it may be necessary to ventilate the area using intrinsically safe fans.

Downed Power Lines. A relatively small percentage of bus crashes involve downed power lines. However, if they are involved, they add another potentially life-threatening dimension to the incident. One of the most frustrating and most dangerous vehicle extrication scenarios is that in which an injured vehicle occupant can be seen through the vehicle's windows but rescuers cannot touch the vehicle because it is in contact with a downed power line. Because rescue personnel are trained to help those in need, the temptation to assume that the power line is no longer energized — or to attempt to move the power line off the vehicle — becomes almost overwhelming. But it *must* be resisted!

WARNING!

Until power has been shut off by utility service personnel, rescuers must assume that all power lines are energized. DO NOT attempt to move downed power lines for any reason before power has been shut off.

While waiting for utility service personnel to arrive at the scene, rescuers should cordon off the area of the downed power line to protect themselves and others at the scene. The presence of a downed power line should be announced over the radio to alert all emergency personnel and over public address systems or bull horns to alert others.

Bus on Side

Obviously, any or all hazards just discussed can be involved in any bus crash, regardless of the position in which the bus comes to rest. However, if a bus comes to rest on its side, many of those hazards — as well as the difficulty of stabilizing the vehicle and accessing its interior — can be harder to manage.

Stabilizing any bus that has come to rest on its side is virtually the same regardless of whether it is a school bus, transit bus, or commercial bus. Because the sides of most buses are large flat surfaces, buses in this position tend to be relatively stable. However, if the crash that caused it to roll over has drastically altered its original shape, or if it came to rest on an uneven surface, a bus on its side may be anything but stable. Just as in any other vehicle extrication incident, the goal is to create as many points of contact between the bus and the surface on which it rests as are necessary to prevent sudden and unexpected movement of the bus in any direction. This stability is usually achieved through the use of cribbing, step chocks, shoring, jacks, or a combination of these. These devices should be installed as described in earlier chapters. The bus may also need to be secured to a solid object with chains, cables, or webbing (Figure 6.51).

Depending upon the dynamics of the crash and other variables in the situation, a bus on its side may leak fuel and other flammable fluids — and access to the means of controlling these and other hazards may be difficult if not impossible. The battery compartment may be on the underside of the vehicle. The fuel supply valve on an LPG- or LNG-fueled vehicle may likewise be inaccessible. These situations make the need for fire protection a very high priority. When fire protection is indicated, it should be no less than two 1½-inch (38 mm) hoselines with foam capability.

Bus Upside Down

Just as with automobiles, most buses have rounded contours along the junction between their roof and

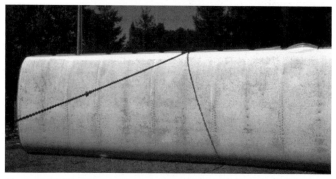

Figure 6.51 The bus may have to be initially stabilized with rigging.

118 Chapter 6 • Bus Extrication

sides. In addition, the roof itself is usually rounded to a greater or lesser extent. Unless its roof was significantly flattened during the crash, a bus that has come to rest upside down on a flat surface may be very unstable. This will require the installation of multiple step chocks or other similar devices along both sides of the bus, and perhaps both ends (Figure 6.52).

The amount of fuel and other fluids leaking from a bus that is on its top may be even greater than that from a bus on its side. Liquid fuels will almost certainly leak from the fuel filler. Engine oil will drain from the crankcase, and battery acid may drain from the batteries. This combination of uncontrolled fluids can drain into electrical components shorting them out and increasing the danger of a fire starting. Therefore, fire protection is a very high priority.

Buses in Other Positions

Just as with automobiles, buses can come to rest in any of a variety of positions other than those already described. A bus may be still on its wheels but on such an angle that it is in danger of falling onto its side — or even worse — rolling over and over down a steep hillside. The lives of those trapped inside the bus may depend upon fast and efficient work by the first rescuers on scene to stabilize the vehicle. Buses in these unusual situations can tax the ingenuity and resourcefulness of these rescuers. The situation will dictate the means by which rescuers can stabilize the bus. Therefore, rescuers must be thoroughly trained in the use — and adaptation — of all available tools and equipment, both from within the agency and from outside sources.

When a bus loaded with passengers has come to rest in an unusual position, rescuers may have to use a combination of cribbing, jacks, shoring, and other devices. They may have to secure the vehicle with

chains, cables, or webbing attached to a secure anchor point. Or, they may have to employ tow trucks or cranes to stabilize the vehicle.

Gaining Access into Buses

Once a crashed bus has been stabilized, rescuers can begin the task of gaining access into the interior of the vehicle. Access is necessary before rescue personnel can perform the remaining functions: victim triage and initial treatment, disentanglement, and extrication. In any extrication incident involving a bus, there are three primary access routes: doors, windows, and other openings.

Doors

Assuming that the bus has come to rest in a position that allows access to the front service door, this is the preferred starting point. When possible, open doors by operating them in the normal manner. Most front doors on buses are designed to operate only from the inside, while rear emergency doors are operable from both the inside and outside (Figure 6.53). Rarely are all doors inoperable following a collision.

Entry may be somewhat difficult if the front door is the "operable door" but is in the closed position. However, the door will often be open because

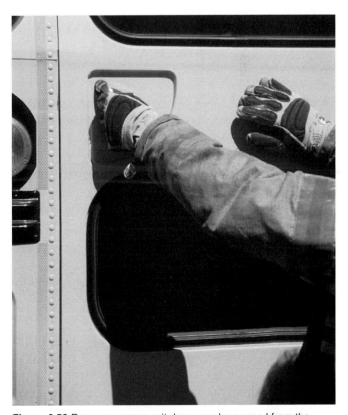
Figure 6.53 Rear emergency exit doors can be opened from the outside.

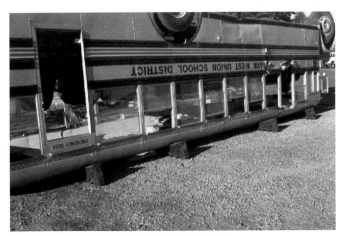
Figure 6.52 Many points of contact may be needed.

passengers will have escaped through it, leaving it open. If it is necessary to force open the front door, there are several methods that may be used.

On buses so equipped, the quickest way to open front doors is to use the emergency opening button located below the center of the windshield (Figure 6.54). On other buses, the fastest way is to create an avenue of access to the center pivot arm control and operate the door in the normal manner. There are two good ways to do this:

• Remove the windshield so that a rescuer can reach through the opening and manually operate the control.

• Reach in through the driver's side window with a pike pole to operate the control.

If the door is operated by an alternate method, such as an air-actuated control mechanism, it can be opened by reaching in through the driver's side window and operating the main switch. This switch is usually located to the left of the driver's instrument console. There will also be a backup emergency release mechanism in the stairwell just inside the door. The readily identifiable release button or switch permits the air lock device to release the door. Then, rescue personnel can manually move the door through its normal path of travel. The air override release mechanism may not be required if there are two operable doors located along the same side of the bus.

If it is necessary to force the doors, any type of power spreading tool may be used. First, identify the type of door by locating the hinges. If there are hinges on either side of the door and an overlapping rubber seal in the middle, it is a center opening door. This type of door can be pried open by inserting a power spreader between the two overlapping seals about

half way up the door and forcing each half to its respective side. It may be necessary to repeat this procedure at the top and bottom of the door to maximize the size of the opening.

A jammed center opening door can also be cut apart, disconnected, or disassembled. It is often possible to remove the door by breaking the hinges (usually piano hinges) that connect it to the bus. This can usually be done by driving the wedge end of a Halligan into the hinge area with a sledgehammer. This will usually fracture the hinge, enabling rescuers to remove the door. The pivot control arm will also have to be cut or detached to completely remove the door.

If the door has hinges in the middle and on one side, during normal operation it will open to the side with the hinges. When using a spreader on this type of door, it should be inserted between the nonhinged side and the frame. The entire door can then be forced toward the hinged side. Depending on the circumstances, it may also be necessary to completely remove the door.

Because of the narrowness of the front door area on some older buses, it may be difficult to maneuver litters and/or immobilized victims through that area. This problem can be alleviated somewhat by widening the front door opening by cutting through the A-post at the top of the windshield opening, and then making a relief cut in the bottom of the A-post at floor level. With these cuts complete, insert an extension ram between the A- and B-posts, parallel to the ground at the top of the dashboard level, and extend the ram to push the front wall forward.

In the event of a rear-end collision, if it is necessary to use the rear emergency exit door for access, it may be necessary to force this door open. The rear exit door is held secure by one or three latch points. The main latch is at the edge of the door near the control handle. The other two latches, if present, are found at the top and bottom of the door, holding fast into the bus body and the floor assembly. This door may be forced open by inserting a prying or spreading tool between the door and the frame and separating the two.

To remove the door, insert a spreading tool on the hinged side of the door and operate it to rip the hinges off the frame. If a spreading tool is not available, the rear door can also be disassembled, disconnected, or cut apart with a variety of other rescue tools.

One reason that removing a rear door is slightly more difficult than removing other doors is that the

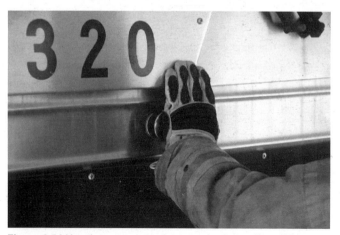
Figure 6.54 Use the emergency door opening button if available.

rear door is normally higher above the roadway surface. This means that rescuers will have to stand on something to effectively operate the rescue tool. Any object that provides solid footing will suffice (Figure 6.55).

Sometimes opening or removing the rear door still does not provide a large enough opening to remove immobilized victims. In these cases, it may also be necessary to remove part of the rear wall of the bus. To open the rear wall, the following steps should be taken:

Step 1: Using power shears or a reciprocating saw, make cuts to the top of the window post nearest the door and along the floor level of the rear wall (Figure 6.56).

Step 2: Make vertical relief cuts just inside the corner post of the bus (Figure 6.57).

Step 3: Once these cuts are made, the end wall can be folded to the side to increase the opening size (Figure 6.58).

It may be necessary to remove the last few rows of seats to take full advantage of this wide opening.

If the bus comes to rest on its side with the hinge side up, it may be difficult for small children to push the rear door open because of its weight. Rescuers should first try to open the door using the handle. Once the door is open, it must be propped open with a pike pole or similar tool. If time permits, remove the door. Removal of the rear wall is a good idea when a bus comes to rest on its side. This eliminates the need to step over the wall every time someone goes through the exit. The procedure for removing the rear wall is the same as that described for upright buses.

Windows

Because of the extensive skeletal structure in the side walls of buses, and the availability of other means of access, gaining access into a bus by breaching the side walls is often too time consuming to be worthwhile. Even though bus side windows are sometimes removed, gaining access through the windshield and/ or rear window is usually preferred.

Windshield Access

Entry through the windshield can be advantageous when the front exit is unusable or the bus has come to rest on its side. Removing the windshield will give rescuers quick access to the interior of the bus and will also provide a route for removing victims.

Unlike automobile windshields, bus windshields are divided into two or more parts, which may be

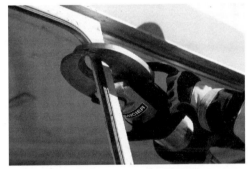
Figure 6.56 Cut the top of the window post.

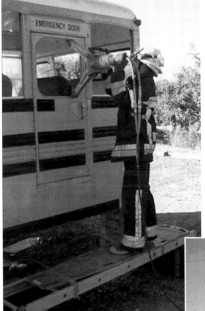
Figure 6.55 A makeshift scaffold may be needed.

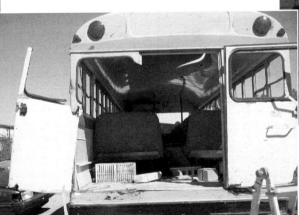
Figure 6.58 Fold the end wall back.

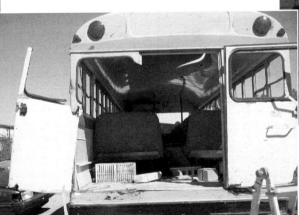
Figure 6.57 Make the vertical relief cuts.

separated by posts. Bus windshields are mounted with gaskets that are somewhat different than those used for automobile windshields, although removal methods are basically the same. To remove a bus windshield, cut the rubber mounting gasket with a knife, baling hook, or other similar tool.

Once the gasket is removed, remove each piece of the windshield. If no rescuer is inside the bus yet, rescuers can sometimes reach through the gasket gap with the end of a baling hook and gently pull the glass toward them. If a rescuer is already inside the bus, a gentle push on the glass should loosen it enough that the rescuers on the outside can remove it. After the glass has been removed, removing the center windshield post will provide rescuers with a full width opening through which they can work.

NOTE: Rear windows can be removed in a similar manner; however, it is preferable to use the rear exit door or completely cut away the rear walls whenever possible.

Side Window Access

Gaining access through the side windows may be difficult for two reasons: (1) they are small, and (2) they may be 6 to 8 feet (2 m to 2.5 m) above ground level. This forces rescuers to work from ladders or

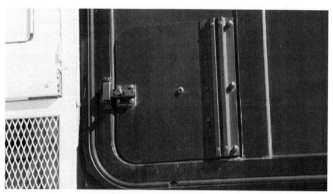
Figure 6.59 The emergency access hatch.

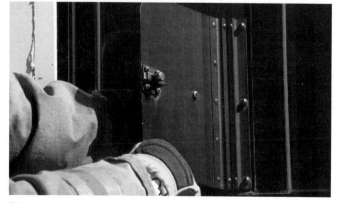
Figure 6.60 A rescuer reaches through the hatch.

platforms and that makes it more difficult to handle tools and victims.

Even with the positive latching systems found on many transit and commercial buses, the side windows can be pried open from the outside with a screwdriver or other rescue tool. Many buses have a small access hatch that rescuers can reach through to open a window from the inside. This hatch is usually level with the bottom of the last window on the passenger side of the bus (Figure 6.59). On commercial buses, it is located directly outside the restroom. It will be necessary for the rescuer to stand on a ladder or other object to reach this hatch (Figure 6.60). Once the hatch is opened, the rescuer can reach in and operate the window latch to open the window. Then, rescuers can enter and open more windows as necessary.

Most school buses have side windows that only slide down part way. They provide an opening of about 9 x 22 inches (225 mm by 550 mm), which is too small to be useful. Therefore, it will be necessary to enlarge the window opening. To double the size of the window opening, break the glass and remove the aluminum frame from the opening. Remove the glass using standard techniques described in Chapter 4. Almost any cutting tool can be used to cut away the soft aluminum window frame.

If the size of the window opening is still too small, it can be made even larger. This can be done by removing two adjacent windows and the post between them, and then removing the section of sidewall (Figure 6.61). If necessary, more windows can be removed and the posts cut. However, be careful not to remove so many posts that the structural integrity of the bus is compromised.

Access by Other Means

If removing the windshield, rear window, and/or the side windows still does not provide adequate access

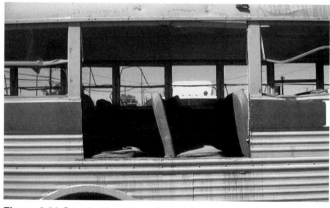
Figure 6.61 Opening the sidewall provides good access.

to the interior of a crashed bus, or if these window openings are inaccessible, some other means must be found. The most common of these alternative means of access are through the side wall, through the roof, and through the floor.

Side Wall Access

Even though forcing entry through the sides of a bus can be time consuming because of the extensive amount of skeletal structure and the obstructions posed by the seats, it may sometimes be necessary. It becomes necessary when the bus has remained upright but the front and rear exits are unusable. If the proper equipment is available, a large hole can be cut that will provide maximum access to the passenger area.

Forcible entry through the side of a bus will require considerable work to cut a usable opening. The heaviest beams in bus construction are located on the floor, where the seats bolt to the wall, and above and below the windows. The seats should be removed before opening a side wall.

If time allows, the seats can be unbolted from the floor. If not, the steel tube seat frame can be cut with any number of cutting tools. Cutting the legs or supports may leave sharp stubs, and they should be covered with duct tape to prevent additional injuries.

Once the seats have been cleared away and the windows and posts removed, cutting on the side wall may begin. The best tool for this operation is the reciprocating saw with a 6-inch (150 mm) metal cutting blade. This combination will cut through any of the structural components found in the side wall of the bus. To cut through the side wall of a bus:

Step 1: Cut away the widow frame (Figure 6.62).

Step 2: Make vertical cuts straight down from two window posts. The cuts should extend down only as far as the floor level (Figure 6.63).

Step 3: At the floor level, make short horizontal relief cuts, 1 to 2 inches (25 mm to 50 mm) long, toward the center of the portion to be laid down (Figure 6.64).

When these cuts have been made, the wall section can be pushed/pulled down to create an opening in the side wall.

Another way to remove a portion of the side wall is to remove entire sheets of metal by using an air chisel to pop the rivets or welds that hold the sheets. Once the sheets are removed, the individual beams in the side of the bus can be cut. However, this method is

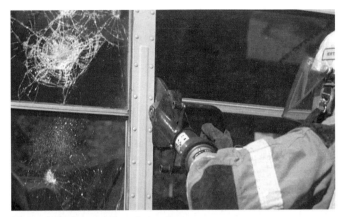
Figure 6.62 Remove the window frame.

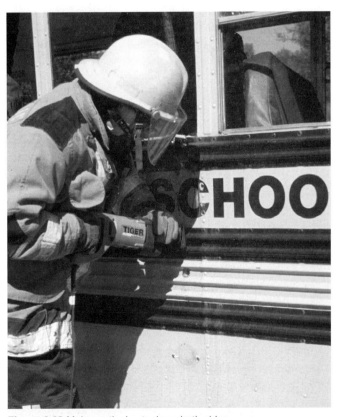
Figure 6.63 Make vertical cuts down both sides.

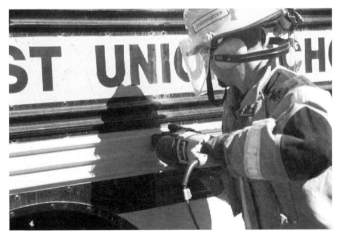
Figure 6.64 Make horizontal relief cuts at the floor level.

considerably slower and noisier than using a reciprocating saw and should only be used as a last resort.

Roof Access

In some cases, it may be necessary to gain access through the roof of a bus. A roof opening may be needed when a bus has come to rest on its side, and occasionally on an upright bus. When a bus lands on its side, the front door may be virtually useless. It will either be under the bus, making it inaccessible, or it will be on top, making it difficult to use for evacuation purposes. Access may still be possible through the rear emergency door or windshield; however, these openings may not be sufficient or may themselves be blocked. Any of these situations may require rescuers to make entry through the roof.

The first choice for removing victims through the roof should be to use any roof escape hatches with which the bus may be equipped. These hatches are easy to force from the outside. Most can be pried off with any standard prying tool or power spreading tool. However, these hatches only provide a clear opening of up to about 2 feet (0.6 m) square. They may be too small to allow the removal of immobilized victims. This will require rescuers to enlarge the opening.

Before beginning to cut, rescuers must determine the best location for the roof opening. This will be determined by the location of the victims inside the bus, the position of the bus, and the type and amount of damage to the bus. If there are victims located throughout the entire length of the bus, the opening should be cut where it will be most effective. Each situation will dictate where the best location is.

Cutting an opening in the roof of the bus can sometimes be difficult and time consuming. However, the overall benefits can easily justify the time involved. Cutting an opening in the roof can provide rescuers with more or less complete access to the interior of the bus. However, cutting an opening in a bus roof can be time consuming because of the multiple layers of materials that are used in the roof's construction. The roof is comprised of two layers of sheet metal with supports, insulation, and wiring sandwiched between them.

While an air chisel can be used if that is all that is available, it is not ideal. Because an air chisel can only cut one layer of metal at a time, the layers have to be cut one at a time. This virtually doubles the amount of time needed to cut the opening.

The most effective tool for cutting roof panels is a reciprocating saw with at least a 6-inch (150 mm) blade. The reciprocating saw will produce a smooth cut through all layers of material at one time, and with little chance of igniting any flammable vapors in the area. To cut an access opening in the roof of a bus, take the following steps:

Step 1: Create an access hole near a row of rivets with either a pick-head axe or the point of a Halligan tool (Figure 6.65).

Step 2: Insert the saw blade into the hole and make a horizontal cut across one row of rivets, but stopping short of the second row (Figure 6.66).

Step 3: Make vertical cuts from the ends of the horizontal cut down to ground level (Figure 6.67).

Step 4: Fold the flap of roof down to the ground (Figure 6.68).

The foregoing procedure is specifically for cutting an access opening in the roof of a school bus. The

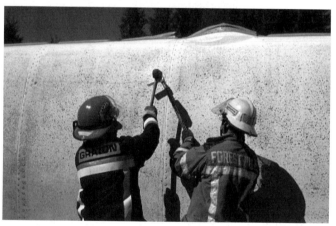

Figure 6.65 Create a starter hole in the roof.

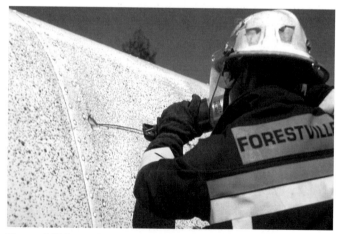

Figure 6.66 Insert the saw blade and make the top cut.

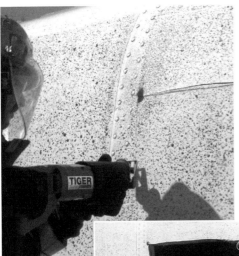

Figure 6.67 Cut down both sides from the ends of the top cut.

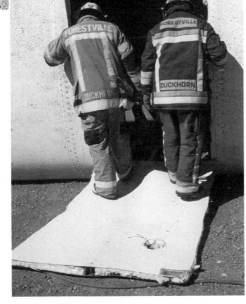

Figure 6.68 Fold the roof flap down.

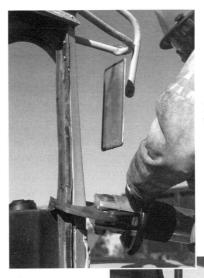

Figure 6.69 Cut the three front posts.

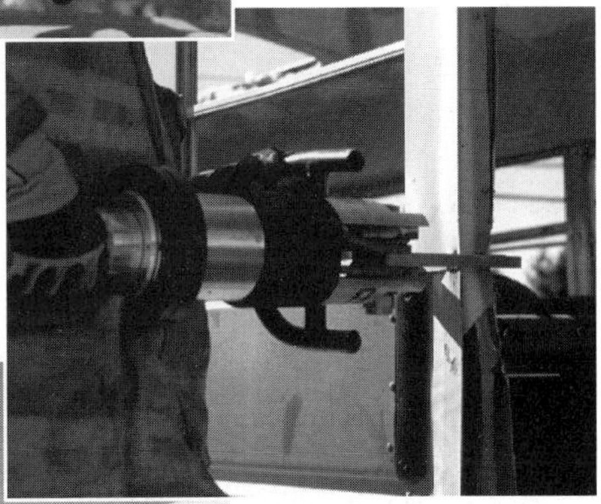

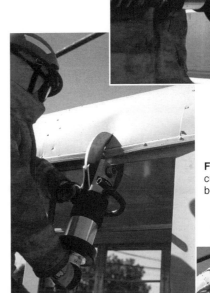

Figure 6.70 Cut both B-posts.

Figure 6.71 Make relief cuts aft of the B-posts on both sides.

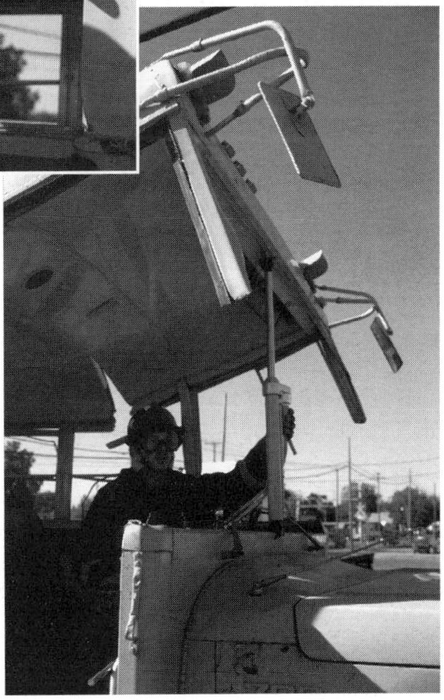

Figure 6.72 Push the roof up with an extension ram.

same procedure can be used with transit and commercial buses except that commercial buses have overhead storage bins along each outside wall. To avoid these bins, rescuers must cut access openings as near the centerline of the roof as possible.

Sometimes access through the front of the bus is needed. In these cases, it may be useful to flap a portion of the roof backward. While this procedure is possible with the proper equipment, it will be difficult. To perform this evolution, take the following steps:

Step 1: After removing the windshield, cut the three front window/roof posts (Figure 6.69).

Step 2: Cut the B-posts on each side (Figure 6.70).

Step 3: Make relief cuts into the roof slightly aft of the B-posts (Figure 6.71).

Step 4: Position an extension ram in the middle of the windshield opening and push the roof up (Figure 6.72).

Floor Access

Gaining access through the floor of a bus should only be considered as a last resort. Fortunately, this will rarely be necessary. Any attempt to breach this area will require a considerable amount of time because of the many layers of materials that are combined to construct the floor. Bus floors consist of a heavy frame to support the entire bus, plus sheet metal, plywood, and a vinyl or rubber floor covering. The beams and other framework are often placed as close as 9 inches (225 mm) apart. One factor helping rescuers is the fact that, depending on the manufacturer of the bus, only every third or fourth beam is a solid, supporting member. The beams in between are only welded to the underside of the floor and provide little support or hindrance to rescue operations. Because through-the-floor access is likely to be attempted only when the bus is on its side or roof, the fuel tank, which is mounted under the vehicle, will be inverted and probably leaking fuel near the cutting area. This makes the risk of a flash fire very high.

WARNING!

Take extra care when attempting to breach the floor of a bus due to the danger of flash fire. Keep charged hoselines manned and ready at all times.

Regardless of the type of bus, the steps involved in cutting an access opening are virtually the same. After identifying the two adjacent main supporting beams between which the opening will be made, take the following steps:

Step 1: Using an air chisel or power shears, make two cuts in the end of each of the non-supporting beams that lie between the main supporting beams. The first cut should be at the end of each beam, and a second cut should be at least 3 inches (75 mm) inside the first cut (Figure 6.73).

Step 2: Using a sledgehammer or similar tool, knock out the small section of beam between the cuts (Figure 6.74).

Step 3: Using an air chisel or other tool, cut an access hole in the floor of the bus (Figure 6.75).

Step 4: Insert the blade of the reciprocating saw into the access hole and cut the floor (Figure 6.76).

Step 5: When three sides of a square or rectangular opening have been cut, fold back the flap of flooring to create the access opening (Figure 6.77).

Because of the massive understructure associated with transit buses and commercial buses, access through the undercarriage and floor is a difficult and

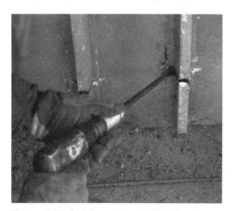
Figure 6.73 Cut the nonsupporting beams.

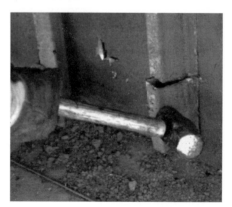
Figure 6.74 Knock out the small sections.

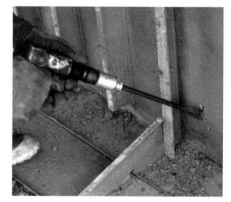
Figure 6.75 Make an access hole for the saw.

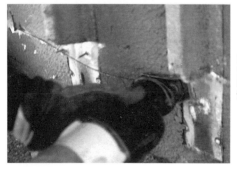
Figure 6.76 Insert the saw blade and make the cuts.

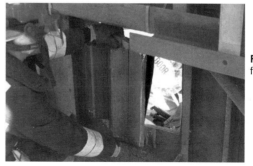
Figure 6.77 Fold the flap of flooring back.

tedious job. An additional problem with commercial buses is the storage area between the bottom of the bus and the actual underside of the floor. This requires cutting an access opening through the storage area floor and the main floor of the bus. The other methods of gaining access previously described in this section should be used as alternatives to access through the floor of a bus.

Bus Extrication Process

Once a crashed bus has been stabilized and access has been gained, rescuers can enter the bus for triage, disentanglement, and extrication of the victims trapped inside. While many of the required tools and techniques are the same regardless of the position of the bus, the extrication process is discussed with the bus upright, on its side, on its roof, and in other positions.

Bus Upright

When a bus has been involved in a front-end collision, the driver is sometimes trapped by the steering wheel. This is often caused by the driver having to tilt the steering wheel into his lap after he takes his seat. This virtually traps the driver if a collision prevents him from moving the steering wheel. Pulling the steering column and steering wheel on buses involve the same dangers as described in Chapter 5 for automobiles. Therefore, this technique is not recommended. Just as in an automobile, tilting the steering wheel or cutting the steering wheel ring puts the driver at less risk of being injured by the end of the steering column pivoting into his torso. In many cases, it is possible to free the driver by simply tilting the steering wheel toward the windshield. In some older buses, cutting the brace between the steering column and the front wall of the bus may be necessary. Otherwise, cutting the steering wheel ring may be the next best option.

The steering wheel on a bus is constructed in a manner similar to that of an automobile. A hardened steel ring is molded inside a covering of rubber or plastic. The quickest method of freeing the victim is to cut away the bottom half of the steering ring. While a hacksaw or reciprocating saw can be used to cut the ring, a power shear is the tool of choice (Figure 6.78). Often, this alone will free the driver, thus eliminating the need for further action.

However, if cutting the steering wheel ring is not possible, or if cutting it does not free the driver, it may be because the driver's seat is pneumatically controlled. These seats automatically adjust to

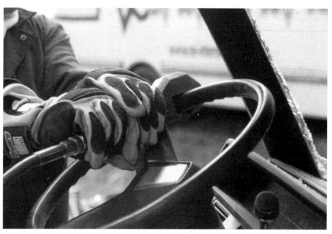

Figure 6.78 The steering wheel ring may have to be cut.

changes in weight or pressure on them, and this can hold the driver against the steering wheel and make him appear to be trapped. Operating the seat adjustment control may release enough air to lower the seat and free the driver. If this does not free the driver, the seat may have to be unbolted from the floor and moved rearward. It may also be necessary to remove the partition behind the driver's seat to create enough room to lay the driver's seat back.

Removing Interior Obstructions

As just described for freeing the bus driver, it may be necessary to move or remove interior features of the bus to facilitate removal of victims. The narrow aisles in buses create a limited working space. Most litters and backboards are too wide to fit in the aisle and have to be placed on the top of the seat cushions or across the tops of the seat backs. Seat frames are easily bent during a collision and can entrap a victim.

Deciding whether to simply move a seat or to remove it will depend on the position of the victim and the rescuers' need for operating space. In many cases, it is advantageous to remove the seat and get it out of the way. There are several effective ways to do this. The seats may be pulled from their moorings by using a winch, come-along, or power spreader. This should not be done if any victims are still trapped close to the seat being pulled because the seat may suddenly dislodge and aggravate their injuries.

There are several good methods for removing seats. One method is to use a power spreader to dislodge the legs connected to the floor and then break the seat-to-wall connection. Another method is to cut the legs of the seats. The legs are made of tubular steel and can be cut with power shears (Figure 6.79). The legs should be cut as close to the floor as possible and the sharp stubs taped or covered with duct tape.

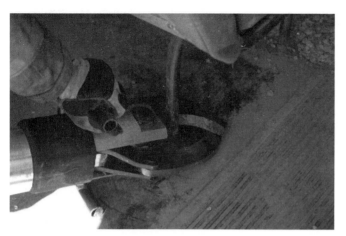

Figure 6.79 Seat legs may have to be cut.

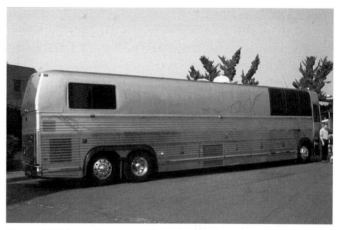

Figure 6.80 Some bus conversions are obvious.

Many school buses also have partitions in front of the first row of seats, on either side of the aisle. These dividers are usually made only of thin sheet metal attached to a tubular steel frame. The whole unit is connected to the bus in a manner similar to the seats. These partitions can be removed in the same manner as a seat.

Likewise, most of the objects inside of transit or commercial buses are either seats or partitions. Both of these assemblies are bolted to the floor. Partitions may also be connected to the ceiling. If it becomes necessary to remove either of these objects, it is best to unbolt them and remove them from the bus. If time does not permit them to be unbolted, most can easily be cut with any number of cutting tools. The legs or supports are generally constructed of tubular steel that can easily be cut. Cutting these legs or supports will result in sharp stubs being left behind and, if possible, rescuers should cover them as described earlier.

Commercial buses also have overhead storage bins. If it is necessary to remove them to facilitate extricating immobilized victims, rescuers may need to cut or chop them out. Any type of saw or air chisel will work. If a saw is not available, a crash axe or standard fire axe may be used. Rescuers should be cautious when chopping inside of a bus as the space will be very confined and the potential for striking oneself or another person is high. They should use short, controlled strokes. To reduce the slip and fall hazard for those working inside of the bus, debris should be removed as soon as it is cut or chopped away.

As mentioned earlier in this chapter, some motor coaches are not designed to transport large groups of people. Rather, they have been converted into mobile living quarters and/or offices. They are used as campers

or mobile living quarters by entertainers on tour and others whose jobs require them to relocate frequently. It is usually easy to distinguish these vehicles from commercial buses by their blacked-out windows and sometimes ornate cosmetics on the vehicle's exterior (Figure 6.80). The interior layout of some of these vehicles will vary considerably from that of standard motor coaches. Some of these vehicles may have fully equipped galleys for meal preparation and may carry one or more LPG tanks for cooking and for heating water. All of these alterations can complicate the disentanglement and extrication processes.

Bus on Side

When an occupied bus has come to rest on its side, the occupants will be concentrated on the bottom side. Their general condition will depend upon the event that caused the bus to roll over and whether it slowly rolled onto its side or if it rolled over several times and came to rest on its side. In either case, access from either end of the bus will be extremely difficult because the center aisle is now vertical and movement within the bus will involve climbing over each row of seats. Therefore, it may be more efficient to cut a large opening in the roof of the bus near its middle. Such an opening reduces the distance that occupants need to travel in order to escape and that rescuers need to travel to reach trapped victims.

The cost/benefit of removing seats and other interior obstructions will be affected by the number of trapped victims, their locations within the bus, and their conditions. If it is determined that the benefit of removing these objects outweighs the time and resources needed to do so, the techniques described in the previous section can be used.

Even though most bus passengers do not wear seat belts, the likelihood of them being ejected in a rollover is relatively low. However, bus rollovers may still result in passengers being trapped beneath the vehicle when it comes to rest. There are two primary methods for removing a person trapped beneath a bus. First, if the bus is resting on soft ground, it may be possible to dig the victim out. The second and most common method of removing a victim from beneath a bus is to lift the bus off the victim. Any one of a number of lifting tools can be used to perform the actual lifting. Regardless of the tool used, the method for performing the rescue will be essentially the same.

The rescue device best suited to perform this operation is the pneumatic lifting bag. The flatness of the uninflated bag allows it to be inserted beneath the bus in a position to achieve the maximum lift possible. To use high-pressure pneumatic lifting bags to free a victim trapped beneath a bus, take the following steps:

Step 1: Insert at least one pneumatic lifting bag beneath the bus on each side of the victim (Figure 6.81). Center the middle of each bag beneath a roof truss support. These supports are clearly marked by rows of rivets across the roof structure. If more air bags are available, a small one can be stacked on top of a larger one when they are put into place. This increases the height that can be achieved.

Step 2: While the bags are being pushed into place, assemble cribbing or place step chocks on either side of the victim (Figure 6.82). The cribbing or chocks are used to shore up the bus as the bag(s) are inflated.

Step 3: Once everything is in place, begin lifting (Figure 6.83). Build up the box cribs or adjust the chocks as the lift progresses. This will minimize the risk to the rescuers and victim if the lifting bag fails. Because the roof of a bus is curved where it meets the side wall, it may be necessary to use wedges to maximize the contact between the cribbing and the bus, or invert the step chocks and use them as large wedges (Figure 6.84).

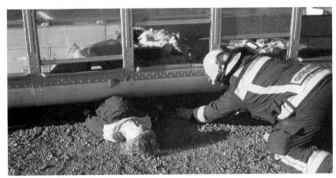
Figure 6.81 Insert a lifting bag on each side of the victim.

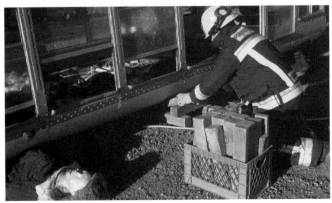
Figure 6.82 Gather cribbing materials.

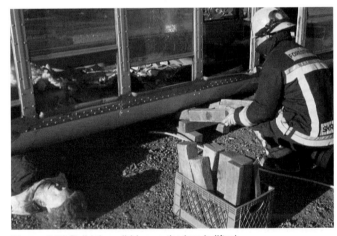
Figure 6.83 Build the cribbing as the bus is lifted.

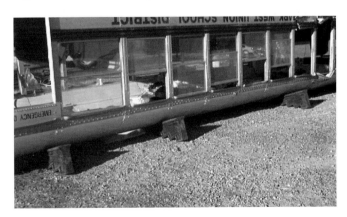
Figure 6.84 Maximize contact with the bus.

If low-pressure bags are used, they should be placed in the same locations as high-pressure bags would be. However, when using low-pressure bags, it is not necessary to stack the bags.

As mentioned earlier, other tools may be used to do the lifting if pneumatic lifting bags are not available. Power spreaders or hydraulic jacks can be used to lift a bus. When lifting on soft ground, it will be necessary to place a board beneath the bottom tip of the spreader or the base of the jack. Because of the overall height of most jacks, it may be necessary to dig a hole beneath the intended lifting area in order to place the jack. Once a jack is in position, one rescuer can operate it while the other rescuers concentrate on building the box crib or adjusting the chocks.

Bus on Roof

When an occupied bus has come to rest on its roof, the occupants will be concentrated on the ceiling because that is now the lowest point. Just as in the preceding discussion, how the bus came to be in that position will largely dictate the condition of the occupants. If the bus rolled over several times, there can be significant distortion of the seats, partitions, and other interior features. The dynamics creating this distortion can result in many occupant injuries and entrapments.

Unlike a bus on its side, one on its roof can allow easier movement within the bus — provided that the roof did not collapse in the rollover. If the roof is still more or less intact, removing the windshield and the rear and side windows will allow uninjured passengers to crawl out and rescuers to crawl in. Ultimately, it may be advisable or necessary to open up a side wall and to remove seats and other features to facilitate movement inside the bus, but this will be dictated by the specific situation.

Buses in Other Positions

In every vehicle extrication operation involving a vehicle in a position other than those already discussed, the ingenuity and resourcefulness of the on-scene rescue personnel can be severely tested. However, regardless of whether the bus was teetering on the edge of a precipice, dangling from a bridge or overpass, or partially submerged in a body of water, the work of stabilizing the vehicle and gaining access to its interior has already been done. What remains are the critical tasks involved in triaging and treating the trapped victims, disentangling them, and extricating them from the wreckage. Therefore, the tools, equipment, and techniques described in the preceding sections apply equally to buses in any position, however unusual.

Summary

There are a number of different types and sizes of buses traveling the streets and highways throughout North America. They range from school buses to local transit buses to commercial buses that travel great distances. These vehicles all share certain characteristics, but each type is also unique in some ways. Conducting safe and efficient extrication operations at bus collisions depends largely upon the extent to which rescue personnel know these vehicles and what to expect when they are faced with a collision involving one.

Collisions involving an occupied bus can present rescue personnel with the same physical and psychological challenges associated with any other vehicle extrication incident — compounded by the possibility of a massive number of victims. However, if rescuers remain calm, view the situation objectively, and apply their training and experience to the situation at hand, they will almost always conduct a successful extrication operation.

Chapter 7

Medium and Heavy Truck Extrication

Many thousands of medium and heavy trucks travel the streets, roads, and highways throughout North America each day. They range from local delivery vans to massive highway tractors pulling up to three huge trailers. This number includes tanker trucks carrying everything from combustible and flammable liquids to highly toxic or corrosive substances to exotic cargoes such as molten sulfur. There is also a variety of highly specialized trucks such as cement mixers, refuse haulers, and fire apparatus.

There are laws that limit the number of hours a driver can operate a commercial truck without a break, and vehicle safety inspections are conducted at weigh stations along major highways. However, considering the number and variety of trucks on the road, it is not surprising that some become involved in collisions with other vehicles, bridge abutments, or a host of other objects. Because of their size and weight, medium and heavy trucks fare better in collisions with smaller vehicles, so there are fewer times when truck drivers are trapped in their vehicles. For these same reasons, air bags are not required in long-haul trucks that fall under federal safety regulations, but seat belts have been required in trucks manufactured in the U.S. since September of 1989.

This chapter discusses the different classifications of medium and heavy trucks and their anatomy. Also discussed are the elements in properly sizing up an extrication incident involving a medium or heavy truck. Finally, how to stabilize collision-damaged trucks in a variety of positions is discussed, along with the steps involved in gaining access into them and extricating victims from them.

Classification of Medium and Heavy Trucks

There are several different classifications of medium and heavy trucks. The most common are straight trucks and tractor/trailer combinations, including tankers, grain transports, and auto transports. There are also a number of specialty trucks within this size range, including cement mixers, refuse haulers, ambulances, and fire apparatus. Medium trucks are Class 3, 4, or 5 with a gross vehicle weight rating (GVWR) between 10,000 pounds (4 540 kg) and 19,499 pounds (8 853 kg). Heavy trucks are Class 6 with a GVWR of 19,500 pounds (8 853 kg) to 29,000 pounds (13 166 kg) (beverage trucks, two-axle vans), Class 7 with a GVWR of 29,001 pounds (13 166 kg) to 33,000 pounds (14 982 kg) (fuel trucks, refuse haulers, and two-axle highway tractors), and Class 8 with a GVWR of 33,001 pounds (14 982 kg) or more (three-axle dump trucks, cement mixers, and three-axle highway tractors).

Straight Trucks
This is perhaps the most common of all the truck types — those built on a rigid frame and not intended to pull a trailer (Figure 7.1). Most have either two or three axles and a GVWR between 10,000 pounds (4 540 kg) and 40,000 pounds (18 160 kg). Some have large, rather boxy bodies, and are used as local delivery vans. Others have either flatbeds or large box bodies mounted on their frames.

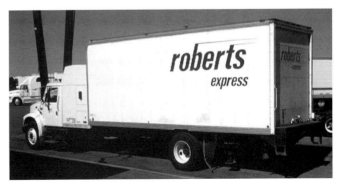
Figure 7.1 A typical straight truck.

Truck/Semitrailer Combinations

These heavy combinations consist of a highway tractor and one or more separate trailers (Figure 7.2). The tractors may have either two or three axles and may weigh up to 18,000 pounds (8 172 kg) by themselves. The entire tractor/trailer combination may weigh up to 140,000 pounds (63 560 kg). The trailers may be flatbeds, enclosed box trailers, tankers (in any of a variety of shapes), or any of a number of specialized types such as grain transports and vehicle transports. While some of these vehicles will be labeled or placarded to indicate the nature of their cargo, others will not — and they may be carrying almost any commodity, including up to 440 pounds (200 kg) of hazardous materials (Figure 7.3).

Specialty Trucks

Specialty trucks are differentiated only by their unique purposes. Otherwise, they may have the same configuration as any of those already described, and they are likely to weigh as much as any other truck of the same type and size. As mentioned earlier, *specialty trucks* can include everything from cement mixers,

refuse haulers, tow trucks, and grain transports, to ambulances and fire apparatus (Figure 7.4). There are countless others.

Truck Anatomy

As with automobiles, light trucks, and buses, medium and heavy trucks all have certain characteristics in common and others that are unique. The most distinguishing characteristic of all types of medium and heavy trucks is that they are relatively big and often extremely heavy. Their sheer size and weight can complicate an otherwise routine extrication problem and necessitate the use of specialized resources such as booms, cranes, or other massive lifting devices.

Cabs

Except for delivery vans, all medium and heavy trucks have a cab of some sort. In delivery vans, the cab is merely the front portion of the vehicle's body, separated from the cargo area only by a bulkhead on either side of the center aisle. The two most common types of cabs are conventional and cab-over units.

Conventional Cabs

In a *conventional cab*, the passenger compartment is located aft of the engine compartment (Figure 7.5). A

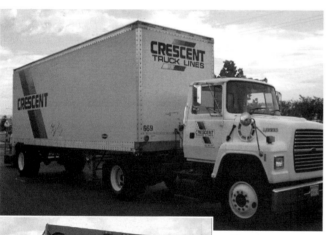

Figure 7.2 A typical truck/semitrailer combination.

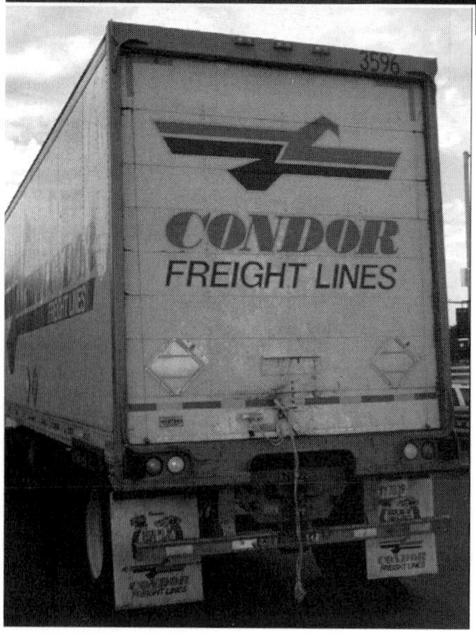

Figure 7.3 Vehicle signage may or may not reveal what the cargo is.

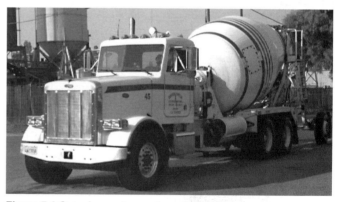

Figure 7.4 One of many types of specialty trucks.

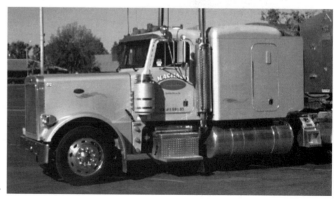

Figure 7.5 A conventional cab.

conventional cab is longer from front to back than is a cab-over model, and the cab does not tilt forward to provide access to the engine. The engine is accessed by raising the sides of a hood that is hinged down its midline, or the hood and front fenders may be a molded fiberglass unit that tilts forward (Figure 7.6). The remainder of a conventional cab is usually made of steel, aluminum, or a combination of fiberglass panels over a steel framework.

Cab-Over Units

In this design, the engine is located directly under the midline of the passenger compartment, roughly between the seats. The *cab-over unit* is designed to tilt forward to allow access to the engine (Figure 7.7). Generally, the cab is attached to the chassis at three points — in the center behind the cab (latch point) and by a hinge at the forward end of each frame rail. As with conventional cabs, cab-over units may be made of steel, aluminum, fiberglass, or a combination of these materials.

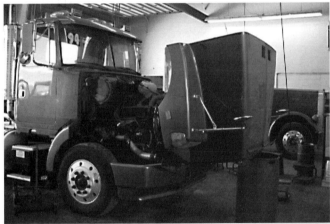

Figure 7.6 Some trucks have molded fiberglass front ends.

Sleepers

Because many long-haul trucks drive from coast to coast, and the law limits the number of hours a driver can operate a commercial vehicle without a rest period, many heavy trucks are equipped with a small sleeping compartment in or behind the cab. This feature allows a driver to sleep in relative comfort at highway rest stops without the expense of renting a room. It also allows a two-person team to drive continuously, stopping only for fuel and meals. One driver operates the truck while the other sleeps, and they trade places when the driver reaches his legal driving limit.

The vast majority of sleepers are merely an extension of the cab and not a separate unit, so access into these units is through the cab or by forcing entry through the required exterior door. In those units that are separate compartments, they must have an intercom between the sleeper and the cab. The access door to the sleeper may be on either side of the unit (Figure 7.8).

The fact that a truck has a sleeper attached to the cab should alert rescue personnel to check there for another possible occupant during the size-up of an incident involving one of these rigs. Since the occupant of a sleeper is not required to be restrained, rescuers should expect to find an injured victim in the sleeper following a collision.

Cab Doors

The forward doors on most delivery vans are pocket doors that slide rearward into the vehicle's side wall to open (Figure 7.9). These doors have a single latch point at the center of the front edge of the door.

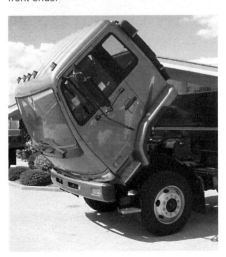

Figure 7.7 Cab-over units are designed to tilt forward for engine service.

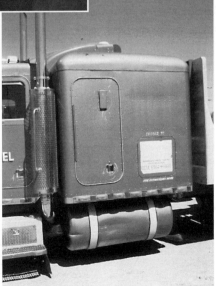

Figure 7.8 The access door may be on either side of the sleeper.

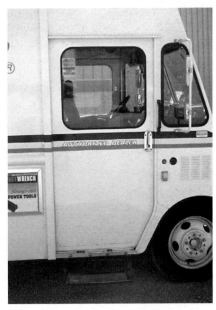

Figure 7.9 A typical sliding door.

The doors on both conventional and cab-over units are much heavier and stronger than those on automobiles and light trucks. They are equipped with either conventional or piano-type hinges. Most have a single latch with a two-step locking action. Because of the height of the doors above the ground, the door latch handle is usually located in the lower rear corner of the door (Figure 7.10).

Cab Windows

The windshields and rear windows of medium and heavy trucks are made of laminated safety glass, and they are set in center-bead rubber gaskets. The cab side windows are made of tempered glass that is heavier than that used in automobiles and light trucks.

Cab Roofs

The cab roofs of most medium and heavy trucks are usually covered with the lightest gauge metal or fiberglass on the vehicle, and the skin is supported by two or more ribs running from front to rear. Many heavy trucks have a large fiberglass fairing (wind deflector) mounted on the roof, behind which are often an air horn and an air-conditioning unit (Figure 7.11).

Batteries

Medium and heavy trucks have either a 12-volt or 24-volt electrical system supplied by one or more banks of batteries. The battery banks may be in more than one location on the vehicle. Those with 24-volt systems normally have four 6-volt batteries in series, with a negative ground.

Fuel Systems

Most medium and all heavy trucks operate on diesel fuel, rather than gasoline. This reduces, but does not eliminate, the danger of a flash fire following a collision. While the flashpoint of diesel fuel varies from 126° to 204° F (52° C to 95° C) it can easily be heated to that point if it leaks onto exhaust system components or even very hot pavement. The diesel fuel is usually contained in large external saddle tanks attached to either side of the frame (Figure 7.12). The capacity of these saddle tanks may vary from 50 to 300 gallons (200 L to 1 200 L) each. Some saddle tanks are

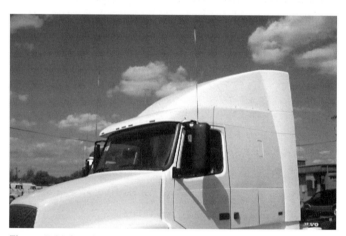

Figure 7.11 A typical roof-mounted fairing.

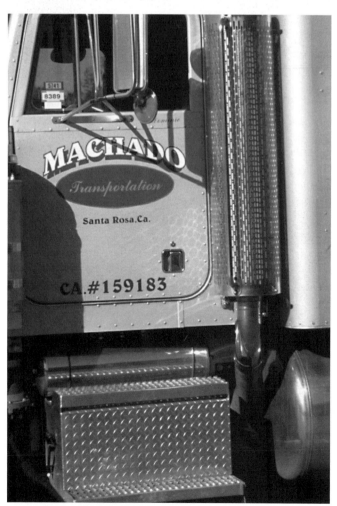

Figure 7.10 Door handles are within easy reach.

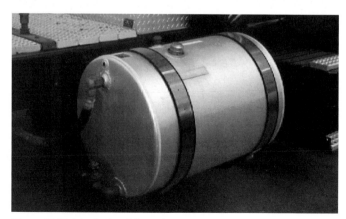

Figure 7.12 A typical saddle tank.

interconnected by a small tube that equalizes the volume of fuel in both tanks. At one or both ends of this tube is a small valve that can be used to isolate the tanks from each other if one tank is leaking. This will limit the amount of fuel that can escape.

Just as with buses and some light trucks, some medium and heavy trucks operate on alternative fuels — either liquefied petroleum gas (LPG) or compressed natural gas (CNG) (Figure 7.13). A small number of trucks now operate on liquefied natural gas (LNG) or hydrogen. Decals or other signs should be visible to alert rescue personnel that a particular vehicle uses an alternative fuel. The locations of the fuel tanks vary considerably.

> **WARNING!**
> Leaking fuel may present more than fire and explosion hazards. Contact with LPG and LNG can cause frostbite to exposed skin.

Brake Systems
Medium and heavy trucks are equipped with either hydraulic brakes, air brakes, or a combination of the two. The hydraulic brake systems are similar to those in automobiles and light trucks, but they are heavy-duty. Some trucks have hydraulic brakes that are assisted by air pressure. In the air brake systems, compressed air is used to apply the brakes under normal operation (Figure 7.14). Under abnormal conditions, such as a complete loss of air pressure in the braking system, heavy-duty springs automatically apply the rear brakes.

Because the trailers on tractor/trailer rigs also have air brakes, the trailer's air system is connected to that of the tractor by a breakaway valve (commonly called glad-hand connections) at the rear of the cab. The flexible air line connecting the tractor and trailer is often supported on a vertical stand (sometimes called a pogo stick) mounted on the rear of the tractor or by some other securing device (Figure 7.15).

Both trucks and tractor/trailer combinations with air brakes have air brake chambers mounted under each axle. The double chambers (called piggyback chambers) under the rear axles contain large compressed springs that are designed to apply the brakes mechanically for parking or if there is a loss of air pressure. The parts of each double chamber are held together with a metal clamp — and rescue personnel should *never* loosen this clamp (Figure 7.16).

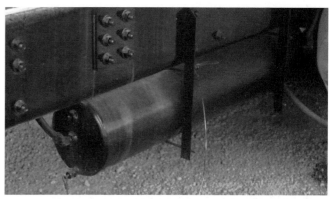
Figure 7.14 A typical brake system compressed air tank.

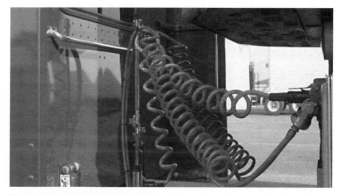
Figure 7.15 A typical pogo stick.

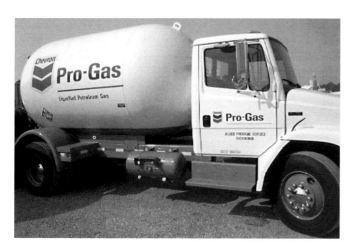
Figure 7.13 Some trucks use alternative fuels.

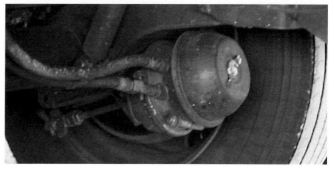
Figure 7.16 Clamps hold the brake chamber components together.

Suspension Systems

Most medium and heavy trucks have conventional heavy-duty suspension (i.e. leaf and/or coil springs). However, a growing number of heavy trucks are equipped with air suspension systems. In these systems, the conventional metal springs are replaced with compact rubber air bags that are somewhat similar to a bellows (Figure 7.17). At each wheel, there are air suspension bags — two on each axle. An on-board compressor maintains the air pressure within the bags as high as 120 psi (840 kPa). Depending upon the load of the vehicle and the condition of the road, the pressure within each bag is automatically increased or decreased to maintain the vehicle in a level state.

If the pressure in an air suspension bag is lost because of damage to the bag or its associated piping, the truck chassis can suddenly drop several inches without warning.

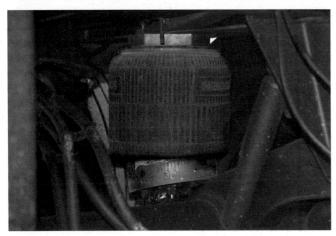

Figure 7.17 A typical air suspension bag.

Fifth Wheel

Mounted on the rear of every highway tractor is a heavy-duty circular steel plate called a *fifth wheel* (Figure 7.18). The fifth wheel is capable of rotating horizontally more than 90 degrees from center in both directions, and on some vehicles, it can be adjusted fore and aft. The fifth wheel has a wedge-shaped slot in its rear aspect to receive the trailer's king pin. When the king pin reaches the center of the fifth wheel during coupling, the pin is locked into place by two spring-loaded jaws. A pull handle on the driver's side of the tractor opens the jaws to allow the trailer to be uncoupled from the tractor (Figure 7.19).

Trailer Anatomy

Trailers are available in a wide variety of shapes and sizes — depending upon their intended use. There are flatbed trailers used for hauling virtually anything that can be lashed to the bed. There are trailers with bottom-dump capability used for hauling sand, gravel,

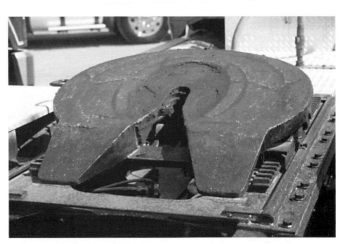

Figure 7.18 A typical fifth wheel.

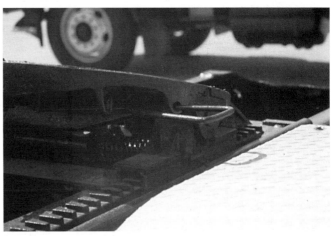

Figure 7.19 A pull handle opens the fifth wheel jaws.

grain, and other dry products (Figure 7.20). There are long cylindrical tankers in a variety of styles depending upon what they are intended to carry (Figure 7.21). There are trailers for carrying cryogenic materials (Figure 7.22). Probably the most common trailers seen on the highways are the huge box trailers used for hauling almost anything that will fit inside the box (Figure 7.23).

Regardless of whether the trailer is a flatbed, box, or tanker, they are all designed in one of two basic styles: trailers or semitrailers. A *trailer* is a freestanding unit with wheels front and rear. The front axle on a trailer is connected to a turntable that can be turned from side to side for better tracking, and the rear axle is fixed. A trailer couples to a tractor or another trailer with a long tow bar, often called a dolly (Figure 7.24). *Semitrailers* only have wheels at or near the rear end, and the front end is supported by the tractor when locked into the fifth wheel described earlier (Figure 7.25). When a semitrailer is not coupled to a tractor, its front end is supported by a pair of small wheels or plates (sometimes called landing gear) that are attached to the underside of the trailer by two struts (Figure 7.26). When not in use, the trailer's landing

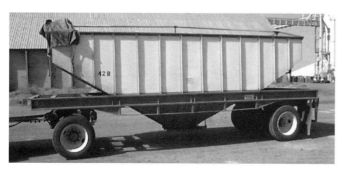

Figure 7.20 A typical bottom-dump trailer.

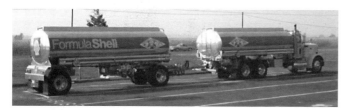

Figure 7.21 Tankers carry a wide variety of products.

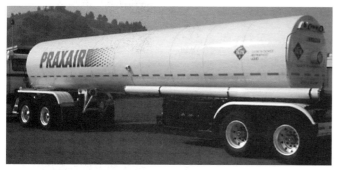

Figure 7.22 A typical cryogenic materials tanker.

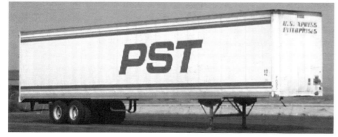

Figure 7.23 The most common type of highway trailer.

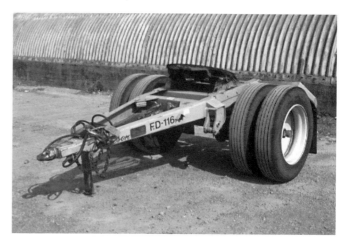

Figure 7.24 A typical trailer dolly.

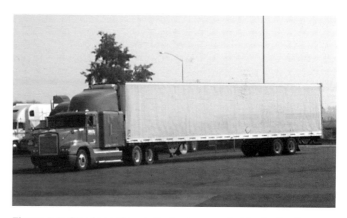

Figure 7.25 The front of a semitrailer is supported by the tractor.

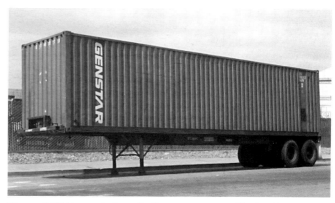

Figure 7.26 Uncoupled semitrailers are supported by landing gear.

gear can be lowered with a hand crank (Figure 7.27). On many of these trailers, the hand crank has two speeds — push in and crank for slow raising or lowering, pull out and crank for fast raising or lowering. The landing gear can be used for additional temporary stabilization, but not for lifting the trailer.

Many trailers and semitrailers are equipped with air suspension systems as described earlier in the section on truck anatomy. The same precautions apply to working under these trailers as apply to working under trucks with similar suspension systems.

Box Trailers

With the exception of refrigerated trailers that have heavily insulated walls and roofs, most box trailers have a relatively lightweight metal frame that is covered by metal or fiberglass or a combination of the two. There may be rub rails along the inside walls of the box

to protect it and add shear strength. The roof of the box is the area most easily penetrated because the covering material is thinnest and there are the fewest structural members. While there are many exceptions, most box trailers have 110 inches (2.8 m) of vertical clearance inside, from front to rear (Figure 7.28).

Cargo Doors

The rear cargo doors on box trailers may be one of two types: swinging or roll-up. Trailers with swinging doors usually have two single-leaf doors that latch near the middle and swing outward on conventional or piano-type hinges. Most roll-up doors on trailers are constructed in sections similar to a garage door (Figure 7.29). All types of roll-up doors latch in the center at the bottom of the door (Figure 7.30).

Livestock Trailers

While not as numerous as the types of trailers already described, livestock trailers bear mentioning because unlike most other trailers on the highway, they often contain a significant life hazard (Figure 7.31). Horses or other livestock that are already frightened and upset

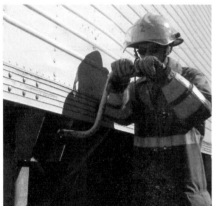

Figure 7.27 The landing gear can be lowered with a hand crank.

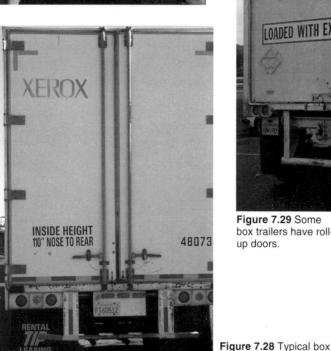

Figure 7.28 Typical box trailer dimensions.

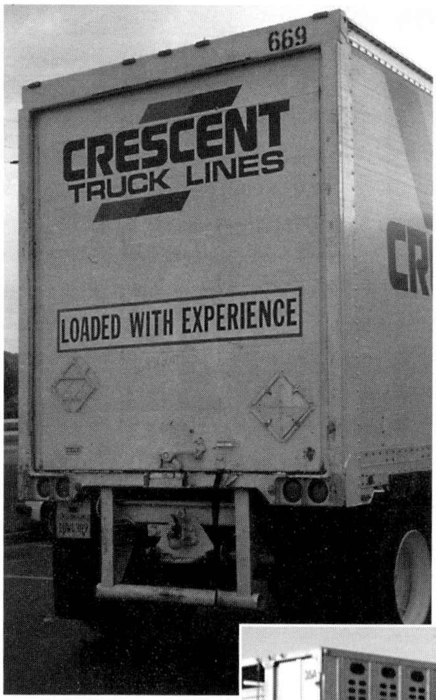

Figure 7.29 Some box trailers have roll-up doors.

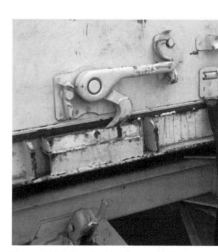

Figure 7.30 A typical latch on a roll-up door.

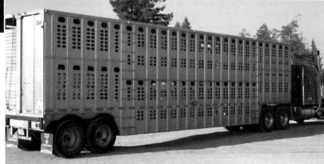

Figure 7.31 A typical livestock trailer.

because of the collision can be further agitated by the sounds of power tools being used in the extrication operation. In their panic, they can seriously injure themselves, other animals, or rescue personnel. It may be possible to calm the animal by blindfolding it and/or restricting its hearing. If this is not successful, it may be best to free the animal as quickly and as quietly as possible. However, be aware that a frightened animal that is freed from the confines of a wrecked trailer may bolt and attempt to flee. This can create a traffic hazard for other motorists and may result in harm to the animal. It is sometimes advisable to call a veterinarian to the scene to tranquilize any animal that cannot be extricated quickly.

Medium and Heavy Truck Extrication Size-Up

As described in Chapter 5 on sizing up automobile extrication, sizing up an incident involving a medium or heavy truck is done in steps. The first step is assessing the scene, followed by an assessment of the vehicles involved. Finally, the victims must be assessed along with the extrication requirements. As always, size-up continues until the incident is terminated.

Scene Assessment

During this step in the size-up process, rescuers should observe the weather and the day/date/time of the incident and factor these variables into their decision making. As described earlier, weather can adversely affect the response of emergency vehicles, and it can add the dangers of hyperthermia and dehydration or hypothermia to the trauma already suffered by trapped victims. The day, date, and time of the incident can greatly affect the volume of vehicular and pedestrian traffic in the area.

One of the potentially most important parts of assessing the scene of an incident involving a medium or heavy truck is identifying the cargo that the truck is carrying (Figure 7.32). In addition to the other hazards that may be present — fuel leaks, downed wires, incipient fires, etc.—the cargo itself may be hazardous. 49 CFR 171 allows up to 440 lbs. [200 kg] of hazardous cargo without placarding.

WARNING!

Before approaching a crashed medium or heavy truck, stop a safe distance away and use binoculars to look for hazardous materials labels or placards.

If any labels or placards are seen, follow agency protocols for the material indicated. These protocols will usually follow the recommendations contained in either the DOT Emergency Action Guide or CANUTEC.

Pedestrians fleeing the scene may be the first indication of the need to stop and assess the scene before approaching. If people are running from the scene with a look of panic on their faces or if pedestrians have collapsed in the area of the crashed vehicles, it would be imprudent to jeopardize rescue personnel by approaching the scene without taking the necessary precautions.

If it appears that an airborne contaminant has been released in the collision, use public address systems or bull horns to instruct those near the scene to vacate immediately. A hazardous materials response team should be called, and all incoming units informed of the situation. They should be instructed to stage uphill and upwind of the incident scene. Wearing SCBA and full PPE, rescue personnel should cordon off the scene and deny entry until the haz mat team arrives.

However, even if the cargo is labeled as hazardous, it may be contained and represent no immediate threat. The cargo area should still be cordoned off until a hazardous materials specialist can assess the situation, but the balance of the operation can proceed. All nonessential personnel and spectators should be kept upwind of the scene in case of a subsequent release. The adjacent highway should be closed to all but emergency vehicle traffic. Emergency vehicles should stage uphill and upwind.

If the truck driver is conscious, he may be able to tell rescue personnel what the cargo is and if it needs any special handling to maintain safety. If not, rescuers should attempt to locate the bill of lading (cargo

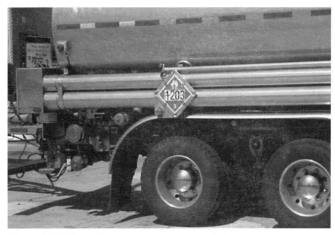
Figure 7.32 Identifying the cargo is extremely important.

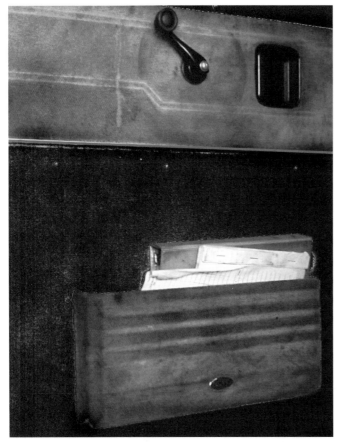
Figure 7.33 The bill of lading is often carried in a pouch on the door.

manifest) which is usually carried in a pocket on the driver's door (Figure 7.33).

Vehicle Assessment

The second step in the initial size-up of an incident involving a medium or heavy truck is a more detailed assessment of the vehicles involved than was done as a part of scene assessment. Each vehicle involved in the collision must be assessed in terms of its position, stability, and condition.

In what position is each vehicle — upright, on its side, or upside down? What will be required to stabilize each vehicle? Are those resources available on scene? In what condition is each vehicle — accordioned, crumpled, leaking fuel or other fluids, or smoking? Did the vehicles roll over one or more times? Have the roof posts collapsed? Each of these considerations will affect the need for extrication resources to mitigate the incident.

Victim Assessment

Perhaps the best thing that can be said about incidents involving medium or heavy trucks is that there is usually a small number of occupants who can become trapped in the wreckage. Most medium and heavy trucks are occupied by the driver only, the driver and a helper, or two drivers. However, regardless of how few or how many victims are involved, a quick but thorough assessment of their number and condition is critical to their survival.

As described earlier, this step is usually done in two phases — before the vehicles have been stabilized and again after they have been stabilized. The initial assessment — before the vehicles have been stabilized — is a somewhat cursory triage done by looking through the windows and other openings without touching the vehicles. No attempt should be made to enter the vehicles until they are stabilized. Once they are stabilized, rescue personnel can enter (at least as far as possible) to more carefully assess the condition of the victims.

Extrication Assessment

The extrication assessment step in the size-up process attempts to determine what actions will be required to extricate those trapped in the vehicles. Are the victims located so far above the roadway that ladders or platforms will be needed to reach them? Do the vehicle's windows and/or windshield need to be removed? Do the vehicle's doors need to be forced open or removed? Does the roof need to be flapped forward or backward or removed all together? The IC must assess the equipment and other resources available to take these actions.

Given all information supplied by the foregoing steps in the size-up process, the IC must make a number of quick decisions. Perhaps the first is what personnel and other resources are needed to provide fire protection. Considering the large quantities of diesel fuel carried by some trucks, foam-making capability may be a high priority. Another decision regards the resources that may also be needed for hazard mitigation, victim care and management, and the required extrication operations. If those resources are not already at the scene or en route, they must be requested *immediately*.

Medium and Heavy Truck Stabilization

As mentioned earlier, before rescue personnel can enter the cab or sleeper of a crashed truck, it is imperative that the truck be stabilized. When the truck has been stabilized, rescuers can conduct a more thorough assessment of the victims inside and properly package them for extrication. Stabilization may be accomplished by creating a sufficient number of points of contact between the truck and a stable surface — the ground or the pavement. While the equipment used remains the same as described in earlier chapters, the techniques employed to stabilize a medium or heavy truck will vary depending upon the position in which the vehicle is found. As always, stabilization includes preventing the vehicle from moving in any direction, shutting off the engine, and disconnecting the batteries. The following sections discuss the stabilization techniques used for a medium or heavy truck that is upright, on its side, on its roof, and in other positions.

Truck Upright

Even though some medium and heavy trucks have a relatively high center of gravity, the majority of trucks involved in collisions will be found upright. However, because a truck is resting on its wheels does not mean that it is stable. The inflated tires allow a certain amount of movement, especially laterally. Also, the vehicle's suspension system is designed to allow the vehicle's chassis to move in various directions. Even these small amounts of bounce and sway are enough to aggravate a trapped victim's injuries. Therefore, the truck must be stabilized as quickly as reasonably possible.

There are major differences between stabilizing an automobile or pickup truck and a medium or heavy truck. First, the vertical distance between the road surface and the bottom of the chassis is significantly greater in medium or heavy trucks than in other vehicles — and this raises the truck's center of gravity significantly. And second, medium and heavy trucks generally weigh much more than the smaller vehicles.

In some cases, a four-point box crib installed under the front bumper and both sides of the truck frame is needed. Large wheel chocks, such as those carried on fire apparatus, should be used to prevent the vehicle from rolling forward or backward. On cab-over units,

the cab should be secured with rope, webbing, or chains to prevent it from tilting forward unexpectedly during extrication operations (Figure 7.34). Once these measures have been taken, the truck should be stable enough for rescuers to start the victim assessment phase of the operation.

Truck on Its Side

A medium or heavy truck on its side can sometimes be easier to stabilize than other smaller vehicles. This is because the weight and shape of these trucks often make them relatively stable when they come to rest. However, a truck on its side may behave differently if it is fully loaded than it would if it were empty. In the case of a tractor/trailer, the tractor's center of gravity is different than the trailer's. Therefore, if someone uncouples the tractor from the trailer, the tractor may suddenly shift back toward the upright position while the trailer remains on its side. As with automobiles and other vehicles, chocks or other supports should be installed at the cab's door posts. Because of the roundness of the cab's roof edge, it may be advisable to invert the step chocks before sliding them under the vehicle. Depending upon how stable the truck is after the cribbing is installed, it may be advisable to shore the underside of the truck to prevent any possibility of it rolling back onto its wheels (Figure 7.35). Securing the truck with rope, chain, or webbing can also be used to prevent it from rolling back onto its wheels. However, if rapid extrication is needed, removing the cab's windshield may be the best course of action.

Truck on Its Roof

A truck on its roof can be even more of a challenge to stabilize than one on its side. The roofs of most truck cabs are rounded and offer few if any positive purchase

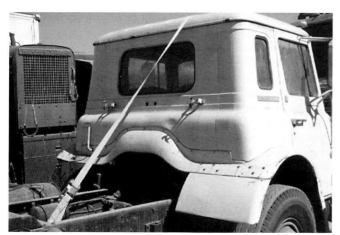

Figure 7.34 Cab-over units should be secured.

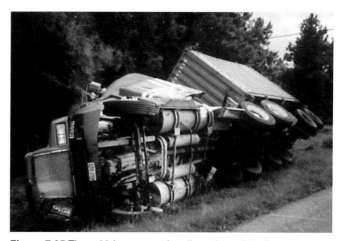

Figure 7.35 The vehicle must not be allowed to roll back onto its wheels. *Courtesy of Michael Hughes.*

points. However, inverted step chocks installed at the door posts and box cribbing or hi-lift jacks installed under the front bumper will often suffice. In some cases, it may be necessary to crib the truck's bed to prevent the truck from rocking fore and aft. Again, depending upon the situation, it may be practical to stabilize these trucks with ropes, chains, or webbing.

Trucks in Other Positions

Stabilizing trucks found in positions other than those already described will test the ingenuity of rescue personnel assigned to perform this task. However, regardless of what technique is used to stabilize a truck, the emphasis must be on safety. While speed and efficiency are highly desirable, the security and effectiveness of the stabilization measures are far more important. A rapidly installed crib that fails is far worse than one that takes longer to install but does the job.

When deciding how to stabilize a truck that has come to rest in an unusual position, rescue personnel should remember the discussions in Chapter 4 regarding center of gravity, mass, and vehicle integrity. These basic physical principles will dictate how a truck is likely to move when its components are manipulated or removed during extrication operations. If a truck is on a steep slope or hanging over the edge of a bridge or cliff, shoring and/or rigging can be used to offset the forces of gravity and secure the vehicle in place. If the vehicle is wedged under another vehicle or other object, the goal is to limit if not eliminate the vehicle's reaction when the overlying object is removed. Exactly how this is done will be dictated by the specific situation.

Gaining Access into Trucks

Once a crashed truck has been stabilized, the next step is to gain access to the interior of the cab. This may be as simple as opening the doors in the normal way — as in all forcible entry, *try before you pry*. However, in many cases, the doors are either locked or jammed, or both.

Windows

If the cab doors are either locked or jammed, removing the side windows to allow access to the door locks/handles is often necessary. The windows can be removed using the tools and techniques described in Chapter 4. Once the windows have been removed, the door lock/handle can be reached through the window opening. Depending upon the specific situation, it

may or may not be necessary to remove the windshield. If it is, it should be done using the tools and techniques described in Chapter 4.

Doors

When the cab door has been unlocked, the door handle should be tried. If that allows the door to be opened, the door handle can be held in the open position by inserting a short piece of angle-iron, cut specifically for this purpose, between the handle and the door handle recess. Holding the door handle in the open position prevents the door from latching again if it closes when released. If operating the exterior or interior door handle does not open the door, it sometimes helps to operate both of these handles simultaneously.

If the doors are jammed, they will have to be forced open using the tools and techniques described in Chapter 4. Whether the doors need to be removed or merely opened will be dictated by the specific situation.

Third-Door Conversion

As described in Chapter 4, this technique involves using shears and air chisels (or other suitable substitutes) to flap the side panel of a vehicle. This technique may be needed in a truck collision only if the sleeper area is an extension of the cab and not a separate compartment. In this case, the side wall of the cab aft of the door is flapped rearward. Otherwise, the tools and techniques described in Chapter 4 apply.

Roof Removal

When victims are trapped inside a truck that has come to rest on its side, one of the fastest and most efficient ways of gaining access is by opening the door that is on the top side of the vehicle. However, this is usually not the best route to use for extricating the victims. This is more often done by removing all or part of the vehicle's roof (Figure 7.36).

Again, as described in Chapter 4, shears or other suitable cutters can be used to cut through those door/roof posts that are accessible, depending upon how the vehicle is laying. If the vehicle is lying on its side, but the door/roof posts are accessible, all of the posts can be cut and the entire roof removed. If the vehicle is lying on the door/roof posts on one side of the vehicle, the other posts can be cut and the roof flapped down to the ground. Or, depending upon the situation and the tools and equipment available, it may be best to use an air chisel to cut around the edge of the roof and remove the sheet metal and any cross members, leaving the door/roof posts and the roof frame intact (Figure 7.37).

Medium and Heavy Truck Extrication Process

Once the truck has been stabilized and access to the cab's interior has been gained, the trapped victims must be disentangled and removed from the vehicle. As mentioned earlier, the techniques and procedures involved in medically stabilizing and properly packaging an injured victim for extrication are beyond the scope of this manual. Therefore, in the extrication techniques that follow, it is assumed that medical stabilization and packaging have been or are being done. As with the other phases of the process, the extrication techniques used will vary depending upon the position of the truck.

Truck Upright

Regardless of where the trapped victims are located within the cab, rescuers must focus their efforts on disentangling the victims — that is, *removing the vehicle from the victims*. And, they must do so in a way that will not aggravate the victims' injuries. This means that the extrication team must closely coordinate their efforts with those who are stabilizing and packaging the victims.

Disentanglement may involve cutting the brake and/or clutch pedals or bending them out of the way to free the driver's feet. It may involve removing the seat backs or the entire seats. Or, it may involve removing or flapping the roof. These operations, too, can be done using the tools and techniques described in Chapter 4.

Once the vehicle has been removed from the victims and they have been properly packaged, the extrication

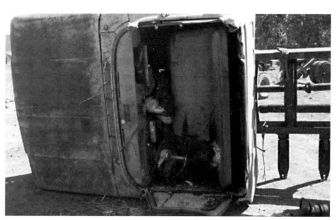
Figure 7.36 It may be necessary to remove the roof.

team should work with the medical team to secure each victim to the appropriate-sized backboard. Then, working together, the team members carefully lift each victim and remove them from the wreckage. Once clear of the wreckage, the victims can be transferred to those responsible for transporting them to a medical facility.

Truck on Its Side

Disentangling and extricating victims from a truck on its side can sometimes be very challenging. However, because the victims may be piled on top of each other at the bottom of the wreckage, the greatest challenge may be for the medical team responsible for stabilizing and packaging the trapped victims. Roof removal is probably the best option for creating a clear opening through which the victims can be extricated — provided that it can be done without compromising the vehicle's stability. Given a well-trained and equipped extrication team, the roof of a truck's cab can be flapped down or removed in less than a minute.

If the truck's stability cannot be maintained if the roof is flapped down or removed, then cutting through the roof and leaving the roof frame intact is the only remaining option. Using an air chisel to cut around the edge of the roof and removing the sheet metal and

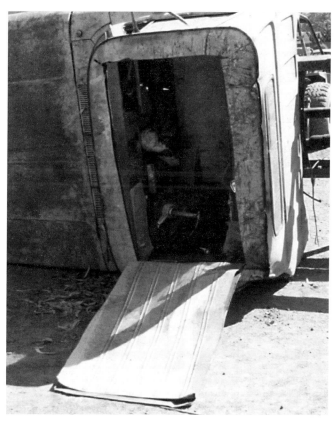
Figure 7.37 Cutting through the roof has little effect on its structural integrity.

any cross members will create a relatively large opening through which victims can be extricated. However, compared to roof removal, cutting through the roof takes considerably longer.

Truck on Its Roof

When a truck has come to rest on its roof, the occupants may be in dire need of extrication — and as quickly as safely possible. The possibility of the vehicle catching fire is greater than when in other positions because of the fuel and other flammable fluids that are almost surely to be leaking from the vehicle. Therefore, time is of the essence.

Depending upon the structural condition of the vehicle, members of the extrication team may be available to assist the medical team in freeing victims and with packaging them for extrication. As in all extrication operations, rescue personnel must work together cooperatively for the good of those in need of their help.

Disentanglement and extrication from a truck on its roof may be complicated by the fact that removing door posts or other components may weaken the cab's structural integrity. This could cause the cab to suddenly and unexpectedly move in some way, perhaps aggravating the victim's injuries. Therefore, rescue personnel must anticipate the consequences of each action before it is taken. If removing a structural component will weaken or destabilize the vehicle, steps must be taken to counteract those effects, or another option must be considered. Otherwise, disentangling and extricating victims from a truck on its roof are no different than from vehicles in the positions already discussed.

Trucks in Other Positions

When a truck has come to rest in a position other than those already discussed, rescue personnel may have to use all of their ingenuity and skill to safely and efficiently disentangle and extricate the victims trapped inside. For example, if the victims are trapped in the cab of a truck that is wedged under a collapsed bridge or other structure, the working room inside the cab may be extremely limited. The space limitation may render the most reliable extrication techniques impractical if not impossible to perform. Members of the medical and extrication teams may have to work in either the prone or supine position inside the cab. They may also have to take turns working inside. However, regardless of how innovative the situation forces rescuers to be, they must never forget that the techniques employed must be safe for them to apply and as safe as possible for the victims. While the goal of extricating all victims without doing further injury still applies, these unusual situations may not allow that to happen. In some extremely rare instances, it may be medically necessary to sacrifice a limb to save a life. Such a decision must be made according to local protocols and through consultation between the IC and a physician at the scene.

Incident Termination

Once all trapped victims have been extricated, the emergency phase of the incident has ended. What is left is still very important, but there is no longer a need for speed nor to put rescue personnel in jeopardy. Rescue personnel may or may not be involved in righting overturned trucks or trailers and other scene restoration activities. In any case, it is important to follow the incident termination procedures described in Chapter 5.

Summary

Extrication incidents involving medium or heavy trucks can be extremely challenging for rescue personnel. Therefore, if they are to function safely and efficiently at these incidents, personnel must be familiar with the nomenclature and anatomy of these sometimes massive vehicles. Regardless of the size of truck involved, rescue personnel must keep in mind that their role is to protect themselves and others from harm, to protect the trapped victims from further harm, and to free those victims as safely and as quickly as possible.

Chapter 8

Railcar Extrication

Of all forms of land-based transportation, passenger trains have the greatest potential for large-scale extrication operations. Large passenger trains may carry hundreds of people at a time. When in motion, the size and weight of a railcar can produce tremendous inertial forces. These forces tend to create an accordion effect in collisions and derailments. The cars often come to rest in a characteristic zigzag pattern with the forward cars stacked upon each other. When you add to this scene the cries for help from trapped and injured passengers and the hysterical screams of horrified onlookers, the emotional control of the first-arriving rescue personnel can be severely tested. An incident involving a loaded passenger train can challenge the resources and abilities of even the most capable emergency response organizations because of the potential for mass casualties and the difficulty involved in accessing the trapped victims.

When assessing the need to be prepared for train incidents, the parameters are clear. Unlike automobiles, trucks, and buses, which can be found in virtually every area, a jurisdiction either has rail lines or it does not. If the jurisdiction has no rail lines, there is no need to be prepared for incidents involving trains, unless responding to rail incidents on mutual aid is anticipated. On the other hand, if passenger trains regularly travel through the district, rescue personnel should be familiar with them and the techniques required for removing people from the railcars should a collision or derailment occur. The importance of thorough pre-incident planning, followed by realistic training exercises, cannot be overemphasized.

While the information in this chapter is based primarily on Amtrak passenger trains, it is applicable to most rail transportation systems and vehicles. The information on locomotives applies to all locomotives regardless of what type of cars make up the consist. The information on passenger cars, all-electric units, and electrical systems also applies to equipment used in local commuter transportation systems. For the most part, this information will also apply to subway systems, although the construction of some subway cars may differ slightly.

Fires and other emergency incidents that occur in railway tunnels, on elevated tracks, or in trams suspended high above the ground are among the most hazardous that rescuers may encounter. Because of these hazardous environments, such incidents are considered to be technical rescue incidents and are beyond the scope of this manual. NFPA 1670, *Standard on Operations and Training for Technical Rescue Incidents* (1999) requires fire and rescue organizations having such exposures within their jurisdictions to make provisions for handling these emergencies. The standard allows agencies to train and equip their own personnel to perform these tasks, to enter into automatic aid agreements with other agencies that are trained and equipped to handle these incidents, or to contract with another public or private entity for these services. Planners can obtain information on tunnel emergencies from *Amtrak Train Emergency Response (1999)* available from the National Railroad Passenger Corporation (Amtrak).

This chapter describes the classification of trains and train anatomy. Also discussed are rails and roadbeds. Size-up of train incidents is discussed along with train car stabilization, height considerations, gaining access, and extrication techniques. Finally, special situations involving trains are discussed.

Train Classifications

In general, trains can be classified into two broad categories — passenger trains and freight trains.

Within each of these classifications, many different types of cars may be used. In passenger trains, there may be baggage cars and various types of passenger cars in addition to the locomotives (engines). In freight trains, there may be any of a variety of cars such as flatcars, boxcars, tank cars, and others.

Passenger Trains

Whether long or short, main line or local, all passenger trains consist of one or more locomotives or self-propelled cars and a number of passenger cars (Figure 8.1). Passenger trains vary from relatively slow-moving local commuter trains (light rail) to high-speed express trains that travel up to 150 mph (240 km/h) (Figure 8.2).

Also in this classification are trams and cable cars (Figure 8.3). These small vehicles are designed to carry a few passengers (rarely more than two dozen) a relatively short distance (usually less than a mile [1.6 km]). The motive power for trams may be all-electric, diesel, or hoist cable.

Freight Trains

Like passenger trains, freight trains are composed of one or more locomotives and a string of cars (Figure 8.4). As mentioned earlier, freight cars include flatcars,

boxcars, hopper cars, tank cars, and a number of other specialized cars. In addition to hauling lumber and similar products, flatcars are also used to carry semitrailers and huge intermodal shipping containers. With the exception of the locomotive, extrication is likely to be needed only if a freight car has come to rest on top of a railroad passenger car or an occupied highway vehicle (Figure 8.5).

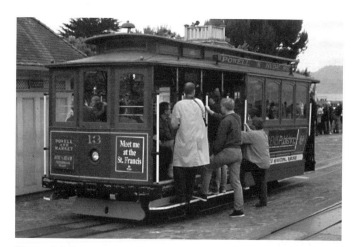
Figure 8.3 Trams and cable cars also carry passengers.

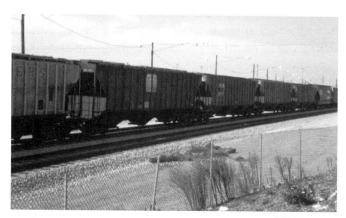
Figure 8.4 Freight train incidents usually involve a small number of victims.

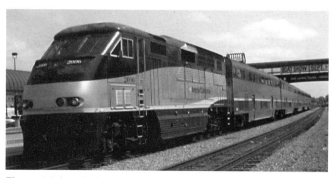
Figure 8.1 A typical Amtrak passenger train.

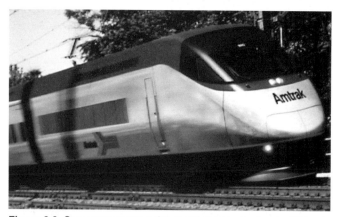
Figure 8.2. Some passenger trains travel at speeds of up to 150 mph (240 km/h).

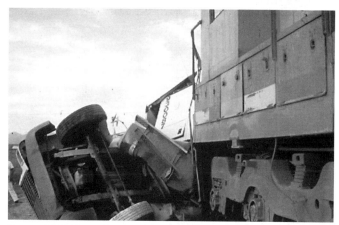
Figure 8.5 Other vehicles add to the number of victims. *Courtesy of Steve Taylor.*

However, the contents of freight cars and shipping containers can greatly complicate any incident in which they are involved. Obviously, a derailed tank car that is leaking a flammable, corrosive, or toxic liquid is a threat to rescue personnel, trapped victims, and the environment. Even if the load is not hazardous in itself, if tons of lumber or thousands of boxes or other containers are strewn about the scene, it can make all phases of the operation much more difficult, dangerous, and time consuming.

Types of Railcars

Amtrak operates a wide variety of railcars. There are several different types of locomotives, passenger coaches, dining cars, and lounge cars as well as specialized cars such as auto carriers. These cars are organized in different fleets that have common characteristics and styling. These fleets are named *Heritage, Superliner* I and II, *Amfleet* I and II, *Viewliner, Horizon, Turboliner,* and *Talgo* (Figure 8.6). Rescue personnel who serve in areas where rail travel is common should familiarize themselves with the various types of railroad equipment common to their area. However, most rescue personnel cannot be expected to know and remember the intricacies and variations of all these various types of cars especially under emergency conditions. Therefore, only general information about railcars and railcar anatomy is presented here.

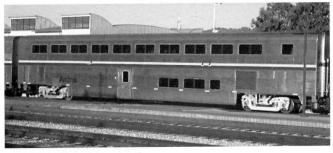

Figure 8.6 Superliner is one of Amtrak's fleets.

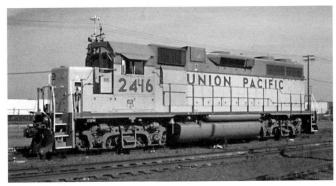

Figure 8.7 Most locomotives are diesel/electric.

On freight trains, the only cars likely to contain a life hazard are their locomotives; therefore, they are the only freight cars to be discussed in the balance of this chapter. Instead, the chapter focuses primarily on railroad passenger cars and those other types of railroad cars that may involve extrication or body recovery.

Locomotives

Locomotives differ in how they are powered and how they are employed. Most of the locomotives in both passenger and freight service in North America are diesel/electric — that is, diesel engines operate onboard generators that power electric motors on each axle to drive the wheels (Figure 8.7). In addition to those used in main line operations, many of these locomotives are used as switching engines in terminals and shop areas. Diesel/electric locomotives can weigh more than 130 tons (118 tonnes), develop as much as 4,250 horsepower, carry up to 2,200 gallons (8 800 L) of diesel fuel, and have a top speed of up to 125 mph (201 km/h). While running, diesel/electric locomotives generate both high- and low-voltage AC and DC electrical current for train operation.

Some locomotives are powered by diesel engines only. Others are dual-mode units — that is, they have diesel engines but can also be powered by electricity from a 600-volt DC third rail.

Intercity commuter trains with all-electric locomotives serve the Keystone Corridor between Philadelphia and Harrisburg, PA, and the Northeast Corridor between Washington, DC and Boston, MA. (Figure 8.8). Most operate with power from a 12,000 volt AC catenary system of wires suspended above the tracks. A roof-mounted pantograph maintains contact with the over-

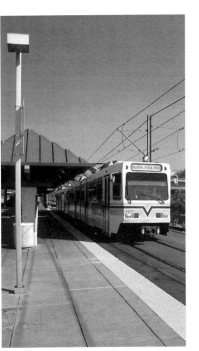

Figure 8.8 Some locomotives are all-electric.

head wires to provide power to the locomotive (Figure 8.9). **NOTE:** Both catenary systems and pantographs are discussed in greater detail later in this chapter. These locomotives weigh as much as 100 tons (91 tonnes), develop as much as 7,000 horsepower, and have a top speed of up to 150 mph (240 km/h).

WARNING!

Do not climb or walk on top of any locomotive or car in a catenary system. Do not attempt to disconnect any jumper cables between the cars and do not touch any electrical equipment. Do not touch the pantograph even if it is not in contact with the overhead wire.

Some Amtrak trains as well as local commuter trains have all-electric locomotives operated by power from an electrically charged third rail between or adjacent to the regular rails (Figure 8.10). As mentioned earlier, this enclosed third rail carries 600 volts DC and must be avoided by all but trained Amtrak personnel.

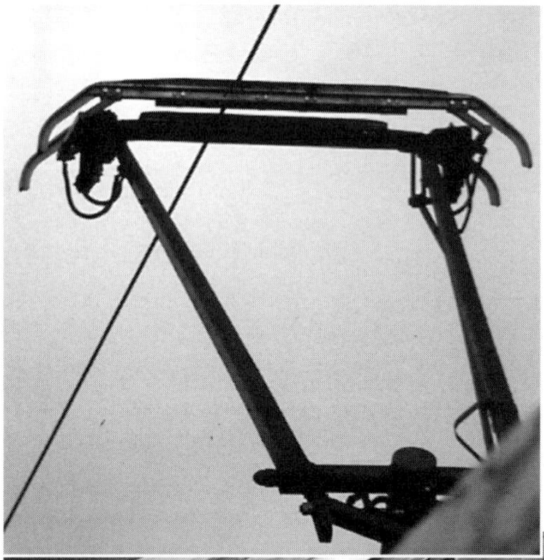

A few steam locomotives are still in service but only as part of local tourist attractions. As mentioned earlier, trams may be all-electric, diesel powered, or cable operated.

Passenger Cars

Amtrak operates a variety of passenger cars, and they are representative of those operated by other rail systems. The construction of railroad passenger coaches is similar to that described in Chapter 6 for commercial buses. The primary difference is that railcars are constructed much more substantially, with heavier material than that used in buses.

Coach and coach dome cars provide passenger seating space. High-level cars provide two levels of coach space for passengers (Figure 8.11). Some coach cars also provide crew sleeping space. Depending on the layout of the cars, they can seat anywhere from 44 to 85 passengers. Both passengers and crew members may be present during train operation. The 85-passenger coaches have seating facilities for passengers with disabilities. These cars are usually the last in the consist, and some contain secondary controls that allow the train to be operated in reverse from the last car without turning the train around.

Sleeper cars provide passengers with seating room and sleeping accommodations (Figure 8.12). Some sleepers also provide daytime private rooms for first-

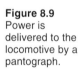

Figure 8.9 Power is delivered to the locomotive by a pantograph.

Figure 8.11 Some passenger cars are double-deckers.

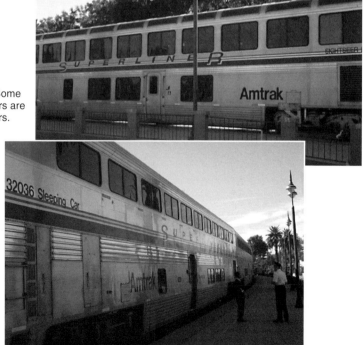

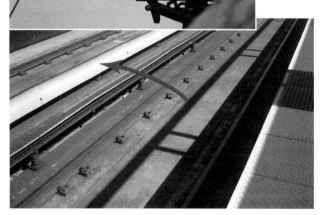

Figure 8.10 Power is delivered to some trains by a third rail.

Figure 8.12 A typical Superliner sleeper car.

class passengers. These cars are normally located either toward the front or rear of the consist. Passengers and crew members may be present in these areas during train operation. All sleeping/bedroom, seating, and toilet areas should be checked for victims during size-up and search and rescue.

Lounge/Food Service Cars

Also known as club cars, *lounge/food service cars* provide food/beverage service and entertainment to passengers aboard Amtrak trains (Figure 8.13). Some dining cars include an upper level dining area for passengers as well as a food preparation area in the lower level of the same car. Some variant configurations also provide limited passenger coach space. Full-dome lounge cars provide food and beverage service for passengers and crew members, as well as a panoramic view. These cars are normally located in the center of the consist. Passengers and crew members may be present in these areas during train operation. All dining, bar, and food storage areas should be checked for passengers and crew members during size-up and search and rescue.

Baggage Cars

With the exceptions of commuter trains and trams, all passenger trains will have one or more baggage cars in the consist. The purpose of the baggage car is to transport passenger baggage. Some coach/baggage cars provide upper level coach space for passengers and space on a lower level for transporting baggage. These cars are normally located directly behind the locomotive at the front of the consist. An assistant conductor may be present in the car during train operation. Therefore, it is essential that all areas of the car, including the toilet room, be checked for crew members during size-up and search and rescue.

Material Handling Cars

These are essentially standard boxcars used for carrying baggage and mail. They are usually located directly behind the locomotive or at the end of the consist. In addition to having side doors only, these cars have plug doors that must be pulled outward before sliding laterally. However, material handling cars are usually unoccupied during train operation.

Railcar Anatomy

Regardless of what type of railroad passenger cars are involved in an incident, they all have certain features and characteristics in common. Of most interest to rescue personnel are those features that either help or hinder them in an extrication operation. The most common features are discussed in the following sections.

Electrical Hazards

All Amtrak cars are equipped with 480-volt electrical circuits charged by power from the locomotive, commonly called head-end power. The power may be supplied to the locomotive by an overhead catenary system or a third rail (both discussed later in this chapter) or from diesel generators aboard the locomotive. Power is s upplied to the individual cars by jumper cables connected between each car (Figure 8.14). Rescue personnel should not remove or attempt to remove these cables. Only trained Amtrak crew members can safely de-energize head-end power, lower locomotive pantographs, disengage third-rail shoes, ground electrical equipment when required, or remove or install power cables.

> ### WARNING!
> All Amtrak cars are equipped with 480-volt electrical circuits. Do not attempt to cut through or remove any electrical cables. Do not touch any electrical equipment. Failure to heed this warning may result in electrocution.

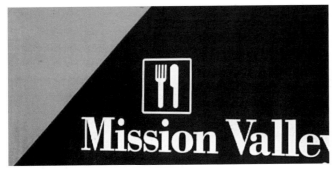

Figure 8.13 Club cars are clearly marked.

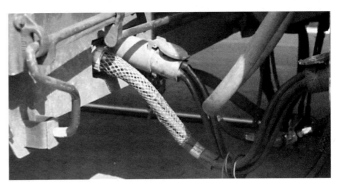

Figure 8.14 Jumper cables connect each car.

Windows

Railroad passenger cars have windows along the full length of both sides of the car, some have an upper and lower row, and they may be any of several different styles. Two different window pane materials are used: Lexan® plastic and tempered glass. The type of pane used will vary on different types of cars.

All Amtrak passenger coaches are equipped with emergency window exits (Figure 8.15). Each car will have at least four of these window exits — two on each side — and some have more. These windows have double panes — the outer pane is either Lexan or tempered glass, but the inner pane is always Lexan.

Doors

All passenger cars have end doors (Figure 8.16). These doors either swing inward or slide sideways to open. Most sliding doors are power assisted — either electrically or electro-pneumatically. In case of power failure, they easily slide open manually. Car end doors are not locked during train operation and function normally while the train is in motion.

Some passenger cars also have side-entry doors located at both ends of each car (Figure 8.17). These are pocket doors that slide sideways into the car body to open (Figure 8.18). Other passenger cars have inward-swinging side-entry doors located in the center of the car. These doors are closed and automatically locked during train operation. Therefore, rescuers may have to force entry through these doors following a collision and/or derailment.

Walls/Roofs

Most Amtrak cars have exterior skins made of 3/32-inch (2.5 mm) stainless steel. Other cars have an aluminum skin (Figure 8.19). In many cases, the wall construction consists of steel framing members and plywood sandwiched between two sheets of stainless steel or aluminum. Heavy-duty framing members are placed 12 to 24 inches (300 mm to 600 mm) on center in the walls, floors, and roof structure.

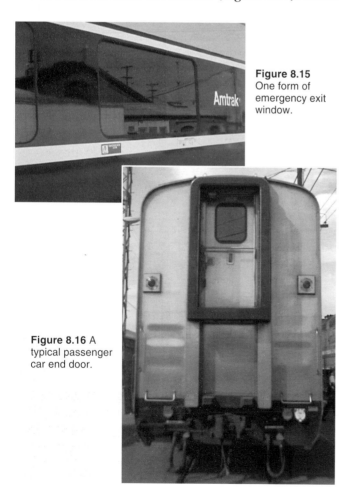

Figure 8.15 One form of emergency exit window.

Figure 8.16 A typical passenger car end door.

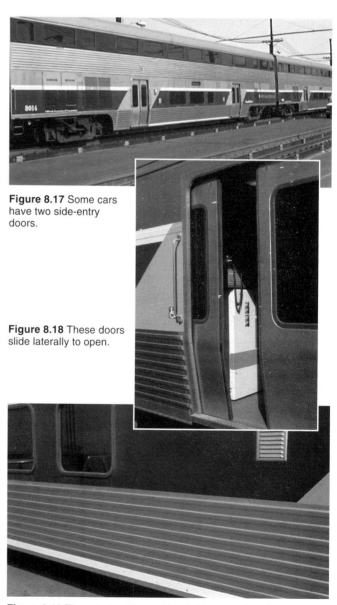

Figure 8.17 Some cars have two side-entry doors.

Figure 8.18 These doors slide laterally to open.

Figure 8.19 The exterior skin may be stainless steel or aluminum.

Brakes

Firefighters and other rescue personnel need to be familiar with the operation of the hand brakes on freight cars. On level tracks, applying the hand brake may be all that is needed to stabilize a car (Figure 8.20).

Rails/Roadbeds

Most trains run on standard-gauge twin-rail beds. Some trams and tourist trains operate on narrow-gauge rail beds. However, from an extrication standpoint, the width of the rail bed is far less important than the electrical hazards associated with some systems. Some Amtrak locomotives and many local commuter trains obtain their motive power from wires suspended above the tracks (catenary systems), while other commuter trains and trams obtain motive power from an energized third rail between or adjacent to the regular rails.

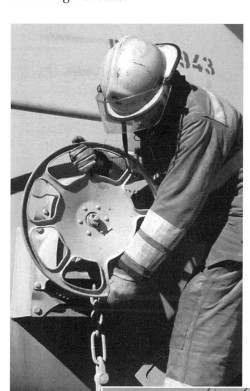

Figure 8.20 The hand brake may stabilize a car on level track.

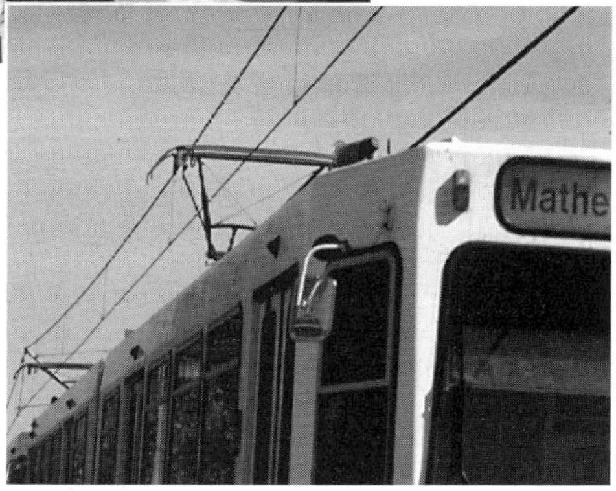

Figure 8.21 The pantograph is supplied with 12,000 volts of electricity.

Catenary Systems

The overhead catenary system consists of longitudinal wires and cables suspended from poles that hold an electrically charged trolley wire in a firm position above the track. The pantograph mounted on top of the locomotive maintains contact with the trolley wires to conduct 12,000 volts, 25 Hz, to the locomotive motors (Figure 8.21).

Catenary poles are 14-inch (350 mm) square steel H-sections weighing 84 pounds per foot (125 kg/m). They range in height from 70 to 170 feet (21 m to 52 m). At the top of each pole is a ground wire located approximately 9 feet (3 m) above the transmission conductors. The ground wire is a return for the propulsion current and protects the transmission line from lightning strikes. Approximately 3 feet (1 m) down from the ground wire are the transmission cross arms, 18 feet (6 m) across, held level by sag rods. Below these cross arms are two transmission lines energized at 138,000 volts (Figure 8.22).

On one side of the pole is a signal power line energized at 6,900 volts, 100 Hz. The signal line is a transmission line between substations to locations along the right-of-way. There, it is transformed into various voltages to feed signals, track circuits, and other equipment.

The trolley wires above the tracks are supported between the body span by three units of 10-inch (250 mm) disk-type insulators. Immediately below the insulators is a longitudinal messenger wire. Below this is an auxiliary messenger wire supported by bronze hanger rods. Below the auxiliary wire is the contact or trolley wire, supported from the auxiliary messenger by clips spaced 15 feet (5 m) apart. All wires and hardware of the catenary system are energized at 12,000 volts.

Under no circumstances should any object be allowed to contact these wires. Materials such as wood, rope, clothing, etc., that might be considered nonconductive at low voltages are not safe for use in close proximity to high-voltage wires.

WARNING!

Due to the high voltage carried by this system, no one should approach or permit any metallic object within 8 feet (2.7 m) of the 138,000-volt transmission lines or within 3 feet (1 m) of the 12,000-volt catenary system or 6,900-volt signal power lines.

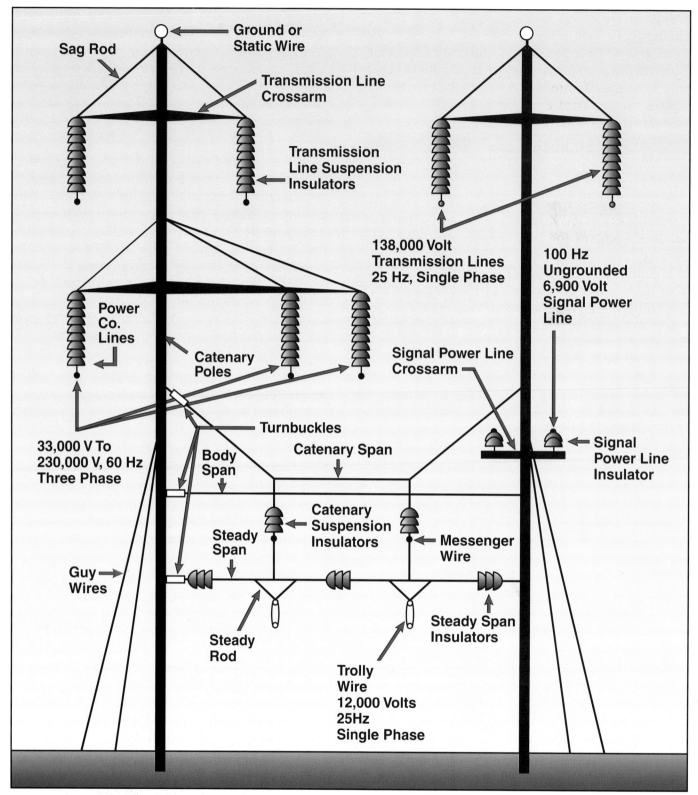

Figure 8.22 A typical catenary system.

Substations on the system are spaced 8 to 10 miles (13 km to 18 km) apart. These substations contain power control apparatus for the 12,000 volt, 25 Hz, catenary system; the 6,900 volt, 100 Hz, signal power line; and the 138,000 volt, 25 Hz, transmission line.

Firefighters and other rescue personnel should not enter these facilities unless accompanied by qualified Amtrak employees.

If there is no obvious electrical hazard following a collision and/or derailment on a catenary line, the overhead power should *not* be disconnected. Electrical power will provide for lighting and electric door operation. When an electrical hazard does exist, the overhead power supply can be disconnected by pressing the "Pantograph Down" button in the locomotive control cab and then grounding the locomotive. This is usually done by Amtrak crew members before emergency responders arrive. If it has not been done, rescuers should see that it is done by properly qualified personnel.

WARNING!
The pantograph on top of each car conducts electrical power from the overhead wires to the car. Do not touch this device even if it is not connected to the power supply.

Third-rail Systems
Third-rail electrical-power distribution systems generally distribute 600-volt DC current. The third rail is usually located slightly above and to the side of the two regular rails on which the train's wheels run (See Figure 8.10). No one should be allowed to touch a third rail or its protective cover. Third-rail power may be de-energized by contacting the appropriate power director/dispatcher or by using emergency switch boxes where installed along the right-of-way. Only personnel from those agencies having direct authority from Amtrak or the local train authority should use these emergency switch boxes.

Roadbeds
Although some percentage of all roadbeds are at grade level, especially in switching yards and loading/unloading areas, much of their length is not. The rails

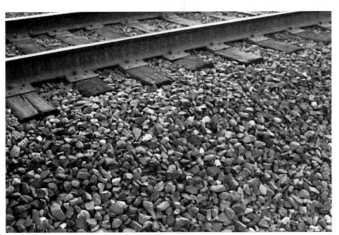
Figure 8.23 Roadbeds are covered with gravel.

and cross ties are set atop a berm that allows the roadbed to be more-or-less level throughout its length. To discourage the growth of vegetation along the roadbed, and thereby reduce the risk of fires, the spaces between the cross ties and down both sides of the berm are covered with coarse gravel (Figure 8.23).

The steeply sloped sides of the roadbed embankment and the loose gravel make traction and footing difficult. Therefore, gaining access and stabilizing the crashed vehicles may be far more difficult than would be the case in other locations. The slope of the embankment and the lack of traction may make it difficult to position rescue vehicles close to the scene. It may be necessary to lay ground ladders on the slopes of the berm to provide secure footing for rescue personnel.

Train Incident Size-Up
As with any other type of extrication incident, those involving trains should be assessed (sized up) in a systematic way. First, the scene is assessed, followed by an assessment of the vehicles involved. Then, the victims are assessed as are the extrication requirements for that particular incident. As always, size-up continues throughout the incident.

Scene Assessment
As discussed in earlier chapters, assessing the scene of a train derailment starts before the first rescue unit arrives. The officer in charge considers the day, date, time, and weather — and how these variables may affect the incident at hand. Approaching the scene, the officer must attempt to get the "big picture" by ascertaining how many and what types of vehicles are involved. Are there collateral hazards such as downed power lines, leaking fuel, or other hazardous materials? Are there incipient fires? Even though Amtrak passenger trains do not carry hazardous materials, some of their locomotives carry considerable quantities of diesel fuel in their tanks — certainly enough fuel to create a large and lethal fire.

The officer must decide what resources are likely to be needed to deal with the obvious problems at hand. In addition to notifying the involved railroad and requesting their emergency response crews, the officer must decide whether the extrication resources already en route are sufficient to handle this situation — or whether more need to be requested. Will additional ambulances or medevac helicopters be needed? Are utility crews needed to handle downed power lines or broken gas mains? Are additional law enforcement personnel needed to control crowds and/or highway traffic at the scene? Is there a need for lighting units to illuminate the scene? Especially with passenger trains where there is a high probability of large numbers of casualties trapped inside the cars, the threat of fire may indicate a need for additional fire apparatus with large-scale foam-making capability. If any additional resources need to be called, they should be requested *immediately*.

Vehicle Assessment

Once on scene, the first-in officer must determine if a legitimate emergency exists. If so, he should assume command of the incident and begin a more thorough assessment of the vehicles involved. As with other types of extrication incidents, the incident commander (IC) must try to determine how many vehicles are involved and their conditions. In the derailment of a long passenger train, this can be a daunting task. With railcars resting at various angles and in various positions along both sides of the track, it can be very difficult to see the entire scene from one location (Figure 8.24). How the cars came to rest — upright, on their sides, upside down — will dictate how much and what types of shoring and cribbing materials will be needed.

As mentioned earlier in this chapter, diesel/electric locomotives can carry up to 2,200 gallons (8 800 L) of diesel fuel in tanks located on the underside of the locomotive. Fuel shutoff devices (clearly marked FUEL SHUT OFF) are located on each side of the locomotive body side rails and also on the firewall of the cab (Figure 8.25). To shut off the fuel supply to the engine,

push and hold the emergency fuel shutoff device for 8 to 10 seconds. The engine will stop running within about one minute.

Victim Assessment

In situations where there is a high likelihood of mass casualties, one of the highest operational priorities is setting up for triage, treatment, and transportation. Prior to the train cars being stabilized, any passengers who have escaped the wreckage should be questioned about the location and condition of others still trapped inside (Figure 8.26). After the cars are stabilized, rescue personnel should be assigned to quickly but thoroughly search all cars and triage the passengers trapped inside. The number and condition of the victims may indicate a need for additional ambulances or medevac helicopters.

Extrication Assessment

Based on the specifics of the crash — the number of cars involved and their conditions and the number of trapped victims and their conditions — a determination must be made regarding how much and what types of extrication resources will be needed. Are there a sufficient number of power spreaders, cutters, and similar equipment available on scene, or do more need to be requested? Is there a need for oxyacetylene cutting torches, plasma cutters, or burning bars? Is there a need for additional personnel to allow more tasks to be performed at the same time or for crew relief if the incident becomes protracted? If the incident becomes protracted, will a full Rehab Unit be needed?

Railcar Stabilization

Because of the size and weight of most railroad cars, they are generally very stable. However, following a

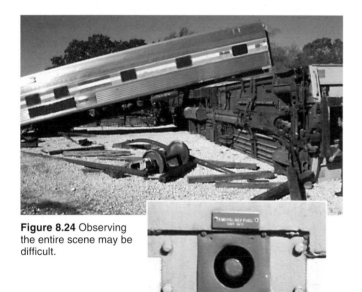

Figure 8.24 Observing the entire scene may be difficult.

Figure 8.25 A typical fuel shutoff device.

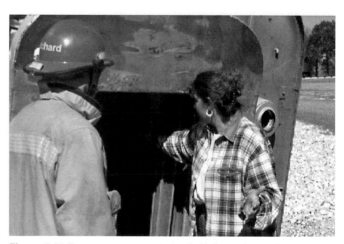

Figure 8.26 Passengers may supply vital information.

collision and/or derailment, some of the cars may have come to rest in unstable positions. They may need to be stabilized to protect trapped and injured victims and to provide a safe working environment for rescue personnel. Considering that much of the equipment used to stabilize highway vehicles will be of limited value when trying to stabilize these massive vehicles, determining how to stabilize railcars can be a tremendous challenge. Simply deciding where to start can be difficult. However, the survival of both the trapped victims and rescue personnel depend upon this critical step being performed quickly and effectively. If railroad ties are available at the scene, they can be used as cribbing for stabilization (Figure 8.27).

Railcar Upright

Because the majority of the weight of most railcars is concentrated in the lower third of their structure, railcars that are upright and still on the tracks are relatively stable. If a car is still upright but off the tracks and subject to sliding or rolling down the side of the roadbed embankment, then extensive stabilization may be required.

WARNING!

It is unlikely that pneumatic lifting bags and cribbing will stabilize a locomotive weighing in excess of 265,000 pounds (120 310 kg) or a passenger car weighing in excess of 100,000 pounds (45 400 kg).

Railcar on Its Side

Unless affected by slope or similar environmental influences, a railcar on its side is very stable. The shape, size, and weight of most railcars make it unlikely that they will move suddenly or unexpectedly when resting on their sides on a stable and level surface.

However, if the car is resting on mud, snow, or unstable soil, rescue personnel must be extremely cautious. Under these conditions, the biggest danger is that the car will suddenly roll back upright without warning. To reduce this possibility, the car should be stabilized with shoring from the underside (Figure 8.28).

Railcar on Its Roof

Because a railcar is top heavy when resting on its roof, this position can be very unstable. Unless its movement is limited by an adjacent embankment and/or leaning against other railcars, a car on its roof may suddenly roll to one side or the other. The car should be secured with webbing, etc., before personnel are allowed close enough to install shoring along both sides.

Railcars in Other Positions

As mentioned earlier in this chapter, the inertial forces involved in many train derailments leave railcars accordioned into a characteristic zigzag pattern, with the forward cars stacked upon each other (Figure 8.29). Stabilizing several cars at the same time can be very difficult. Only the specific situation can dictate which car should be stabilized first and how stabilization should be accomplished. As mentioned earlier, cars may need to be stabilized to prevent them from sliding or rolling down a steep embankment or into a body of water. Cars that have overridden other

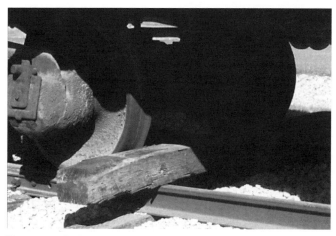

Figure 8.27 Railroad ties make good cribbing.

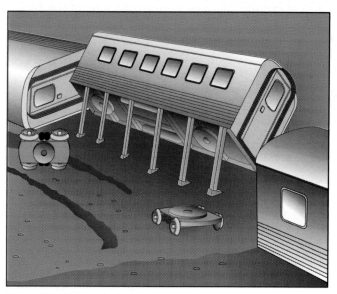

Figure 8.28 Heavy shoring may be needed.

cars may need to be stabilized to prevent them from sliding or falling off the cars beneath them. Unlike highway vehicle extrication incidents, the time that would be needed to install a sufficient amount of rigging and heavy shoring to stabilize these railcars may eliminate this as an option. Instead, if heavy construction vehicles are available, they can be used to temporarily stabilize the railcars by placing their bucket, blade, etc., against the sides of the cars (Figure 8.30).

Gaining Access into Railcars

Once the railcars have been stabilized, rescue personnel can enter the cars for search and rescue. Whenever possible, the best way to enter wrecked railcars is through the doors and windows. The following sections describe these entry points in some detail. If entry through the doors and windows is not possible, rescue personnel may have to force entry through the roof or walls of these vehicles — but this should be attempted only as a last resort. In addition, the height of the roadbed and the individual cars above grade may make it necessary for rescue personnel to use ladders and other means to reach the most desirable access points.

Height Considerations

As discussed earlier, the height of the roadbed above grade, the steepness of the sides of the berm, and the poor footing afforded by the loose gravel covering the berm, may force rescue personnel to lay ground ladders on the sides of the berm just to be able to reach the roadbed. Where a paved road parallels the railroad, it may be possible to position an aerial device on the roadway to allow the use of the main ladder or articulating boom to reach the roadbed. Once on the roadbed, rescuers may need ladders to reach the doors and windows of the railcars (Figure 8.31).

Even when the roadbed is at grade, the height of the railcar doors and windows may make it necessary for rescue personnel to use their ingenuity to create stable working platforms for extrication operations. If immediately available, conventional aluminum scaffolding can be set up beside a railcar and moved along from car to car as needed. Wooden planks between two stepladders can be used as a makeshift scaffold. A flatbed truck or a fire engine positioned beside a railcar can provide a relatively large, stable platform from which to work, and it can be moved from car to car as needed (Figure 8.32). If railcars are stacked one upon the other, ground ladders and/or

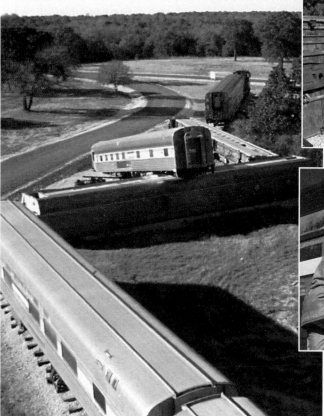

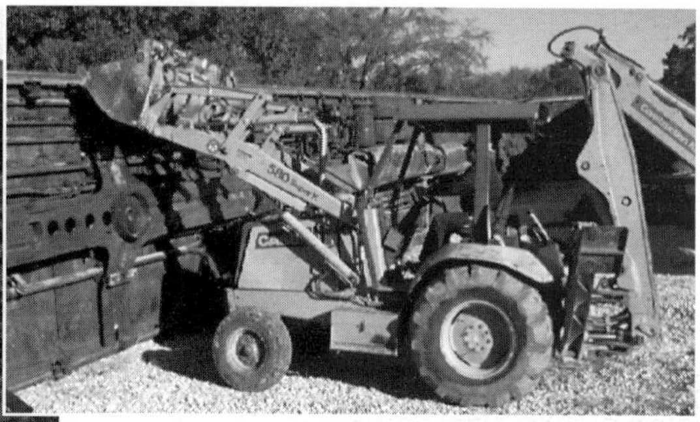

Figure 8.30 Construction vehicles may provide temporary stabilization.

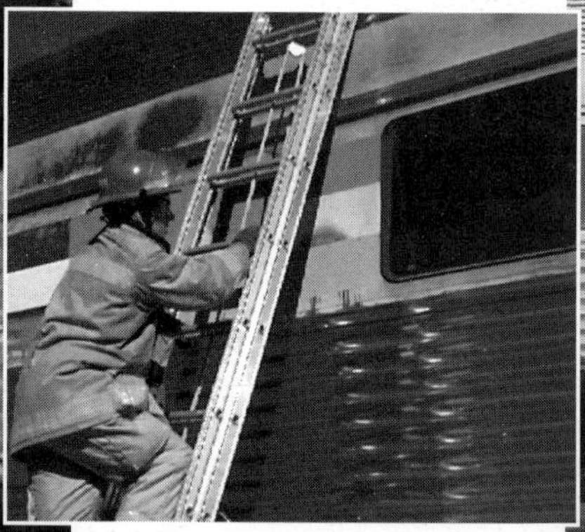

Figure 8.31 Ladders may be needed to reach the windows.

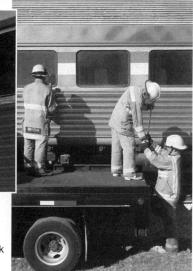

Figure 8.32 The bed of a truck makes a good elevated work platform.

Figure 8.29 A typical derailment scene.

aerial devices may be needed to reach the necessary access points.

Locomotive Entry

Most locomotive cabs can be entered through either of two doors on each side or on some models, through an additional door in the nose. Almost all locomotive cab doors open by turning the door latch and pushing inward. These doors are not locked during train operation, so rescue personnel should not need to force entry following a collision and/or derailment.

If entry is not possible through the doors, the windshield and side windows are the next best access. Some locomotive windshields are single-pane, laminated safety glass; others are Lexan. Side door and sliding cab windows are single panes of either Lexan or tempered glass that slide sideways to open and are not usually locked. If access is not possible through the side windows, remove the windshield protector, if the unit has one, and then remove the windshield.

Passenger Car Door Entry

As mentioned earlier, all railroad passenger cars have end doors, and some have side-entry vestibule doors. These doors are the first points where rescue personnel should attempt entry into these cars.

Passenger Coach End Doors

Passenger coach end doors normally remain unlocked during train operation and are likely to be unlocked following a collision or derailment. If not, the majority have latches that are manually operated. Some end doors are power assisted and have push plates or bars marked "PUSH TO OPEN" or "PRESS" (Figure 8.33) These push plates activate an electric or electro-pneumatic power assist opening device. If this device is not operable, the door can be opened manually by either pushing it inward or sliding it sideways. Power-assisted end doors have power cut-out switches on both sides of the door permitting door operation during malfunctions and emergencies. Lockable end door latches may be unlocked with a standard Amtrak coach key obtainable from a crew member.

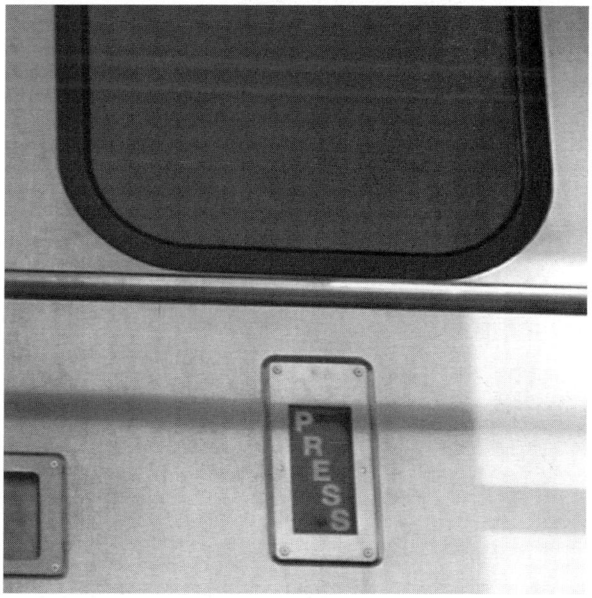

Passenger Car Side-Entry Doors

Some passenger coaches, sleepers, and lounge/food service cars also have side-entry vestibule doors. Some of these doors are manually operated and pneumatically locked. These doors are automatically locked by an inflatable weatherseal that releases automatically when the door handle is pulled, opening the latch. If the seals do not deflate, open the ceiling panel directly above the door on the public address system locker side, and open the door seal cut-out cock. This allows both doors in that vestibule to be opened manually.

Other side-entry doors are electrically actuated and locked. They can be opened by obtaining a standard Amtrak coach key from a crew member (Figure 8.34). If electrical power is still on to the door circuits, the door will slide open. If the power is off, open the door manually by grasping the outside door indentation and pushing it sideways. These doors may be opened from the inside by pulling down on the door lock handle located in a ceiling recess above the door (Figure 8.35). The door can then be opened manually by sliding it sideways.

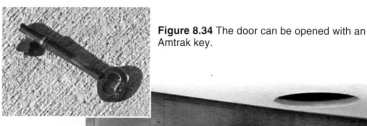

Figure 8.34 The door can be opened with an Amtrak key.

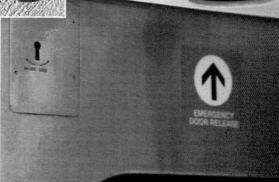

Figure 8.35
From the inside, the door lock handle is accessible.

Figure 8.33 Typical of some end doors.

Some side-entry doors may be opened from outside the car by opening the door seal cut-out cock located under the car adjacent to the door. Preferably, a trained Amtrak crew member should perform this function to ensure that nearby air brake lines remain operative.

While many side-entry vestibule doors slide sideways to open, the side-entry doors on some other cars swing inward to open. These doors are closed and latched during train operation. When unlatched, the door can be opened manually. If the door is jammed, open the door window using the latch handle in the frame.

Interior Door Locks/Latches

Once inside a rail passenger car, rescue personnel will find a variety of locking and latching mechanisms on interior doors. Most are similar to those found in industrial settings and their operation is obvious from their construction. Mechanical locks may require a standard Amtrak coach key obtainable from a train crew member. This section covers only those locks and latches unique to trains or those whose functions may not be immediately apparent.

Toilet Door Latches. The toilet room latch is similar on most models of cars. When the "Occupied" display is showing, assume that someone is inside (Figure 8.36). Insert a screwdriver or similar object into the oval opening in the slide bolt and move the bolt to the left. The door will unlock and open inward. The toilet doors on other models may be unlocked using standard Amtrak coach keys.

Sleeping Car Bedroom Door Latches. Some sleeping car bedroom doors can be opened by removing the two Phillips head cover plate screws. This will expose the keyway. The lock may now be opened using a standard coach key.

Sleeping Car Intercommunicating Door Latches. These doors can be unlocked in one of three ways: Slide bar #1 is opened by using the standard Amtrak

coach key; slide bar #2 is opened by the slide mechanism on one side of the bedroom divider; or slide bar #3 is opened by the slide mechanism on the other side of the bedroom divider (Figure 8.37).

Sleeping Car Room Door Latches. All sleeping car rooms are designed to be locked from the inside. To open locked doors from the outside, remove the two slotted screws on the outside door handle. The pin inside the door is attached to the outside cover plate. When the plate is removed, the latch drops allowing the door to slide open.

Passenger Car Window Entry

As discussed earlier in this chapter, railcar window openings are covered with either tempered glass or Lexan, or both. Since tempered glass is designed to fracture into many small pieces when broken, rescuers and victims may suffer minor scratches and small cuts from contact with these small pieces of glass. Tempered glass is easily broken by striking a bottom corner of the pane with a pointed object, such as the pick end of an axe. Smaller panes can be broken by pressing a spring-loaded center punch into the bottom corner of the window pane.

Lexan is a polycarbonate plastic 250 times stronger than glass and 30 times stronger than Plexiglas®. It will not break when struck with a forcible entry tool. In fact, the tool will bounce off the Lexan, and that could injure the rescuer or others nearby. The only successful methods of dealing with Lexan are to remove the entire pane or to cut through it with a power saw.

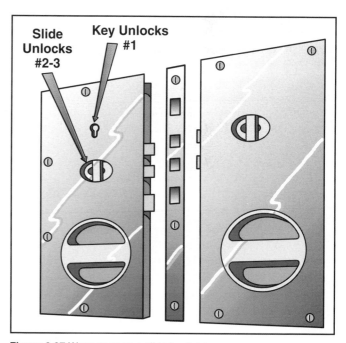

Figure 8.37 Ways to open a slide bar latch.

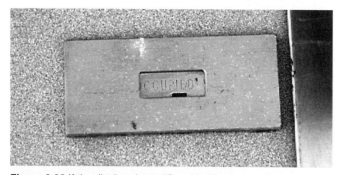

Figure 8.36 If the display shows "Occupied," expect to find someone inside.

The following sections describe the procedures for removing both types of window panes and for opening emergency exit windows from both outside and inside of passenger cars.

Removing Tempered Glass Windows

These window panes are removable from the outside by using the following procedure:

Step 1: Use a small screwdriver or key to pry the zipper strip from the center of the rubber seal surrounding the window unit (Figure 8.38). This zipper strip may be a different color from the seal itself.

Step 2: Pull the rubber strip from around the window (Figure 8.39).

Step 3: Insert a large screwdriver or small pry bar under the corner of the window between the window seal and the car body. Pry down, pulling the window out (Figure 8.40).

Step 4: Continue pushing down on the prying tool, pulling the window outward from the lower edge (Figure 8.41). The window will fall free outside the car.

Removing Lexan Windows

These window panes are removable from the outside by using the following procedure:

Step 1: Grasp the split end of the window rubber molding and pull straight out until all the molding is completely removed (Figure 8.42).

Step 2: Insert a pry bar between the Lexan pane and the window frame at the pry point, and pry out the frame (Figure 8.43). The Lexan pane will fall inside of the car.

Step 3: If prying is not successful, cut out the pane with a power saw, but be prepared for the Lexan to melt onto the saw blade (Figure 8.44).

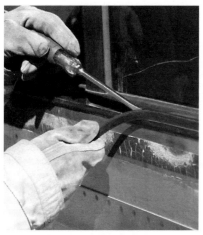

Figure 8.38 Pry out the zipper strip with a screwdriver.

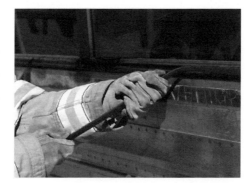

Figure 8.39 Pull the strip from the window seal.

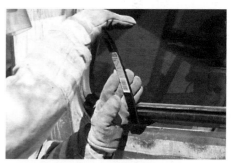

Figure 8.40 Pry the window pane out.

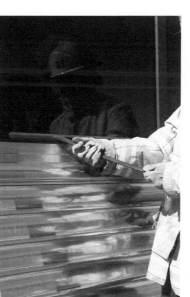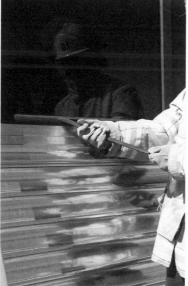

Figure 8.41 Remove the window from the outside.

Figure 8.42 Remove the window molding.

Figure 8.44 If prying fails, cut the window with a power saw.

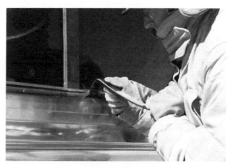

Figure 8.43 Pry out the window frame.

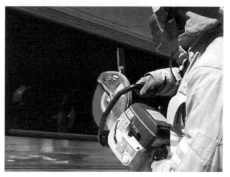

Removing Emergency Exit Windows (Outside)

Emergency exit windows can be removed from the outside of the car. The emergency windows can be identified by a plate with the removal instructions located next to each emergency exit window. These plates are also located at the ends of each car. The following procedure should be used to remove these windows from outside the car:

Step 1: Use a small screwdriver or key to pry the zipper strip from the center of the rubber seal surrounding the window unit (Figure 8.45). This zipper strip may be a different color from the seal itself.

Step 2: Pull the rubber strip from around the window (Figure 8.46).

Step 3: Insert a large screwdriver or small pry bar under the corner of the window between the window seal and the car body. Lift upward and inward (Figure 8.47).

Step 4: Warn passengers inside to stand clear. Push the lower edge of the window firmly to break it loose from the car body (Figure 8.48). Continue to pry until the window falls free to the inside of the car. Cover any sharp edges before making entry.

Removing Emergency Exit Windows (Inside)

Emergency exit windows can also be removed from inside the car. To remove these windows from inside the car, use the following procedure:

Step 1: Pull the red emergency handle in, and remove the rubber molding (Figure 8.49).

Step 2: Use the newly-exposed metal handle attached to the pane to pull the window toward the inside of the car (Figure 8.50). Only one-half of the window is designed to be removed.

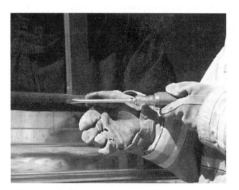

Figure 8.45 Pry out the zipper strip.

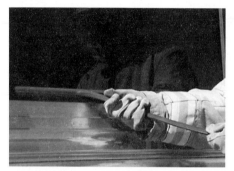

Figure 8.46 Pull the zipper strip from the window seal.

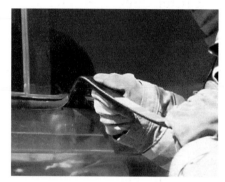

Figure 8.47 Pry the window inward with a screwdriver or pry bar.

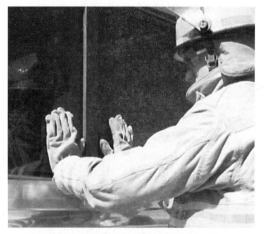

Figure 8.48 Push the lower part of the window inward.

Figure 8.49 Pull the handle and remove the molding.

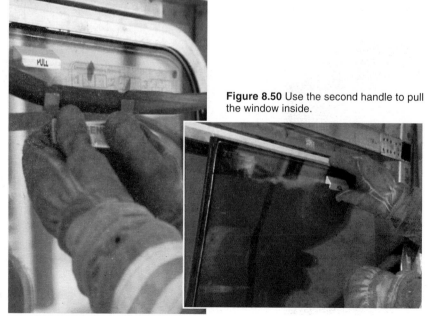

Figure 8.50 Use the second handle to pull the window inside.

Passenger Car Roof/Wall Entry

As described earlier in the section on railcar anatomy, the construction of railroad passenger cars is similar to but much heavier than that used in the construction of buses. The exterior walls are generally reinforced stainless steel designed to resist impact forces. This type of construction resists forcible entry, and it should be attempted only if other means of access are unavailable. Breaching the walls of a railroad passenger car will almost certainly require the use of oxyacetylene cutting torches and/or other exothermic cutting devices.

Unlike buses and heavy trucks, the roof of a railroad passenger car is made of the same gauge material as the walls. Therefore, forcible entry through this area is unlikely to produce positive results.

Lounge/Food Service Car Entry

Entry into lounge cars should be attempted through their side-entry vestibule doors, and if that is not successful, through the end doors. Diner and buffet cars do not have side-entry doors, so the end doors should be used. The kitchen and bar loading doors are locked during train operation, so entry should be made through other doors or windows. If door entry is unsuccessful, entry should be made through the emergency exit windows.

Baggage Car Entry

Entry into baggage cars can be made through the sliding side doors or through the end doors. The side doors are usually locked during train operation. They feature a slide-type lock a few inches above the floor of the car (Figure 8.51). The end doors will usually not be locked if a crew member is inside the car. If entry

through the end doors is not possible and the side doors are locked, the quickest method of entry is through the windows in the side doors. The door window panes consist of a single pane of Lexan that can be removed using the procedure described earlier.

Material Handling Car Entry

Material handling cars have plug doors that must extend clear of the door opening before sliding sideways. The door automatically extends outward when the lever handle or wheel is operated (Figure 8.52). These doors are normally closed and locked during train operation, so forcible entry will be required following a collision and/or derailment. If it is necessary to enter one of these cars, the best way to do so is through the side doors. If the doors are jammed, they will have to be forcibly opened using a rescue saw or power-spreading equipment.

Railcar Extrication Techniques

Because of the relative ease of access and egress, using a railcar's doors is better than using the windows for extricating victims. Even if a railcar is on its side or on its roof, the door openings will still allow the easiest passage into and out of the car. Of course, if all doorways are blocked, then victims will have to be removed through the windows. In the most extreme cases, they can be removed through openings cut in the walls or roof of the car.

Disentanglement/Tunneling

Even though railroad cars are substantially built, the tremendous inertial forces involved in many train wrecks can cause significant damage to the cars. These forces can rearrange the cars' interior configurations

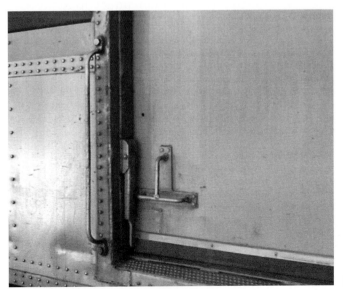

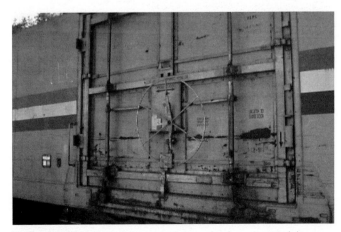

Figure 8.52 One type of door opening mechanism on material handling cars.

Figure 8.51 A baggage car door lock.

and thereby entrap passengers and crew members. The heavy gauge material of which these vehicles are constructed makes the entrapment that much more complete. The same problems involved in disentangling victims trapped in buses are involved in freeing those in railcars, but made more difficult by the heavy construction.

Because of the mass of railroad passenger cars, when they are stacked one upon the other, it may be necessary for rescue personnel to tunnel through the wreckage in much the same way that rescuers tunnel through rubble and debris following structural collapse. And, many of the same tunneling techniques can be used. Before rescue personnel are allowed to work beneath heavy overhanging objects — heavily damaged railcars or parts thereof — these objects must be supported with appropriate shoring. Box cribbing may be sufficient in some cases, but heavy timber shoring or hydraulic/pneumatic shoring is more likely to be needed.

Window Egress
If the doorways are unavailable, properly packaged passengers and crew members can be removed through the cars' side windows (Figure 8.53). While most passenger coaches have relatively small side windows measuring 29½ inches wide by 16½ inches high (737 mm by 412 mm), the Talgo coaches have larger side windows that measure 5 feet 3 inches wide by 39 inches high (1.6 m by 1 m). With the glass

completely removed, these windows offer adequate clearance for most backboards and litters. Because the cab doors on most locomotives are too narrow to accommodate many standard litters, the best option for extricating injured crew members may be to remove the locomotive windshield or side windows and pass them out through the opening. The techniques for removing passenger car windows and locomotive windows and windshields were described in the section on gaining access.

Special Situations
As mentioned earlier, extrication incidents that occur in tunnels, on elevated railways, on railroad bridges, and in similar high-hazard environments are considered to be technical rescue problems that are beyond the scope of this manual. However, there are still numerous special situations with which firefighters and other first responders must be prepared to deal. Some of them are incidents that occur at passenger loading platforms, those involving a train and a highway vehicle, and those involving a train and a pedestrian.

Loading Platform Incidents
These incidents most often involve one or more individuals who, in one way or another, have left the platform and are on the roadbed. They may be in close proximity to a third rail, lying on tracks used by high-speed commuter trains, or under a standing railcar. In most cases, railway personnel will be on the scene when rescue personnel arrive — in fact, they may have initiated the 9-1-1 call. In these cases, a unified command made up of the first-in officer and a railway representative is most appropriate (Figure 8.54). In this way, the incident action plan can accurately reflect the expertise, capabilities, and limitations of both

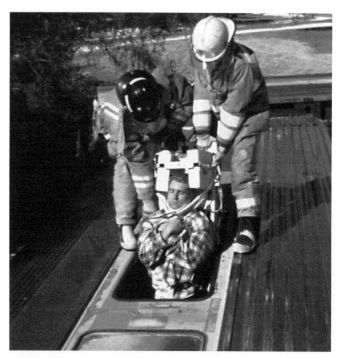

Figure 8.53 Injured passengers can be removed through the side windows.

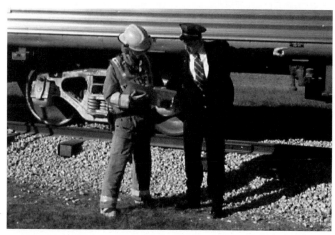

Figure 8.54 Unified command works well in rail incidents.

agencies and is most likely to be a realistic, safe, and effective plan.

If rescue personnel are on the scene before railway personnel, the railway operator should be notified of the situation and asked to send emergency response personnel. Rescue personnel should avoid the third rail (if present), cordon off the area, and deny entry to all but authorized personnel. Depending upon the specifics of the situation, rescue personnel may be able to take effective action to rescue the victim prior to the arrival of railway personnel. However, these actions should only be initiated if they have a reasonable expectation of success and they do not involve unnecessary risk for rescue personnel.

Train Vs. Highway Vehicle

Unfortunately, this type of incident is all too common. Motorists who have their car windows rolled up, the stereo system at high volume, and are perhaps distracted by interaction with others in the vehicle may not hear a train approaching an ungated crossing. Or, as is too often the case, a motorist misjudges the speed of a train approaching a gated or ungated crossing and attempts to cross the tracks before the train arrives. These and other similar scenarios can produce tragic results.

There are two basic types of train vs. highway vehicle incidents: those where the train is derailed and those where it is not. Obviously, those that involve train derailment can be very complex incidents, especially if there are victims trapped in both the highway vehicle and the railcars. This type of incident lends itself to a command structure with two divisions or sectors: one for each mode of transportation and group of victims.

Just because an incident does not involve a train derailment does not mean that it may not be complex. A collision between a train and a highway vehicle carrying hazardous materials can create a very complex incident — especially if it occurs in a densely populated area. A locomotive colliding with a loaded bus or with a truck loaded with farm workers can create mass casualty incidents that will severely tax the resources of many small agencies. Also, these incidents may occur at relatively remote rural crossings that may be many miles from the nearest trauma center or fully staffed emergency medical facility. Fast and efficient on-scene triage, treatment, and transportation — perhaps by medevac helicopter — may be critical to the victims' survival (Figure 8.55).

Train Vs. Pedestrian

These incidents occur in every locality that has one or more active rail lines. Pedestrians put themselves in the path of an oncoming train for a wide variety of reasons. Some, like foolhardy motorists, attempt to dash across the tracks before the train arrives. Others, under the influence of alcohol or other drugs, may fall asleep on the tracks or fall and knock themselves unconscious. And others do so consciously in an attempt to do away with themselves.

Regardless of why a person is hit by a train, unless all or part of the victim is in or under the railcar somehow, it is technically not an extrication incident but merely a medical trauma call that occurred on railroad property. However, if it is an extrication incident involving a train, the goal as always is to use whatever resources are available to save the victim's life and remove him from further harm. Again, working closely with on-scene railway personnel is likely to produce the best result and will increase the victim's chances of survival.

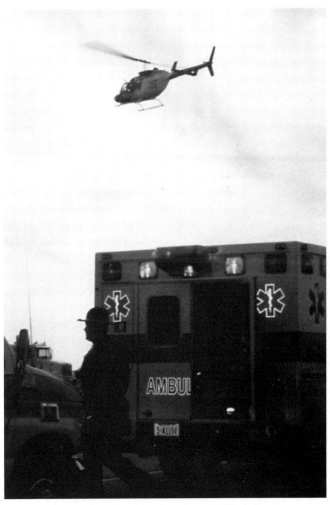

Figure 8.55 Victims may need to be transported by helicopter. *Courtesy of Mike Wieder.*

Trams

Like other classes of transportation vehicles, trams come in a wide variety of sizes and configurations. They range from individual railcars powered by diesel engines or electric motors to cable-drawn vehicles such as the famous San Francisco cable cars (Figure 8.56). There are also cable-drawn trams that travel at a very steep angle on rails set against a mountainside and those that are suspended from a cable high above the ground (Figure 8.57). How incidents involving these vehicles are handled, and who handles them, will vary depending upon the specific situation and on local protocols.

Many trams are like buses or street cars that travel on rails, and extrication operations in them can be handled much the same way as extrication from buses as described in Chapter 6. When dealing with trams that are powered by electricity, either from a third rail or an overhead catenary system, rescue personnel should follow the same safety precautions as those described earlier in this chapter. Extrication incidents involving trams that travel either on elevated tracks or are suspended by an overhead cable — essentially those that are beyond the reach of fire department ground ladders or aerial devices — operate in a hazardous environment. Subject to the dictates of local protocols, these incidents should be handled by technical rescue teams trained and equipped to operate in these environments.

Summary

Extrication incidents involving fully loaded railway passenger cars can be some of the most challenging that rescue personnel may ever face. The potential for large numbers of trapped and injured victims, the often remote incident locations, the size and weight of the railcars themselves, and the difficulty of gaining access into them combine to make these incidents very difficult to handle. Personnel in jurisdictions that have rail lines running through them should familiarize themselves with the various types of railcars that travel through their areas. In areas where trains operate on electrical power, personnel should be especially diligent in their pursuit of knowledge about those systems and the vehicles that operate in them. Also of critical importance is that agencies with the potential for this type of incident follow NFPA 1670 and develop pre-incident plans before the need arises.

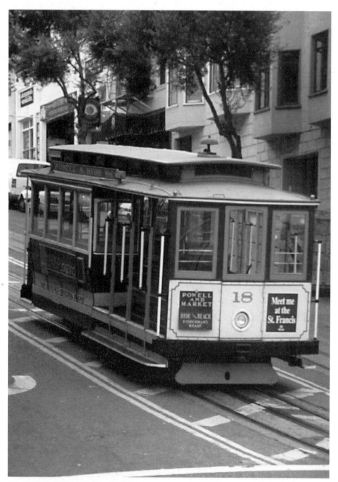

Figure 8.56 One form of tram.

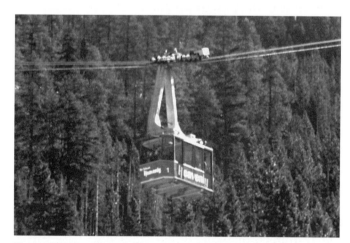

Figure 8.57 Some trams are suspended above the ground.

Chapter 9

Industrial and Agricultural Vehicle Extrication

The variety of shapes and sizes of industrial and agricultural vehicles is almost endless. New types of vehicles and improved models of existing vehicles are continually being introduced. These vehicles are as varied as the tasks that they are designed to perform. Some of them are modern versions of vehicles that have existed for many decades. Others may have never been seen in our society before because the tasks that they have been designed to perform did not exist before. They range from small farm tractors to huge earthmovers used in construction and mining.

To add to the challenge of extrication involving these vehicles, the incident scene may be on a construction site, in an enormous open-pit mine, inside a vast industrial complex, or on a huge corporate farm. In these types of incidents, there is usually only one victim to extricate unless one vehicle collides with or rolls over onto another.

This chapter classifies and describes the most common of the myriad types of industrial and agricultural vehicles in use today. Also discussed are sizing up an incident involving one or more of these vehicles, stabilizing them, and gaining access into them. Finally, the chapter concludes with a discussion of terminating an incident involving an industrial or agricultural vehicle.

Classification of Industrial and Agricultural Vehicles

As mentioned earlier, these vehicles are as varied as their intended purposes. But, like automobiles and other types of vehicles, they also have many characteristics in common. Some of these vehicles have enclosed cabs, others do not. Some of them are two-wheel drive while others are all-wheel drive. Some have no wheels at all because they are tracked vehicles.

Tractors

Tractors are used in a variety of industrial and agricultural settings. Some are used at airports and on construction sites, while many others are used on farms and ranches. Like other types of vehicles, tractors come in many different sizes and configurations. There are two broad classes of off-road tractors: wheel tractors and tracked vehicles, commonly called crawlers or tracklayers.

Wheel Tractors

Typical wheel tractors have very large rear wheels (normally up to 50-inch [120 cm]) and smaller front wheels (normally up to 38-inch [95 cm]), with rubber tires (Figure 9.1). Depending upon the specific use to which a tractor is put, the front wheels may be set the same distance apart as the rear wheels or they may be very close together. Some wheel tractors are two-wheel drive and others are all-wheel drive. The front and rear tires on all-wheel drive tractors have heavy traction treads (Figure 9.2). Only the rear tires on two-wheel drive tractors have traction treads, and the front tires are grooved for lateral purchase. Because these tractors are relatively light in weight and are often used to pull very heavy loads, large cast-iron weights are sometimes bolted to the wheels, and/or the tires are filled to approximately 90 percent with a solution of calcium chloride or ethylene glycol and water to improve traction. In other cases, tractors are equipped with multiple front and/or rear wheels for the same purpose (Figure 9.3).

Regardless of how individual wheel tractors are configured, they all tend to have a rather high profile and are more prone to rolling over than other types of vehicles. Their relatively narrow track (horizontal distance from 60 to 100 inches [144 cm to 240 cm] between wheels on the same axle) and their high ground clearance make them susceptible to lateral rollovers. Therefore, OSHA requires that all wheel tractors manufactured after October of 1976 be equipped with seat belts and roll bars — officially known as roll-over protection systems (ROPS) (Figure 9.4).

On flat, level ground, the center of gravity of these tractors is along their centerline roughly half way between their front and rear axles. When a wheel tractor is traversing a hillside, its center of gravity shifts toward the downhill wheels. If the downhill wheels drop into a depression or the uphill wheels hit a slight bump, or both, it may cause the tractor to roll over laterally (Figure 9.5). Likewise, if a wheel tractor is climbing a steep slope, its center of gravity shifts to the rear axle. If the front wheels hit a large enough bump while the rear wheels are in a depression, it can cause the front wheels to leave the ground and the front end to rotate around the rear axle, with the unit coming to rest upside down — perhaps pinning the

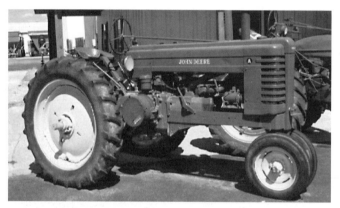
Figure 9.1 A typical two-wheel drive tractor.

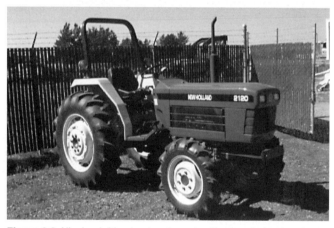
Figure 9.2 All-wheel drive tractors have traction treads front and rear.

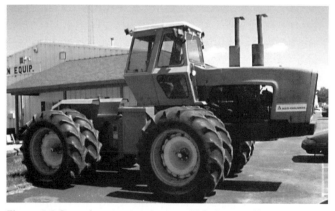
Figure 9.3 Some farm tractors have multiple front and/or rear wheels.

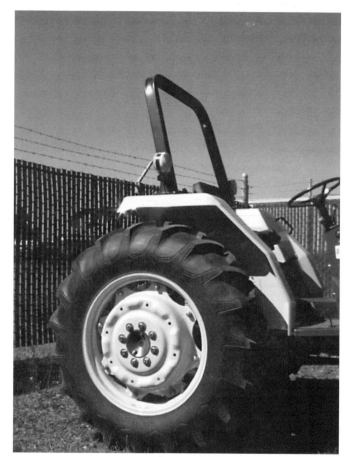
Figure 9.4 A typical tractor ROPS.

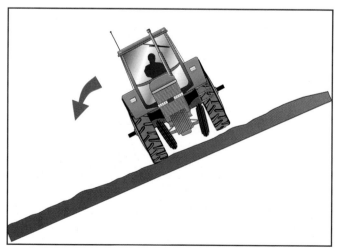
Figure 9.5 Traversing a hillside can be dangerous.

operator beneath it (Figure 9.6). To reduce this possibility, some wheel tractors are equipped with up to 1,400 pounds (635 kg) of cast iron weights attached to the front of their chassis (Figure 9.7).

Crawlers

As mentioned earlier, some tractors have no wheels at all because locomotion is provided by steel or rubber tracks. These tractors are generally larger and heavier than most wheeled tractors, have a wider track, and a lower profile (Figure 9.8). Therefore, crawlers are less susceptible to rollover than are wheel tractors.

Attachments/Implements

In addition to pulling heavy loads, tractors are designed to accommodate a wide variety of attachments and implements. *Attachments* are those auxiliary appliances, such as front-end loaders, backhoes, and scraper blades, that are more or less permanently attached to the chassis of the tractor. *Implements* are those appliances that are temporarily attached to, and usually towed by, the tractor. Typical farm implements are planters, manure spreaders, hay rakes, and balers. Attachments are important to rescue personnel because these devices can affect a tractor's stability and sometimes result in tractor rollovers.

While some wheel tractors are equipped with a scraper blade on the front or rear for snow removal and light-duty grading, heavy-duty grading and excavation is done by crawlers equipped with massive steel blades on their front ends. Some crawlers also have trenching attachments, huge rippers, or other

attachments on the rear of the vehicle. Crawlers are sometimes used at airports, especially during inclement weather, to tow aircraft from one point to another. These vehicles are often equipped with rubber tracks or rubber pads on steel tracks to avoid damaging the taxiway surface. As with wheel tractors, the number and variety of attachments and implements for crawlers is virtually endless.

Forklifts

While the OSHA regulations in 29 CFR 1910.178 refer to forklifts as "powered industrial trucks," they are also known as lift trucks or fork trucks. Forklifts are found in a variety of working environments such as

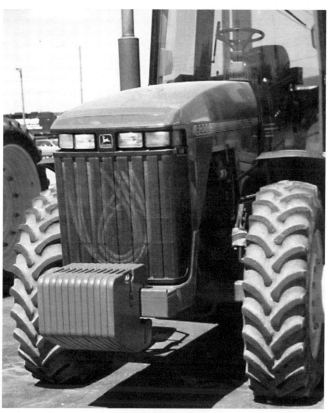
Figure 9.7 Weights help reduce the risk of rollover.

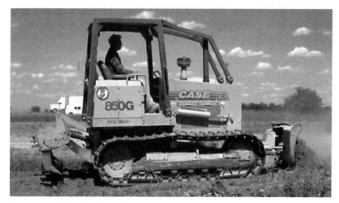
Figure 9.8 A typical crawler tractor.

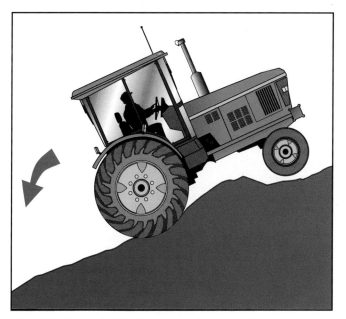
Figure 9.6 The front of the tractor can rotate around the rear axle.

warehouses, lumberyards, construction sites, and many other locations where relatively heavy objects need to be lifted and transported over relatively short distances. They are also used by urban search and rescue (US&R) teams in structural collapse incidents (Figure 9.9). While lifting capacity varies with the manufacturer and the model of the vehicle, most forklifts are capable of lifting from 2,000 to 80,000 pounds (4 400 kg to 176 200 kg). Some forklifts operate on rechargeable lead-acid batteries of either 24, 36, or 48 volts. Others have internal combustion engines that operate on gasoline, diesel, or LPG. Some have dual fuel systems that can operate on both gasoline and LPG.

Most forklifts are equipped with two broad lifting forks, approximately 4 feet (1.2 m) long. The forks can be moved laterally to adjust to the width of a particular load. Some forklifts are equipped with more specialized lifting devices for lifting unique loads. Regardless of what type of lifting device is used on the front of the vehicle, the device is attached to a horizontal cross beam that can be elevated or lowered on rollers that travel in a pair of vertical tracks called the *mast*. These masts can be deflected from five to seven degrees from vertical to increase control of the load. Some masts are designed to also telescope to increase vertical lift range. Forklifts equipped with a four-stage telescoping mast have a vertical lift range of up to 30 feet (10 m) (Figure 9.10). However, the higher the lift, the greater the chance of the unit falling over because of the increase in leverage at the top of the lift mechanism. As with fire department aerial devices, when these high-lift units are extended in close proximity to power lines, there is the additional danger of the mast or the load coming into contact with the power lines.

The design of forklift chassis vary with the manufacturer and the intended purpose of the vehicle, but all have a relatively low profile and are made of very heavy material. The bulk of the weight of a forklift chassis is concentrated at the end opposite the lift mechanism to act as a counterweight. Some forklifts have additional counterweights added to the end of the chassis. Many forklifts, especially those operated in warehouses and other areas with concrete floors, have small solid rubber tires mounted on 12-inch (300 mm) to 21-inch (525 mm) wheels (Figure 9.11). Forklifts intended for outdoor use generally have either pneumatic tires or "cushion" tires (Figure 9.12). All of these design features are intended to increase the stability of these vehicles and decrease the chances of them turning over.

All forklifts have some form of overhead operator protection system designed to ward off falling objects. Most are heavy-gauge wire screen or a steel grille over a steel frame. Forklifts that routinely operate outdoors are sometimes equipped with a fully enclosed cab. The enclosure usually consists of the standard operator

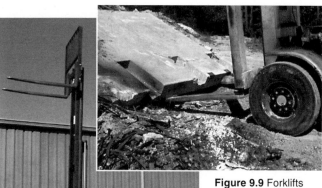

Figure 9.9 Forklifts may be used by US&R teams.

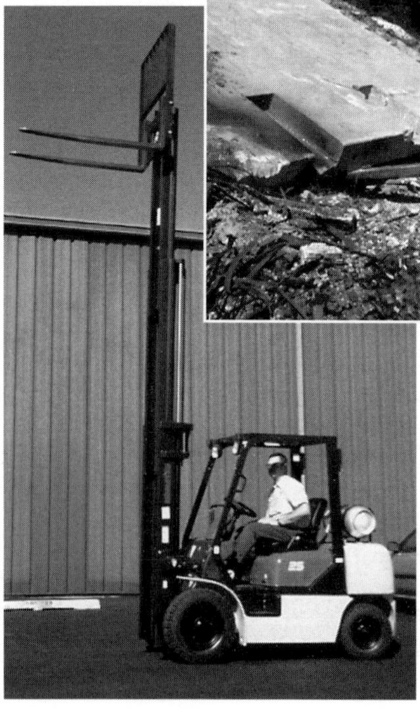

Figure 9.10 Some masts are designed to extend up to thirty feet (10 m).

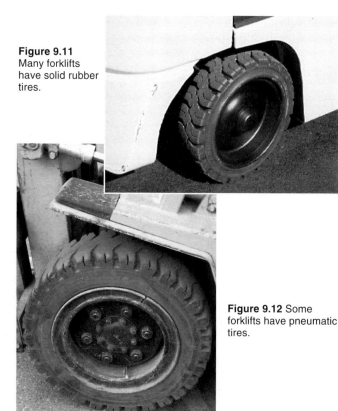

Figure 9.11 Many forklifts have solid rubber tires.

Figure 9.12 Some forklifts have pneumatic tires.

protection system enclosed with Plexiglass® panels or window panes and a laminated safety glass windshield.

Maintainers

Also called graders, these road maintenance vehicles may be found anywhere that unsurfaced roads are common or where highway construction is being done (Figure 9.13). Despite the ability to cant their front wheels, given a sufficiently steep slope and enough lateral force, these vehicles can roll over. Their enclosed cabs are similar to those on tractors and other industrial or agricultural vehicles.

Other Industrial and Agricultural Vehicles

As mentioned earlier in this chapter, the types of industrial and agricultural vehicles are many and varied. Unlike highway vehicles that are often designed for flexibility and versatility, many industrial and agricultural vehicles are designed for a single purpose. In the construction industry, a variety of booms, cranes, and other lifting vehicles are used. In agriculture, harvesters, combines, and other similar vehicles are used by themselves and in combination with trucks, tractors, and other vehicles.

Booms

These are some of the most versatile of this class of vehicle. They consist of a vehicle-mounted boom that can telescope more than 40 feet (12 m) and lift from 7,000 to 10,000 pounds (3 200 kg to 4 500 kg). The end of the boom may be fitted with forks for lifting material on pallets, a platform or basket similar to those on fire service aerial devices, or a bucket as is used on front-end loaders (Figure 9.14). Many of these vehicles not only have all-wheel drive but also have all-wheel steering. Some have fully enclosed cabs similar to those described in the section on forklifts.

Like fire department aerial devices, when booms are operated in close proximity to power lines, there is a danger of them coming into contact with the power lines. These vehicles often operate on unsurfaced construction sites where the soil may be uneven and/or unstable. When the boom is fully extended vertically, these conditions make the boom vulnerable to turning over — especially if there is a strong crosswind.

Cranes

These massive vehicles may have large pneumatic tires and can be driven from site to site, or they may be crawlers that must be transported from site to site on low-boy trailers (Figure 9.15). Regardless of their means of locomotion, these vehicles are subject to the same hazards as the booms just described.

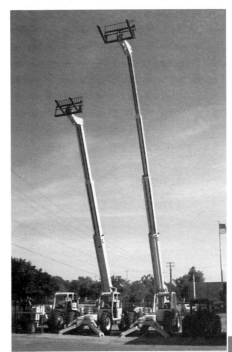

Figure 9.14 Boom vehicles are very versatile.

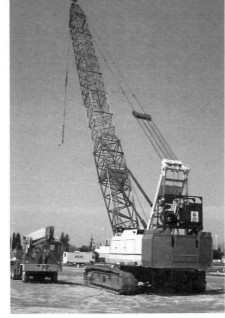

Figure 9.15 Some cranes must be transported from site to site.

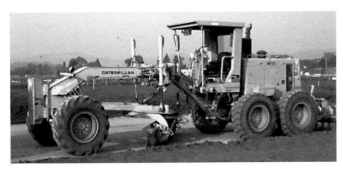

Figure 9.13 A typical maintainer.

Harvesters

Sometimes called combines, these vehicles are wide, have a relatively low center of gravity, and are usually very stable (Figure 9.16). However, like crawler tractors, given a sufficiently steep slope and enough lateral force, these vehicles can roll over. Many harvesters are designed to discharge the grain being harvested into a truck or trailer following the harvester. If farm workers enter the truck bed or trailer to manipulate the material inside, they can become trapped in the grain and suffocate if not extricated in time. In addition, some harvesters discharge the grain into a following vehicle by means of an enclosed auger (Figure 9.17). Many farm workers have had an extremity pulled into these augers when their clothing became entangled in the mechanism.

Anatomy of Industrial and Agricultural Vehicles

Some of these vehicles can be differentiated by their means of locomotion — two-wheel drive, all-wheel drive, or tracklayers. Others are differentiated by their configuration — articulating booms, telescoping booms, etc. Still others are differentiated by their sheer size.

Two-Wheel Drive Vehicles

Many wheel tractors and similar vehicles have two-wheel drive. In most of these vehicles, the driving wheels are at the rear of the vehicle and the steering wheels are at the front. However, most forklifts are configured the other way around — the front wheels are the driving wheels and the rear wheels do the steering. Regardless of which wheels provide locomotion, poor traction makes two-wheel drive vehicles prone to rollovers on hillsides and other slopes. A two-wheel drive vehicle attempting to move obliquely up and across a slope may begin to slide sideways and then down slope. If it hits an obstruction while moving in this way, the vehicle may roll over.

All-Wheel Drive Vehicles

Four-wheel or all-wheel drive vehicles are much better equipped to handle situations involving poor traction and steep slopes. Some of these vehicles have all-wheel steering as well. These are especially agile vehicles that are capable of some extraordinary maneuvers. However, because all-wheel drive vehicles are so capable and so maneuverable, their drivers can be lulled into a false sense of invulnerability. Such a cavalier attitude can cause the operator to take imprudent risks — sometimes resulting in a rollover.

Tracked Vehicles

Unlike wheel tractors that use a steering wheel, the direction of tracked vehicles is controlled by manually operated levers or pedals that apply or release a separate brake for each track. However, because the tracks spread the weight of the vehicle, some crawlers exert a ground pressure of as little as 2.5 psi (35 kg/cm^2). The same physical laws apply to crawlers as to wheel tractors. Considering the extreme environments in which they are often used, if the angles involved are steep enough, tracked vehicles are vulnerable to rollovers (Figure 9.18). And, once rolled

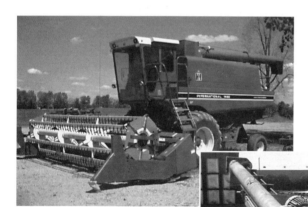

Figure 9.16 A typical harvester.

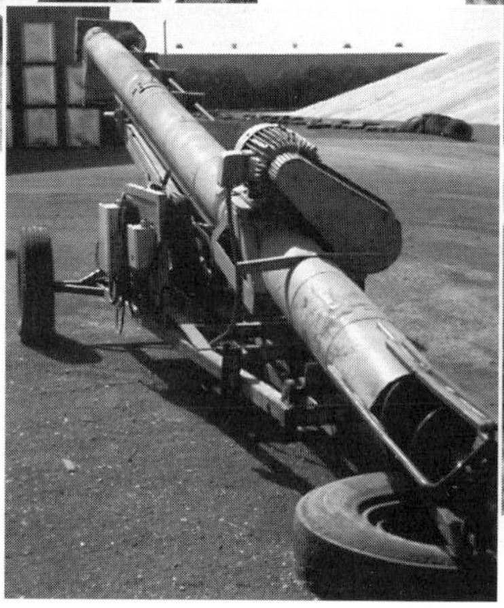

Figure 9.17 A typical grain auger.

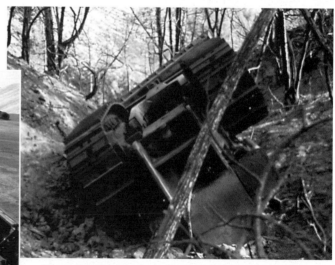

Figure 9.18 Despite their stability, crawler tractors can be turned over. *Courtesy of National Interagency Fire Center.*

over, their size and weight can make extrication much more difficult than with most wheeled tractors.

Articulating Vehicles

The most common articulating vehicles are large earthmovers (Figure 9.19). Normally quite stable because of their huge wheels and low center of gravity, earthmovers can be rolled over if all the elements are present — steep slope, unstable soil, and sufficient lateral force. Other examples of articulating vehicles are all-wheel drive farm tractors, log skidders, large front-end loaders, rough-terrain forklifts, and large dump trucks.

Oversized Vehicles

Perhaps the most common of the oversized vehicles are massive dump trucks used in strip mining and similar activities (Figure 9.20). In this application, they are most often used to haul ore from the mining site to the smelter. Similar types of vehicles are used in heavy construction, such as in building earth-fill dams, where they are used to haul huge boulders and aggregate fill material. Given the environments in

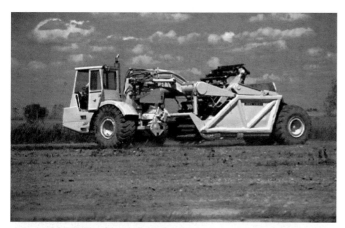

Figure 9.19 One type of articulating vehicle.

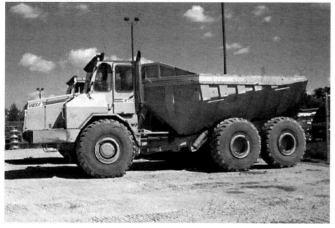

Figure 9.20 One of the largest land-based vehicles in the world.

which these vehicles operate, rock slides, cave-ins, and similar events can cause these vehicles to overturn.

Operational Controls

Industrial and agricultural vehicles employ a variety of control devices. Some of these are steering devices, and others are used to increase a vehicle's stability. Still others are used to power or control auxiliary devices. Regardless of what type of device, most use similar operational controls (Figure 9.21).

Brakes

As mentioned earlier in this chapter, crawler tractors and other tracked vehicles use brakes for changing direction — steering (Figure 9.22). When the operator of one of these vehicles wants to turn left, he pulls a lever or steps on a pedal that applies a brake to the left track, slowing or stopping it. Since the left track is at least momentarily moving slower that the right track, the vehicle veers to the left. The greater the difference in the speed of the right and left tracks, the faster and more abrupt the turn will be. A fully applied brake to one track or the other will cause the vehicle to spin around a fixed point.

Jacks

Also called stabilizers or outriggers, these hydraulically-operated devices, similar to the stabilizing jacks on a fire department aerial device, extend from both sides of a vehicle so equipped. As the name implies, these devices are intended to stabilize a tractor or other vehicle that is operating an attachment such as a backhoe or a boom. When applied, stabilizing jacks normally lift the vehicle's wheels clear off the ground, and the jacks bear the full weight of the vehicle. This makes the vehicle quite stable — unless something goes wrong. If one or more of the jacks suddenly loses hydraulic pressure, the vehicle can lurch to one side. If the vehicle were positioned across a slope and the downslope jacks failed, the vehicle could easily topple over. Also, if the ground under the jacks on one side of the vehicle collapsed into an excavation, the vehicle may roll over.

Auxiliary Power Sources

To increase their versatility, some tractors and similar vehicles are equipped with one or more auxiliary power sources. They may have power take-offs that can be used to operate implements such as portable grain augers or conveyor belts or chains (Figure 9.23). They may have hydraulic pumps that can be used to raise or

New farm tractors, combines, and other self-propelled agricultural equipment have universal operator control symbols so that farmers can readily locate and operate the various controls. These symbols could also assist rescue personnel in an accident. Being able to locate the fuel shut-off or operate a remote hydraulic system might contribute to a successful rescue.

NOTE: These symbols are generally not found on older agricultural equipment.

DASHBOARD CONTROLS

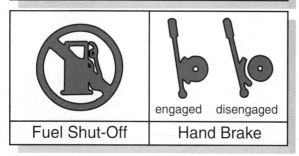

Fuel Shut-Off	Hand Brake
	engaged disengaged

SAFETY ALERT

The safety-alert symbol is often used with signal words to draw attention to potentially unsafe areas.

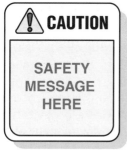

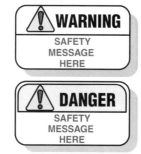

Signal Words

CAUTION is used for general reminders of good safety practices or to direct attention to unsafe practices.
WARNING denotes a specific potential hazard.
DANGER denotes the most serious potential danger.

OPERATIONAL CONTROLS

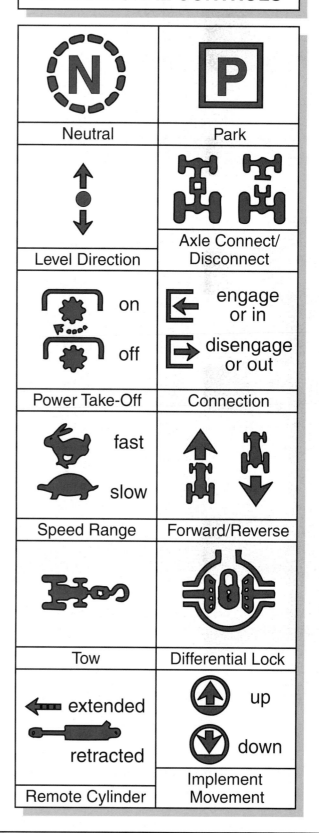

Figure 9.21 Standard farm equipment control symbols.

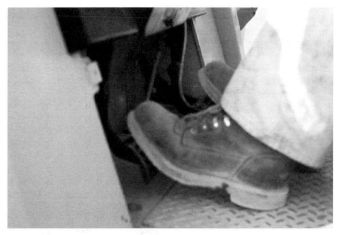

Figure 9.22 A lever or pedal controls each brake.

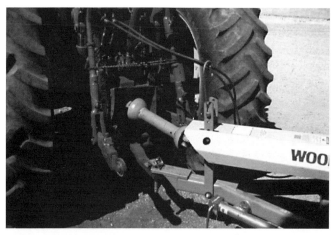

Figure 9.23 Power take-offs operate a variety of implements.

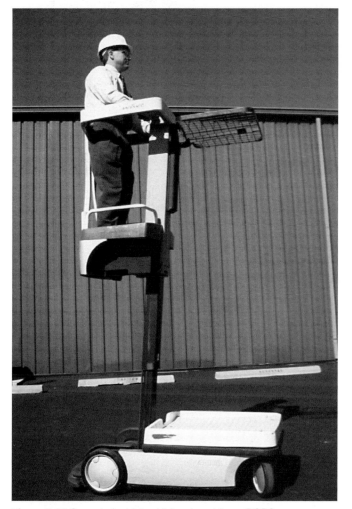

Figure 9.24 Some industrial vehicles do not have ROPS.

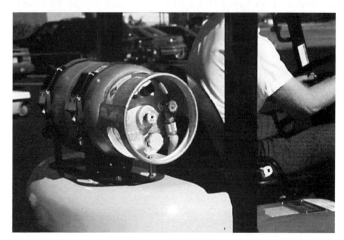

Figure 9.25 Many vehicles operate on LPG.

Roll-Over Protection Systems

As discussed in the section on tractors, OSHA requires a roll-over protection system (ROPS) on every industrial and agricultural vehicle except those in which the operator stands (Figure 9.24). Even in vehicles not covered by the OSHA regulations, ROPS are often installed by the manufacturer for liability reasons. Sometimes ROPS are required by the operator's insurance carrier.

Fuels

As mentioned in earlier sections of this chapter, industrial and agricultural vehicles operate on a variety of fuels. Many of the largest and heaviest vehicles operate on diesel fuel and carry up to 100 gallons (378.5 L) in their tanks. Other industrial and agricultural vehicles operate on gasoline and/or LPG, usually propane (Figure 9.25). Still others operate on compressed natural gas (CNG). Finally, some forklifts and other vehicles are powered by electricity from banks of rechargeable wet-cell batteries.

lower any number of farm implements such as plows or mowers. As with any power source, if the proper guards are not in place or if the operators fail to exercise appropriate caution when using the devices, parts of their clothing can become entangled in the mechanism and this can pull the operator into the machinery.

Vehicles that operate on liquid or gaseous fuels add the danger of fire to the other hazards associated with collisions, rollovers, and other extrication incidents. Part of the size-up process must be to assess the need for Class B foam to suppress flammable vapors and/or flammable or combustible liquid fires. Flammable gases must be shut off at the source or allowed to burn out.

Tires

As mentioned in the earlier discussions on tires, industrial and agricultural vehicles may be equipped with pneumatic or solid rubber tires, depending upon the use to which the vehicle is put and the environment in which it works. Pneumatic tires are to be found on vehicles as small as converted golf carts used as runabouts in warehouses and industrial complexes and as massive as the huge earthmoving vehicles used in mining and heavy construction. To improve the traction of drive wheels with large pneumatic tires, it is common practice to fill the tires to about 90 percent with water or some other inert fluid, and then inflate the tires to their normal operating pressure with air.

Some forklifts and similar vehicles have what are called cushion tires. These are solid rubber tires that look like the pneumatic tires used on automobiles and light trucks. One obvious difference between a cushion tire and a pneumatic tire is the absence of a valve stem on the cushion tire. Other solid rubber tires on forklifts are quite obvious for what they are. They generally are smaller in diameter than either cushion or pneumatic tires, and they usually have no traction treads.

Industrial and Agricultural Vehicle Size-Up

As described in the earlier operational chapters, the size-up of an extrication incident involving an industrial or agricultural vehicle should be done systematically beginning with an assessment of the scene. This should be followed by an assessment of the vehicles involved, the trapped victims, and the extrication requirements of the particular incident. As always, size-up continues throughout the incident.

Scene Assessment

As described in earlier chapters, the first-responding officer must factor the effects of time, day, date, and weather into his assessment before ever reaching the incident scene. For example, if an incident involving an industrial vehicle is reported during normal working hours, on a week day, in the summer, how are these variables likely to affect the incident? Will the scene be congested with curious coworkers? Will some of them try to extricate their fellow worker, perhaps causing the victim further harm and making the situation worse? Will the prevailing weather expose rescuers and trapped victims to extremes of temperature and/or humidity?

On the other hand, if the incident is reported during the graveyard shift (between midnight and 8:00 a.m.) or on a holiday when the bulk of the workforce is likely to be absent, will there be enough technical support or should company management and/or special equipment operators be asked to respond? Will additional lighting be needed?

If the incident involves an overturned farm vehicle or entrapment in some other piece of farm machinery, is the incident location clearly known and readily accessible, or will rescue personnel have to search for the scene? Is the trapped operator the only person at the scene who is familiar with the operation of the machine, and will a farm advisor or other expert be needed? Will the remoteness of the scene require that a medevac helicopter be called?

Finally, as the officer nears the scene, he should look for anything unusual that might indicate other collateral problems. Is smoke (especially that with an unusual color) or steam rising from the scene? Will fire protection be a higher than normal priority because of a known flammability hazard? Will large-scale foam-making capability be needed? Will a hazardous materials team be needed because of a known release or a high potential for the release of a pesticide or other IDLH (immediately dangerous to life or health) substance? What additional resources will be needed to control and mitigate the known and potential hazards in this incident? Whatever those resources are, they should be requested *immediately*.

Vehicle Assessment

Once on the scene, if there appears to be a legitimate emergency, the first-in officer should assume command of the incident by calling the communications center (dispatch) and naming the incident, giving a brief description of the situation, and calling for any additional resources that may be needed. In addition, he can begin to make a more detailed assessment of the vehicles involved.

To make a thorough assessment, the officer must attempt to answer a number of critical questions. Is there more than one vehicle involved? Was there a collision, or did one vehicle roll over onto the other?

What type of vehicle is involved? What is its position? Was the vehicle lifting or carrying some heavy load — and if so, is the load a hazard to rescuers, trapped victims, or others? Are there potential hazards because of springs, cams, or weights that are a part of the vehicle or in close proximity to it? Is the vehicle leaking flammable or combustible liquids or other hazardous materials? Does the scene need to be cordoned off, or is it sufficiently isolated to reduce the need to control access to the scene?

Victim Assessment

As mentioned earlier, in most incidents involving industrial and agricultural vehicles, there will only be one occupant in each vehicle. However, the size and weight of these vehicles may make extricating one victim more challenging and time consuming than extricating several from more conventional vehicles. As always, this phase of the size-up process involves looking for victims to determine how many there are, where they are, and what their medical conditions are. Even though an industrial or agricultural vehicle may seem very stable in its present position, rescuers must attempt to assess the trapped victims without jostling the vehicle — especially the vehicle's cab.

Extrication Assessment

Once all trapped victims have been located and their conditions assessed, a decision must be made about how they can be extricated from the vehicle in the safest, fastest, and most efficient way. This means assessing the types of extrication tools and equipment that are likely to be needed to free the trapped victims. Are there a sufficient number of power spreaders, cutters, and other similar tools on scene, or do more or different types need to be requested? Will oxyacetylene cutting torches, plasma cutters, or exothermic burning bars be needed? Is there a sufficient number of rescue personnel on scene, or will more be needed?

Industrial and Agricultural Vehicle Stabilization

Because of the size and weight of many of these vehicles, they are generally quite stable. However, following a collision or rollover, these vehicles must be assumed to be unstable. Like any other vehicle from which one or more victims must be extricated, an industrial or agricultural vehicle must be stabilized before rescue personnel can enter to assess, stabilize, package, and disentangle trapped victims. As with other types of vehicles, the techniques and equipment

used to stabilize an industrial or agricultural vehicle may vary depending upon how the vehicle came to rest — upright, on its side, on its roof, or in some other position.

Vehicle Upright

Unlike automobiles and light trucks, when an industrial or agricultural vehicle is upright following a collision or other destructive event, it is likely to be very stable vertically. This is because of the extremely heavy suspension, or absence of suspension, on many of these vehicles. However, because the destructive event may have damaged or destroyed the vehicle's suspension system (if any), the same vertical stabilization measures described in earlier chapters should be applied. In addition, the vehicle should be stabilized horizontally using chocks, wedges, etc., to immobilize the wheels.

Both vertical and horizontal stabilization may involve the usual equipment and techniques — four-point or six-point cribbing, timber shores or pneumatic shores, installed at the appropriate points. In addition, wheel chocks, wedges, and/or webbing and chains may be needed to provide horizontal stability. How and where these techniques are applied will depend on the specifics of the situation.

Vehicle on Its Side

Just as with train cars and heavy trucks, once industrial or agricultural vehicles roll onto their sides they may appear to be very stable. However, as with the other types, if the vehicle has come to rest on a slope or on unstable soil, there is the ever present danger of it suddenly and unexpectedly rolling back onto its wheels or tracks, or onto its top. Therefore, to create a safe working environment for rescue personnel, it may be necessary to first secure the vehicle from the top with webbing and/or chains attached to a bombproof anchor point. Then, with that antiroll protection in place, shoring can be installed on the underside of the vehicle.

Vehicle Upside Down

Since many industrial and agricultural vehicles do not have roofs, the vehicle may be resting on a roll bar or on its fenders. Regardless of what part of the vehicle is supporting the rest of it, an industrial or agricultural vehicle in this position is likely to be very unstable. This is because the vehicle's center of gravity is relatively high in this position. Therefore, it is imperative that the vehicle be effectively stabilized as soon as possible.

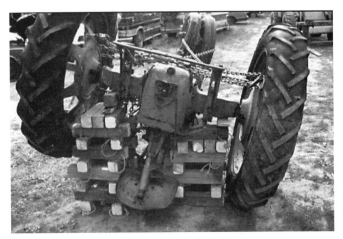
Figure 9.26 Cribbing may be needed to stabilize the vehicle.

Stabilizing an upside down industrial or agricultural vehicle may involve installing cribbing, shoring, and/ or pneumatic struts at various points. Wheel tractors and similar vehicles may require box cribbing under the rear axle, one stack on each side between the differential and the wheel (Figure 9.26). Other types of vehicles may require four-point or six-point cribbing depending upon the situation. Because of the unusually heavy weight of many of these vehicles, it may be necessary to build solid cribbing stacks to provide adequate support.

Other Stabilization Situations

Other stabilization situations involving industrial and agricultural vehicles may include vehicles that have come to rest in positions other than those just discussed. These situations may also include those where equipment operators and others have become entrapped in industrial or agricultural machinery.

Vehicles in Other Positions

As described in earlier operational chapters, stabilizing vehicles that are in positions other than those already discussed can test the ingenuity and innovative thinking of the most skilled and experienced rescue personnel — and the same is true of industrial and agricultural vehicles. Very often, the vehicles come to rest at odd angles and in precarious positions. These unusual angles can dictate that extraordinarily long shoring be used or that the vehicle be stabilized from the top side with webbing and/or chains or cables. If timber shoring is used, a shoring system similar to those used to stabilize weakened building walls may have to be constructed. As always, the goal is to create as many points of contact between the vehicle and a stable surface as are necessary to stabilize the vehicle.

Machinery Incidents

Industrial and agricultural workers often work in close proximity to moving conveyor chains or belts, augers, or gears. If the OSHA-required guards are not in place and if a worker wears loose clothing, the clothing can become entangled in the operating machinery and that can pull the worker into the machine. In some cases, the worker can be freed simply by cutting the clothing free of the machine or having the worker slip out of the entangled clothing.

In most machinery entrapments, power to the machine will have been shut off before rescuers arrive — either by an overload switch being triggered when the machine jams or by a coworker using an emergency shutoff. If not, power to the machinery may need to be left *on* until the machine is stabilized. If so, a guard should be posted by the control switch to prevent anyone from shutting it down prematurely.

Leaving the power on may be necessary to protect the trapped worker by preventing the machine from completing its normal cycle when the power is shut off. Power may also be needed if the mechanism must be moved to extricate the victim. The mechanism may have to be stabilized with rescue tools, wedges, cribbing, chocks, webbing, chains, or cables as necessary to prevent any movement or only allow for controlled movement. Rescuers may have to rely on the knowledge and expertise of the victim's coworkers to help them decide where and how to place the stabilization equipment if they are not familiar with the machinery in which the victim is trapped.

Gaining Access into Industrial and Agricultural Vehicles

Once an industrial or agricultural vehicle has been stabilized, crews can safely work on gaining access into the vehicle's cab. Unless the cab is crushed beneath the upside down vehicle, the tools and techniques used to gain access into the cab are no different than those used to gain access into other vehicles.

Window Entry

The tools and techniques used to remove the windshield and/or windows from the cab of an industrial or agricultural vehicle will vary depending upon the materials used in the windows. Some of these vehicles have Plexiglass in the side and rear windows, with tempered glass or laminated safety glass in the windshield. Others have tempered glass in the windshield as well as in the side and rear windows.

Some of the windows are mounted in rubber frames (Figure 9.27). Others are held in place with industrial adhesive. Still others are bolted to steel hinges or brackets attached to the frame of the cab (Figure 9.28). In most cases, the tools and techniques used to remove the windshield and/or windows are the same as described in Chapter 4 for each type of material.

Door Entry

The cabs of most industrial and agricultural vehicles have outward swinging doors with a window that may or may not be designed to open. Those that open may be of the split-pane type that slide horizontally to open or of the type designed to swing open either partially or fully (Figure 9.29). Because the cabs of these vehicles are usually 4 feet (1.2 m) or more above the ground, the door latches are located near the bottom of the door panel (Figure 9.30).

If the door is jammed and must be removed, the hinge pins are exposed on the outside of the cab and can be cut off with a rotary saw equipped with a metal-cutting blade or with an oxyacetylene torch (Figure 9.31). Once the hinges are cut through, the door can be lifted or pried off manually or with a power spreader.

Roof Entry

If no other route of entry into the cab of an industrial or agricultural vehicle is accessible, then roof entry is feasible. Since the roof panel is part of the ROPS, it is made of rather substantial material — usually steel — so entry through the roof can be a slow process. However, some roof panels gain strength from stamped-in contours, so they can be made of metal thin enough to be cut with most standard extrication tools such as air chisels or rotary saws. Depending upon the manufacturer, there may be one or more steel cross members under the panel. These cross members will have to be removed by cutting them with either power shears or an oxyacetylene cutting torch.

Industrial and Agricultural Vehicle Extrication Process

As always, the goal during the process of extricating the operator of an industrial or agricultural vehicle is to remove the vehicle from the victim without causing further injury. Likewise, if a victim is caught in some piece of machinery, the machinery must be removed from the victim — not the other way around.

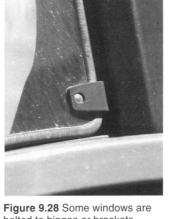
Figure 9.28 Some windows are bolted to hinges or brackets.

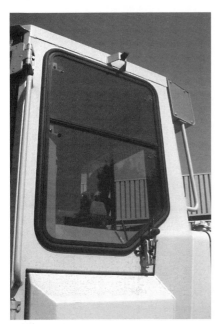
Figure 9.27 Some windows are mounted in rubber frames.

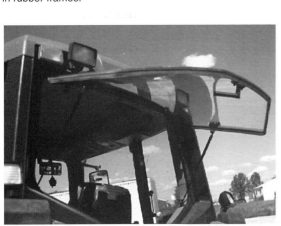
Figure 9.29 Some cab windows open fully.

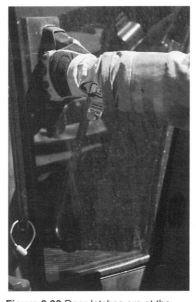
Figure 9.30 Door latches are at the bottom of the doors.

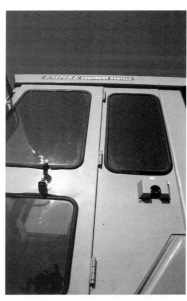
Figure 9.31 Exposed hinges can be cut to remove the door.

Disentanglement

Because the vehicle's cab is essentially the ROPS designed to protect the operator, the strength of the structure can make freeing the operator extremely challenging. When sufficient force has been applied to these structural components to deform them enough to entrap the operator, rescuers may have to apply an equal amount of force to disentangle the victim. Otherwise, the cab or ROPS may have to be dismantled. To do this, power spreaders, shears, and extension rams are most often needed. These devices should be applied as described in Chapter 4.

If the victim is not in the cab of the vehicle but pinned under it or is caught in some piece of machinery, the tools and techniques used will be dictated by the specifics of the situation. Whether the victim is caught in a conveyor chain, an auger, or in some other piece of equipment, the equipment must be dismantled to the point that the victim is freed.

WARNING!

Unless you are _sure_ it is safe to do so, never reverse the machinery in an attempt to free the victim. To do so may cause serious additional injury to the victim.

Victim Removal

Removing an injured victim from inside of the wrecked cab of an industrial or agricultural vehicle can be very difficult because of the limited working room within the cab. There may only be enough room for one rescuer to enter the cab of the vehicle to assess, treat, stabilize, and package the victim for removal. In this situation, it may be faster (and less traumatic for the victim) to simply dismantle the cab before attempting to extricate the victim.

Incident Termination

Once the trapped operator and any other victims have been extricated and loaded for transportation to a medical facility as needed, the emergency phase of the incident has ended. Depending upon the situation and local protocols, rescue personnel may or may not be involved in righting overturned vehicles or other scene restoration activities. In any case, it is important to follow the incident termination procedures described in Chapter 5.

Summary

Extrication incidents involving industrial or agricultural vehicles can be extremely challenging for rescue personnel. Therefore, if they are to function safely and efficiently at these incidents, personnel must be familiar with the anatomy and nomenclature of the types of vehicles and machinery that are common to their response areas. Regardless of the size or type of vehicle or piece of machinery involved in a particular incident, rescue personnel must keep in mind that their role is to protect themselves and others from harm, protect the trapped victims from further harm, and to free those victims as safely and as quickly as possible.

Chapter 10

Special Extrication Situations

While the preceding chapters discussed the more common types of vehicle extrication situations, this chapter focuses on those at the opposite end of the spectrum — the most unusual types of vehicle extrication situations. Some firefighters and other rescue personnel handle vehicle extrication incidents virtually every day, others less often but with some regularity. Because they deal with these more or less routine incidents so often, they become quite adept at handling them. However, there is a danger of these rescuers becoming complacent and overconfident. Regardless of how skilled and experienced rescuers are at handling routine incidents, when the situation is clearly unusual, they may find that they are less than fully prepared. Therefore, it is imperative that adequate pre-incident planning be done and that the appropriate level of training and equipment be provided. Pre-incident planning should identify resources available within and outside of the agency that might be needed during special extrication situations and how these resources can be obtained when needed.

Regardless of how unusual the situation, the steps involved in handling an unusual incident safely and effectively are essentially the same as those in any other vehicle extrication incident: make an assessment of the situation, assume command of the incident, develop an incident action plan, and implement the plan. An incident action plan outlines the incident goals and objectives and specifies how the available resources are to be organized and deployed. The operational units within the incident organization then determine how to deal with hazards at the scene, stabilize the vehicles involved, stabilize and package the trapped victims, and extricate them from the vehicles. Finally, the plan specifies how the scene is to be restored and the incident terminated.

This chapter focuses on pre-incident planning for the most unusual types of vehicle extrication incidents — those that may be special because of the environment in which they occurred, the number of vehicles involved, the number of victims trapped, or any of a number of other factors. Also discussed are the size-up of various types of special situations and the processes of stabilizing the involved vehicles, gaining access into them, and extricating victims from them.

Pre-Incident Planning

NFPA 1670, *Standard on Operations and Training for Technical Rescue Incidents* (1999), requires local jurisdictions to survey their response districts to assess their needs for operational capability in the various rescue disciplines, including vehicle extrication. This requirement serves several purposes. First, it is a means by which local jurisdictions can identify their need for various types of rescue services. It also helps individual agencies assess their ability to meet those identified needs. And, finally, it serves as a guide to help the citizens' elected representatives decide what level of readiness is appropriate and what level they are willing to fund.

As discussed in Chapter 1, NFPA 1670 identifies three levels of operational capability — awareness, operations, and technician — in each of several different rescue disciplines. Included in these classifications are rescues from vehicles and machinery, in other words — vehicle extrication. In addition, the requirements for Fire Fighter II in NFPA 1001, *Standard for Fire Fighter Professional Qualifications* (1997), include operating hand and power tools and using cribbing and shoring to extricate a victim trapped in a motor vehicle — *and* helping special rescue teams.

At the operations level, for which this manual is written, it is anticipated that firefighters and other rescue first responders will be trained and equipped to safely and efficiently extricate the majority of all victims trapped in vehicles. They will also be trained to support technician-level rescuers in special extrication situations that are beyond the operations level. Therefore, those agencies charged with being capable of functioning at the operations level must either provide their own personnel with operations-level training and equipment or arrange for another agency to provide these services.

Classification of Special Situations

As mentioned earlier, any number of factors can cause a particular vehicle extrication incident to be considered a "special" situation. Perhaps the most common factor is the environment in which the incident occurred. But that is not the only factor — the number of vehicles involved, the number of trapped victims, fires or the potential for fires or explosions, or the presence of a large quantity of hazardous materials can change an otherwise routine incident into one that is clearly special.

> The first-in officer at a special incident must be able to recognize that the situation is not routine, is beyond the capabilities of the responding rescue resources, and that a technical rescue or other specialized team should be called.

It is also vitally important that the first-arriving officer prevent on-scene personnel from endangering themselves and others in their zeal to rescue trapped vehicle occupants. Regardless of why a particular incident is considered special, those in charge of these incidents must not allow their personnel to develop tunnel vision and rush into the scene before it is safe to do so—thereby adding more victims to the incident.

> It is essential that all rescuers remember that they did not cause the problem, they are not responsible for the victims being in that situation, and they are not obligated to sacrifice themselves in a heroic attempt to save a victim — and especially not in an attempt to recover a body.

What exactly is a special extrication incident? For purposes of this discussion, special vehicle extrication situations are those that involve any of the following:

- Vehicle in a structure
- Vehicle in water
- Multiple vehicles
- Recreational vehicles
- Amusement park rides
- Hanging vehicles

Special Situation Size-Up

Just as in any other vehicle extrication incident, the first step in the size-up process is to assess the scene. This means that during the response to the scene, the first-due officer assesses how and to what extent the day, date, time and weather may affect the operation. Because of the time of the day and the day of the week, is the scene likely to be congested with pedestrian or vehicular traffic, or both? Are curious spectators likely to be in harm's way? Will the response of emergency vehicles be slowed by rush-hour traffic or inclement weather en route to the scene? Is the weather likely to expose rescue personnel and/or victims to extremes of temperature or humidity, or to rain, snow, or strong winds?

Scene Assessment

As the first-arriving officer nears the scene, he should attempt to see the "big picture" — that is, to develop an understanding of the overall situation. He should be especially watchful for anything unusual, such as people fleeing the scene or otherwise behaving strangely, which might indicate the presence of an airborne contaminant or a potential explosion. Such circumstances may suggest the need to stop well away from the scene, notify other responding units, and continue the assessment with binoculars (Figure 10.1). If a commercial truck is involved, the officer should look for labels or placards to help identify the cargo. The presence of a white vapor cloud that hugs the ground may indicate a release of LPG. A vapor cloud of another color may indicate a release of a toxic material. Steam or smoke rising from the scene may indicate an incipient fire. These and any other unusual circumstances may make scene control and security a high priority.

Once on the scene, or close enough to it to make a reasonable assessment of the situation, the first-arriving officer should assume command of the

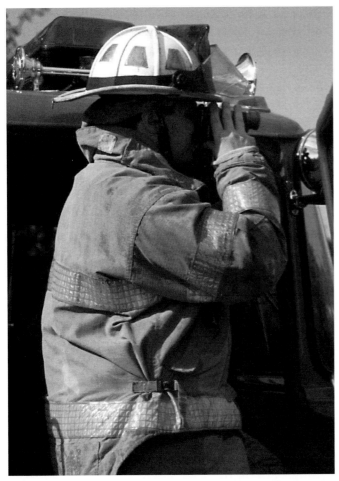

Figure 10.1 Size-up may have to be started from a safe distance.

incident as described in previous chapters. He should attempt to answer one of the most critical questions relating to the incident — Are the resources on-scene and en route sufficient to handle this situation? If not, he should call for the additional resources *immediately.* An important part of answering this question is deciding whether this is a special situation that is beyond the operations level. If so, the appropriate technical rescue team and/or other specialized resources should be requested and the on-scene personnel deployed to establish and maintain control of the scene and to support the technical rescue team when it arrives. Otherwise, the scene assessment is the same as in any other vehicle extrication incident.

Vehicle Assessment

As in any other vehicle extrication incident, once the scene has been assessed and any hazards mitigated, the process of assessing the condition of the involved vehicles can begin. In some special situations, such as those involving multiple vehicles or vehicles in hazardous environments, assessing the involved

vehicles can sometimes be a slow and tedious process if it is to be done safely.

The IC should attempt to determine the number of vehicles involved and their conditions by answering the following questions: Did the vehicle crash into a structure? And, if so, what is the vehicle's condition? Did the vehicle come to rest in a body of water? And, if so, is the vehicle under the water? Are there multiple vehicles involved? And, if so, what types of vehicles and what are their conditions? Will heavy-duty tow trucks be needed? Will cranes, barges, or other specialized resources be needed to handle this incident?

Victim Assessment

Prior to vehicle stabilization, identifying the exact number of trapped victims and assessing their conditions may be extremely difficult — especially a in hazardous environment. Under these circumstances, the most prudent course of action may be to merely confirm that the vehicles contain one or more trapped victims, and delay a more thorough victim assessment until the vehicles have been stabilized.

Extrication Assessment

As discussed in previous chapters, this final step in the initial size-up is intended to identify the methods by which trapped victims will have to be extricated and the tools, equipment, and other resources that will be needed.

Application to Specific Special Situations

Applying the information gathered during size-up to specific special situations can sometimes be a challenge for any emergency response agency. The following sections discuss the application of this information to the various types of special situations listed earlier in this chapter — vehicle in structure, vehicle in water, multiple vehicles, recreational vehicles, amusement park rides, and hanging vehicles.

Vehicle in Structure

In this context, the term *structure* refers to any stationary man-made object into which a vehicle has crashed. The object could be a building, bridge abutment, or tunnel (Figure 10.2).

Size-Up

Scene Assessment. First, the integrity of the structure must be assessed along with the other items normally associated with the assessment of a vehicle extrication

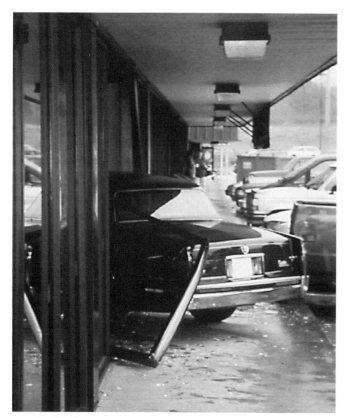

Figure 10.2 A vehicle into a structure may be a special situation. *Courtesy of Mike Wieder.*

scene. The questions to be answered are: Has the structure been damaged to the point that a collapse is likely? If so, would a collapse endanger rescue personnel or others? If the answers are yes, then a structural collapse rescue team should be called in to shore up and stabilize the structure. While waiting for the structural collapse team to arrive, on-scene personnel should be used to establish and maintain control of the scene, and perform any other duties that would not require them to enter the collapse danger zone.

Vehicle Assessment. Once the structure into which the vehicle crashed has been stabilized, the process of assessing the condition of the vehicle may be relatively quick and easy. Or, depending upon the type of vehicle and the type of structure, it may be very difficult and time consuming. If the vehicle cannot adequately be assessed in place, the cost/benefit of pulling the vehicle out of the structure may have to be considered. Since this could be very risky for any trapped victims, it should be considered only in the most extreme situations.

Victim Assessment. Prior to the involved vehicles being stabilized, the assessment of the trapped victims must be somewhat cursory. At this point, all that is necessary is to confirm that there are victims in the vehicles, and what their general conditions are.

Extrication Assessment. The point here is to assess how the victims are entrapped and what will be needed to extricate them. Are they trapped because the structure into which the vehicle crashed will not allow the vehicle's doors to be opened? Or are they trapped by some part of the vehicle having collapsed around them? What sorts of tools, equipment, and other resources will be needed to free the victims?

Vehicle Stabilization

If structural collapse is not a consideration, rescue personnel can begin to stabilize the vehicle. Given adequate space in which to operate, stabilizing a vehicle in a building, regardless of its position, is the same as described in the earlier chapter that focused on that type of vehicle.

If the shoring needed to stabilize the building so restricts the operating space around the vehicle that rescuers cannot maneuver as necessary to stabilize the vehicle, then the cost/benefit of pulling the vehicle from the building must be considered. But as mentioned earlier, moving the vehicle before the occupant is stabilized can be very risky. Therefore, this option should be considered only in the most extreme situations.

Gaining Access

Once the structure and the vehicle have been stabilized, the tools and techniques used to gain access into the vehicle are the same as those described in Chapter 4. However, if the vehicle is inside the building, operating space may be limited and extrication personnel must be careful not to disturb or dislodge any of the shoring that is supporting the structure.

Extrication Process

The same space limitations and other environmental challenges that affected the vehicle stabilization and access processes may also affect the disentanglement and extrication processes. It may be necessary to package victims so that the litters in which they are placed can be manipulated in a variety of ways (even vertically) to avoid the shoring used to stabilize the building. As in the other phases of the operation, rescuers must be careful not to disturb or dislodge the structural shoring.

Vehicle in Water

Even in areas with very arid climates, vehicles sometimes leave the roadway and come to rest in a body of water. The water may be in a swimming pool, canal, river, estuary, lake, or even the ocean (Figure 10.3).

Size-Up

Scene Assessment. If a vehicle has crashed into a body of water, the first question that must be answered is: Can rescue personnel do what must be done to extricate any trapped victims without having to enter the water? If the answer is no, then a water rescue team should be called. On-scene personnel should be used to establish and maintain control of the scene, and perform any other tasks that would not require them to enter the water. This is especially important if the vehicle fell from a great height into the water, or if the vehicle and its occupants have been submerged for more than an hour. Under these circumstances, the operation is almost certainly a body recovery and not a rescue. If the agency has one or more rescue boats, personnel trained in boat-based rescue operations can perform those tasks that can be done from the boat.

Vehicle Assessment. Depending upon the overall situation — the type of vehicle, the nature of the body of water, how much of the vehicle is above the surface of the water, and in what position the vehicle came to rest — the process of assessing the vehicle's condition may be relatively easy or quite difficult. Unfortunately, much of the vehicle damage may be hidden below the waterline. Or, the vehicle may be entirely submerged making damage assessment virtually impossible without entering the water.

Victim Assessment. Depending upon how much of the vehicle is visible above the water, it may be possible to see into the vehicle and determine the number of victims and their conditions. In other cases, it may only be possible to determine that there are victims inside the vehicle and a more thorough assessment of their conditions will have to be delayed until the vehicle is pulled from the water and stabilized.

Extrication Assessment. Once again, the degree to which an assessment of the extrication requirements can be made will depend upon how much of the vehicle is visible above the water's surface. Assessing the extrication problems involved may have to wait until the vehicle is pulled from the water.

Vehicle Stabilization

In most cases, there is little that anyone can do to stabilize a vehicle that is immersed in water except secure the vehicle to the shore with rope, chain, or webbing attached to a secure anchor point. The major challenge may be to prevent the vehicle from sinking to the bottom or being swept downstream. Depending upon the vehicle's position and how much of it is above the water's surface, it may be necessary to pull the vehicle from the water before attempting any other extrication activities.

Gaining Access

If the vehicle is still in the water, there is a remote possibility that the occupants could be surviving by taking advantage of a pocket of air trapped under the roof of the vehicle. If rescuers attempt to cut through the roof or to remove the rear window, any trapped air will escape and allow the vehicle to sink beneath the surface and possibly drown the occupants. Therefore, in this situation, members of a water rescue team should make entry into the vehicle from below the waterline.

If the vehicle has been pulled from the water, the tools and techniques used to gain access into the vehicle are the same as those described in Chapter 4 — with one exception. Electrically powered extrication tools and equipment must be used only where contact with water is unlikely. One additional consideration for rescue personnel in this situation is to make sure that their actions do not cause the vehicle to roll back into the water.

Extrication Process

If the vehicle is still in the water, the disentanglement and extrication of trapped victims should be carried out only by those trained in water rescue. If the vehicle has been pulled from the water, the extrication process is the same as in any other vehicle extrication incident with that type of vehicle.

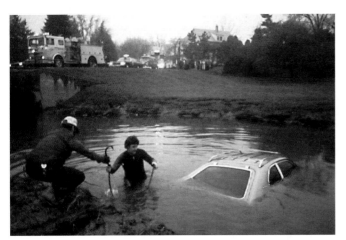

Figure 10.3 An occupied vehicle that is submerged is a special situation. *Courtesy of Steve Taylor.*

Multiple Vehicle Incident

A multiple vehicle incident that qualifies as a special situation is one that involves more vehicles than the responsible agency can handle. If the responsible agency has to call for mutual aid or other outside assistance because of the number of vehicles involved, the incident meets the criteria for a special situation.

Size-Up

Scene Assessment. The first question that must be answered in this type of incident is: Is there anything in the situation that would put rescue personnel or others at greater risk than any other vehicle extrication incident? If so, the needed resources should be called *immediately*. While waiting for the additional resources to arrive, on-scene personnel should be used to establish and maintain control of the scene, and perform any other duties that would not require them to enter the danger zone before the hazard has been mitigated.

Vehicle Assessment. The problems associated with assessing the condition of multiple vehicles involved in a single incident probably have less to do with the environment and more to do with the sheer number of vehicles involved. What is needed is a form of vehicular triage — a sorting of the damaged vehicles into categories of damage. Some may have superficial damage to the front and rear; others may have suffered significant structural damage and deformation that will require major manipulation to provide access to their occupants. In these types of collisions, there is a greater than normal threat of fires being initiated by the uncontrolled release of flammable liquids in close proximity to a variety of ignition sources. Fire crews with portable fire extinguishers, charged hoselines (1½-inch [38 mm] minimum), and foam-making capability should be standing by.

However, the environment cannot be dismissed entirely. Many multiple vehicle collisions are the result of environmental factors — dense fog, heavy rain or snow, or icy roads. These conditions can make damage assessment and other extrication operations much more difficult and dangerous. Under these circumstances, protecting the scene from other oncoming traffic is vitally important.

Victim Assessment. A multiple-vehicle incident is likely to also involve multiple casualties. This may indicate a need for several medical triage teams working at once. Depending upon the number of vehicles involved, weather conditions, darkness, and other factors, simply identifying the exact number of trapped victims may be a challenge. Especially at night, it is critical that this phase of the operation be well organized to reduce the chances of any victim being overlooked.

Extrication Assessment. Depending upon the types of vehicles involved and the rate of speed of the vehicles at the time of the crash, the mechanisms of entrapment may vary from relatively simple to very complex. Also, freeing some victims may be relatively easy, while freeing others may require specialized tools and equipment or personnel with special knowledge and skills.

Vehicle Stabilization

The prospect of having to stabilize a large number of damaged vehicles at the same time can be very daunting. However, based on the results of the vehicular triage performed earlier, the process can be organized and efficient. Each team is only responsible for stabilizing one vehicle at a time. The techniques and equipment described in Chapter 4 should be used to stabilize each vehicle.

Gaining Access

Because these incidents often involve a series of rear-end collisions, access to the front and rear of the vehicles may be extremely limited. Otherwise, the tools and techniques involved in gaining access into many vehicles are the same as those used for gaining access into a single vehicle as described in Chapter 4.

Extrication Process

Disentangling and extricating victims from vehicles involved in a multiple-vehicle incident can be very challenging because the vehicles may be in a variety of positions and environments. Some vehicles may be accordioned between other vehicles at their front and rear. Some vehicles may be wedged under or resting on top of other vehicles. Some vehicles may be in other positions — on their sides or upside down. Some vehicles may have been pushed into a ditch, off of a bridge or cliff, or into a body of water. Each extrication team must focus on one vehicle at a time. Based on the condition of the victims and the vehicle, the team must determine the best way to remove the vehicle from around the victims and to remove the victims from the wreckage. Refer to the earlier chapter that focused on the particular type of vehicle for specifics about the extrication process.

Recreational Vehicles

Incidents involving recreational vehicles are those in which motor homes, travel trailers, etc., have crashed. There may or may not be other types of vehicles involved (Figure 10.4).

Size-Up

Scene Assessment. These incidents may put rescue personnel and others at greater than normal risk if an LPG or other fuel tank or associated piping has been damaged and is leaking. Under these circumstances, on-scene personnel should be used to establish and maintain control of the scene, and perform any other duties that would not require them to enter the danger zone until the flammability hazard has been mitigated.

Vehicle Assessment. Assessing the damage to recreational vehicles involved in collisions may be less challenging than assessing other types of vehicles, unless the recreational vehicle is in one of the hazardous environments already discussed. The structure of most recreational vehicles make them highly susceptible to damage but relatively easy to assess. Most of these vehicles are constructed on a chassis with a rigid frame and are built more like mobile homes than highway vehicles.

Victim Assessment. Motor homes and travel trailers normally have a small number of occupants compared to some other vehicles, but this may or may not be true in any particular incident. If the recreational vehicle was parked when struck by another vehicle, there could be several victims in the recreational vehicle as well as in the other vehicle. In any case, the process of locating all of the victims and assessing their conditions must be as thorough and organized as in incidents involving other types of vehicles.

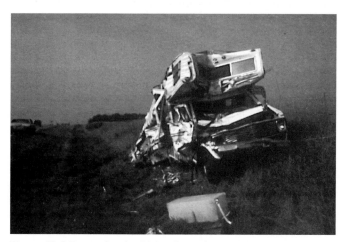

Figure 10.4 Recreational vehicles do not fare well in collisions. *Courtesy of Steve Taylor.*

Extrication Assessment. Because of the relatively lightweight construction of most recreational vehicles, basic extrication tools and equipment are all that are likely to be required. However, because of everchanging vehicle construction technology, and the possibility of alterations made by the vehicle owner, this cannot be assumed. This phase of the operation must also be done thoroughly and conscientiously.

Vehicle Stabilization

Just as with other types of vehicles, the techniques and equipment described in Chapter 4 should be used to stabilize a crashed recreational vehicle. However, stabilizing one of these vehicles may be more like stabilizing a bus than stabilizing any other type of vehicle.

Gaining Access

Again, unless the recreational vehicle has come to rest in some extraordinarily hazardous environment, the tools and techniques described in Chapter 4 can be used to gain access. Because of the relatively light construction of most of these vehicles, entry is likely to be quick and easy.

Extrication Process

Depending upon the type of recreational vehicle involved and other variables in the particular incident, disentangling and extricating victims from these vehicles may be relatively simple or quite challenging. In a collision, the furnishings and other contents of the recreational vehicle may turn its interior into a shambles. This mass of material can make disentangling and extricating the victims much more difficult. Even verifying that all the victims have been located may be difficult.

If a recreational vehicle leaves the roadway and rolls over several times before coming to rest at the bottom of a steep slope, the vehicle may start to disintegrate as it tumbles leaving a trail of objects and occupants on the hillside. However, if the steepness of the slope would require more than low-angle rescue, a technical rescue team should be called in to extricate the victims. Otherwise, extricating victims from recreational vehicles requires the same techniques and equipment described in Chapter 6.

Amusement Park Rides

Amusement park ride incidents may include several different potential dangers for rescuers and others. Many of these vehicles are powered by high-voltage electricity in an electro-magnetic drive system, and others are attached to a gear-driven chain similar to a conveyor. In addition, many of these vehicles travel on or are suspended from elevated tracks that add the element of height to the other potential dangers (Figure 10.5).

Size-Up

Scene Assessment. In amusement park ride incidents, the scene assessment questions that need to be answered are: Has the means of locomotion been turned off, and if not, does the vehicle need to be stabilized before that is done? Also, is the vehicle on an elevated track that is beyond the reach of standard fire service ground ladders or aerial devices? If so, a technical rescue team should be called. In that case, on-scene personnel should be used to establish and maintain control of the scene, and support the technical rescue team when it arrives.

Vehicle Assessment. The uniqueness of these vehicles can make damage assessment difficult. Therefore, pre-incident planning is essential to familiarizing local rescue personnel with the construction of these vehicles.

Victim Assessment. Assessing the condition of the victims of an amusement park ride incident may in some ways be easier than assessing victims in other types of vehicles. The difference lies in the fact that the design of the vehicles used in amusement park rides are usually more open than most highway vehicles, so the victims are often more visible from outside of the vehicle.

Extrication Assessment. Since the tools and techniques of freeing victims from entrapment in an amusement park ride are the same as those used in other types of vehicles, the differences in the extrication assessment may relate more to the environment than the vehicle. If the vehicle is at ground level or close to it, the extrication needs will be the same as those of any other vehicle with a similar passenger load. However, if the vehicle is on an elevated track, the problems are likely to be quite different. If the vehicle is beyond the reach of standard fire service ground ladders or aerial devices, a technical rescue team should be called in to rig the necessary rope rescue systems.

Vehicle Stabilization

The tools and techniques used to stabilize an amusement park ride may be more like stabilizing a piece of industrial machinery than stabilizing a highway vehicle. In other words, it may be necessary to chock the vehicle's wheels and/or secure it in place with ropes, chains, or webbing before de-energizing the means of locomotion. Refer to Chapter 9 for the specifics of stabilizing industrial machinery. However, if the vehicle has derailed and is on the ground, the stabilization tools, techniques, and equipment will be the same as those for any other vehicle of similar size.

Gaining Access

Because of the open design of most of these vehicles, gaining access into them should not be a major challenge unless the crash caused serious deformation of the vehicle or if the vehicle has come to rest upside down. In most cases, the tools and techniques described in Chapter 4 should be sufficient to provide access into these vehicles.

Extrication Process

Considering the open design of most of these vehicles, disentangling and extricating victims may be easier than in other types of vehicles — unless the vehicle is upside down. If the vehicle is upside down, the victims are likely to have suffered massive thoracic, cervical, and cranial trauma due to the lack of overhead protection. The process of packaging and extricating these victims may be protracted. Disentanglement should be no different from that in any other vehicle.

Hanging Vehicles

In this context, a *hanging vehicle* incident is one in which a vehicle has crashed through a guardrail on a bridge, highway overpass, cliff, or an embankment and has come to rest with the cab or passenger compartment hanging above an abyss (Figure 10.6). The goal in this type of incident is to prevent rescue personnel or others, or the occupied portion of the vehicle, from falling to whatever lies beneath it.

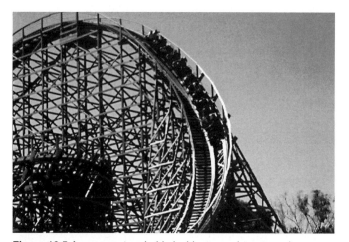

Figure 10.5 Amusement park ride incidents can be extremely dangerous.

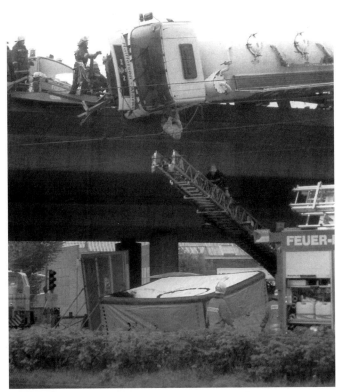

Figure 10.6 Hanging vehicle incidents are among the most challenging. *Courtesy of Ulrich Cimolino.*

Size-Up

Scene Assessment. The first question that must be answered in these incidents is: Can the trapped victims be reached from below with standard fire service ground ladders or aerial devices? If the answer is no, then a technical rescue team should be called in to rig the necessary rope rescue systems. While waiting for the technical rescue team, on-scene personnel should be used to establish and maintain control of the scene.

An important safety consideration during scene assessment, and until the vehicle can be stabilized, is to keep everyone — rescue personnel and all others — out of the area directly below the hanging vehicle. Should all or part of the vehicle come loose before it has been stabilized, anyone below it may be in serious jeopardy.

Another obvious safety consideration is controlling vehicular traffic near the scene. Traffic should be stopped in both directions and detoured around the scene at a sufficient distance that traffic-generated vibration will not affect the stability of the hanging vehicle.

Vehicle Assessment. Getting close enough to assess the damage to a vehicle that is hanging from a high point may be extremely dangerous. The vehicle may be ready to come loose and plunge downward. Or,

that from which the vehicle is hanging may be in danger of collapsing. Assessing the damage to the vehicle may have to be done from some distance away using binoculars.

Victim Assessment. Getting close enough to the vehicle occupants to determine their number and assess their conditions — without putting rescue personnel at serious risk — may be extremely difficult. This, too, may have to be done from a distance.

Extrication Assessment. Determining how the trapped victims will have to be removed from their precarious situation may influence the decisions about what tools and techniques can be used to accomplish that. If rescue personnel will have to work from scaffolding or some other platform — perhaps one suspended from a crane boom — only the types of tools and equipment that are appropriate for use under those conditions should be selected. In most cases, only those tools and equipment that are fully portable and self-contained will be used. Those that require cords, hoses, etc., connected to power units mounted on rescue vehicles may not be safe and effective to use in these situations.

Vehicle Stabilization

Stabilizing a vehicle that is hanging from some precipice may be the most challenging of any vehicle stabilization situation. The height of the vehicle above the ground (or water) can make this potentially one of the most dangerous situations for rescuers and trapped victims alike. When devising a plan to stabilize the vehicle, the type of vehicle involved, the height above the surface below, and the likelihood of the vehicle falling must all be considered.

While there may be variables in the specific situation that would dictate otherwise, initial stabilization may have to be provided by securing the vehicle to bombproof anchor points with as many ropes, chains, or pieces of webbing as can be applied quickly and safely. Complete stabilization may be achieved with the application of shoring and/or cribbing as described in Chapter 4. Again, depending upon the specific circumstances, it may be desirable or necessary to stabilize the hanging portion of the vehicle with a sling suspended from the boom of a crane.

Gaining Access

In these situations, being able to reach the part of the vehicle that is hanging may be as difficult as gaining access into it. Once the hanging part has been reached, a stable platform must be created so that rescue personnel have a safe place from which to work. Under ideal circumstances, such as a vehicle hanging from a highway overpass, rescuers may be able to work from an aerial device positioned on the highway below. In other situations, it may be necessary to suspend a platform from the boom of a crane positioned below the point from which the vehicle is hanging. If the vehicle is hanging from a bridge over a river, estuary, or other body of water, it may be necessary to put the crane on a barge in order to reach the hanging vehicle. As mentioned earlier, if the hanging part of the vehicle cannot be reached with standard fire service ground ladders or aerial devices, a technical rescue team should be called to handle this phase of the operation.

Extrication Process

Once a safe working platform has been created, disentangling and extricating victims from a hanging vehicle may be relatively routine. However, depending upon the circumstances, it may be necessary to provide each victim with fall protection in addition to the normal packaging for extrication.

Incident Termination

Once all viable victims have been extricated and transported to a medical facility as needed, the emergency phase of the operation has ended. The two primary goals of this phase of the operation are to return the emergency vehicles and their crews to operational readiness and to restore the scene to a safe condition, but they may or may not be done in that order.

The highest priority during this phase of the operation is safety. There is absolutely no justification for placing rescue personnel in jeopardy to recover pieces of equipment or the remains of a deceased victim. Body recovery is important, but it is a nonemergency function that should be conducted slowly and carefully — especially in the hazardous environments of some special extrication situations. The operation should be conducted in a way that preserves the dignity of the deceased and respects the feelings of family and friends who may be at the scene.

If necessary, it may be better to abandon pieces of equipment in place, even expensive ones, rather than put rescue personnel at risk by having them reenter a danger zone. Some agencies carry insurance to recover the costs of equipment that was abandoned or destroyed. Also, it may be possible to recover these costs from the insurance carrier of the person found to be responsible for causing the incident. *In any case, no piece of equipment is worth putting anyone in serious danger.*

Otherwise, local protocols and standard operating procedures should be followed during this phase of the operation. These procedures may or may not involve agency personnel in scene restoration beyond that necessary for public safety. However, in most jurisdictions, once an emergency response agency has assumed control of the scene, that agency is legally responsible for the scene until it is released to the owner or other individual or agency normally responsible for it.

Summary

Special vehicle extrication situations are those that are unusual in some significant way. They may be special because of the environment in which they occurred, the number of vehicles and/or victims involved, or because of the presence of hazardous materials or some other threat that could put rescuers or others at greater than normal risk.

As in any other vehicle extrication incident, the key word in special situations is *safety*. Part of maintaining safety in special extrication situations is recognizing that the situation is unusual and that it may be beyond the operational capabilities of those responding to it. Another aspect of conducting these special operations safely is avoiding the tunnel vision that can induce some to exceed their operational limits and put themselves and others in jeopardy, perhaps adding more victims to the incident. If these operations are to be done safely, they must be conducted calmly, methodically, and according to agency protocols and standard operating procedures.

special situations, 181, 183, 184
vehicles in structures, 182
extrication defined, 3
extrication techniques
See also specific components of extrication
for buses, 127–130
for industrial and agricultural vehicles, 177–178
for medium and heavy trucks, 141–144
for passenger vehicles, 95–96
for railcars, 161–162

F

facial hair, facepiece seals compromised by, 24
fifth wheels on medium and heavy trucks, 136
filter masks, 25
fire behavior in luggage compartments, 111
fire hazards at multiple vehicle incidents, 184
fire protection as component of extrication, 14
fire suppression and accidental air bag activation, 54
firefighter safety
See also hazardous conditions
air bags, 53, 83–86
air suspension systems, 108, 116, 136
block and tackle and, 49
brake systems on trucks, 135, 136
bus engine compartments, 117
chains and, 34–35
cheaters, 36
driving to incidents, 13
energy absorbing bumpers, 57, 58
facial hair compromising facepiece seals, 24
glass removal and, 64
jacks and, 43
jumper cables connecting railcars, 149
lifting bags and, 41
opening doors using power spreaders, 70
personal protective equipment, 21–25
power saws and, 45, 46
priorities for, 5
roofs of electrically powered buses, 113
stabilization, 34–35, 41, 43, 49, 60, 129
struts exploding, 57, 58
thermal cutting devices, 47–48
winches, 48–49
first responders, 25. *See also officers, first-in*
flash fire risks, 126, 134
floors
of buses, 103, 126–127
entry through, 77–78
foam used at incidents with fuel leak risks, 61, 174
foot protection, 23
forklifts, 167–169
freight trains, 146–147
fuel leak risks
at bus incidents, 113, 118, 119, 126
foam used at incidents with, 61, 174
at medium and heavy truck incidents, 134, 135, 144
at recreational vehicle incidents, 185
fuel systems
See also power systems
of buses, 113
of industrial and agricultural vehicles, 173–174

of medium and heavy trucks, 134–135
of passenger vehicles, 87
of recreational vehicles, 185
of trains, 154
full size cars, 82–83

G

generators on rescue vehicles, 29
gin poles and A-frames, 28
glass, breaking and removing, 38, 63–68. *See also windows*
glass hammers, 38
gloves, 23
goggles, 22
graders (maintainers), 169
grounding vehicles, 55
group/sector operations
as component of extrication, 18
EMS groups, 9, 18
hazardous materials groups, 139
scene control groups, 6, 18
triage groups, 18, 52, 114
vehicle stabilization groups, 6, 18

H

Halligan tools, 68, 70, 120
hammers, pneumatic, 39–40
hand protection, 23
handling victims. *See victims, packaging and handling*
hanging vehicle incidents, 186–188
harvesters (combines), 169
hazardous conditions
See also firefighter safety
at bus incidents, 113, 116–118, 119, 126
cribbing soaking up liquids, 31
downed power lines, 19, 37, 97, 118
electrical hazards, 55, 113, 152–153, 185–186
fluid leaks, 61
at freight train incidents, 147
fuel leaks
at bus incidents, 113, 118, 119, 126
foam used at incidents with, 61, 174
increasing risk of fire, 174
at medium and heavy truck incidents, 134, 135, 144
at passenger vehicle incidents, 87
at recreational vehicle incidents, 185
liquid formed on crushed bumpers, 57
livestock freed after incidents, 139
at medium and heavy truck incidents, 134, 135, 139, 144
at multiple vehicle incidents, 184
at passenger vehicle incidents, 87
pneumatic tools and compressed oxygen, 39
position of vehicle and, 9, 51
power systems for railcars, 148, 149, 151, 152
repairing before incident termination, 18–19, 97, 144
sparks produced by air chisels, 40
storing oxygen and acetylene for cutting torches, 47
vapors, fumes, smoke and dust, 24
hazardous materials, 18–19, 139, 144
hazardous materials teams, 139
head and face protection, 22
head protection systems (HPS), 56, 84, 86

hearing protection, 22
hoselines, conditions for having charged, 45, 47, 61, 126
hydraulic tools, 42–45. *See also names of specific tools*

I

IMS (Incident Management System), 17–18
incident action plans (IAP), developing, 15, 179
incident command, 11–19
Incident Commanders (ICs), 21, 91
Incident Management System (IMS), 17–18
Incident Safety Officer, 21
incident stabilization, 8
incident termination
    as component of extrication, 18–19, 144
    hanging vehicle incidents, 188
    industrial and agricultural incidents, 178
    medium and heavy truck incidents, 144
    passenger vehicle incidents, 96–98
industrial vehicle extrication
    See also specific types of vehicles
    access to victims, 176–177
    anatomy and construction of vehicles, 170–174
    classification of vehicles, 165–170
    process of, 177–178
    size-up, 174–175
    stabilizing vehicles, 175–176
injuries, kinematics, 6, 87–88, 91
insurance covering costs of destroyed equipment, 188
Insurance Institute for Highway Safety (IIHS), 4
intermediate (midsize) cars, 82
International Association of Fire Chiefs, 4
inverters on rescue vehicles, 29
investigations of safety defects in motor vehicles, 4

J

jacks
    blocking and cribbing used with, 43
    industrial and agricultural devices operated using, 171
    lifting objects from vehicles using, 63
    lifting vehicles using, 130
    overview, 38–39, 43, 60
    on rescue vehicles, 28
    stabilizing trucks using, 142
    stabilizing vehicles on roofs using, 142
    stabilizing vehicles on sides using, 118
    stabilizing vehicles upside down using, 62
    stabilizing vehicles using, 60, 116

K

kick panels, 10, 72–73
knee bolsters, 56, 84
knives, 37

L

ladders used in railcar extrication procedures, 156–157
law enforcement personnel, 9, 97
lift trucks (forklifts), 167–169
lifting bags, pneumatic
    cribbing used as base for, 31–32
    lifting buses from trapped victims using, 129–130
    lifting objects from vehicles using, 63
    overview, 40–41

used as temporary support, 60
lifting objects from vehicles, 43, 62–63
lifting vehicles
    See also moving vehicles
    tools and equipment used for, 28, 38–39, 116
    victims trapped beneath buses, 116, 129–130
lifting/pulling tools, 48–49. *See also names of specific tools*
lights
    emergency light use during extrication, 16, 51–52
    on rescue vehicles, 29
livestock trailers, 138–139
load limits of chains, 34, 35
location of incidents, dispatchers gathering information
    about, 12
locomotives, 147–148
lounge/food service railcars, 149, 161
luggage (baggage) railcars, 149, 161
luggage compartments on buses, 111, 128

M

machinery incidents and disentanglement, 170, 176. *See also*
    industrial vehicle extrication
maintainers (graders), 169
mast of forklifts, 168
material handling railcars, 149, 161
mechanics tools, 39
medical triage groups, 18, 52, 114
medium and heavy truck extrication
    access to victims, 142–143
    anatomy and construction of trucks, 132–136
    classification of trucks, 131–132
    process of, 143–144
    size-up, 139–140
    stabilizing vehicles, 140–142
    trailers, 136–139
minivans, 83
moving vehicles, winches used for, 27–28. *See also* lifting
    vehicles
mutual aid resources, 5–6, 11. *See also* unified command at
    railcar incidents

N

National Highway Transportation Safety Administration
    (NHTSA)
    accidental air bag activation described by, 54–55
    classification of automobiles, 81–83
    overview, 4
    restraint system technology information, 53
National Safety Council (NSC), 4
NFPA (National Fire Protection Association) Standards
    See also titles of specific documents
    1001, 179
    1006 (2000), 7, 13–14
    1500, 22, 23, 25
    1670, 5, 6, 7, 30, 145, 179
    1901, 16
    1971, 22, 23
    1981, 24
    1999, 23
NHTSA. *See* National Highway Transportation Safety
    Administration (NHTSA)

COMMENT SHEET

DATE _____ NAME _____

ADDRESS _____

ORGANIZATION REPRESENTED _____

CHAPTER TITLE _____ NUMBER _____

SECTION/PARAGRAPH/FIGURE _____ PAGE _____

1. Proposal (include proposed wording or identification of wording to be deleted),
    OR PROPOSED FIGURE:

2. Statement of Problem and Substantiation for Proposal:

RETURN TO: IFSTA Editor   SIGNATURE _____
            Fire Protection Publications
            Oklahoma State University
            930 N. Willis
            Stillwater, OK 74078-8045

Use this sheet to make any suggestions, recommendations, or comments. We need your input to make the manuals as up to date as possible. Your help is appreciated. Use additional pages if necessary.

Your Training Connection.....

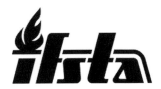

The International Fire Service Training Association

We have a free catalog describing hundreds of fire and emergency service training materials available from a convenient single source: the International Fire Service Training Association (IFSTA).

Choose from products including IFSTA manuals, IFSTA study guides, IFSTA curriculum packages, Fire Protection Publications manuals, books from other publishers, software, videos, and NFPA standards.

Contact us by phone, fax, U.S. mail, e-mail, internet web page, or personal visit.

Phone
1-800-654-4055

Fax
405-744-8204

U.S. mail
IFSTA, Fire Protection Publications
Oklahoma State University
930 North Willis
Stillwater, OK 74078-8045

E-mail
editors@osufpp.org

Internet web page
www.ifsta.org

Personal visit
Call if you need directions!

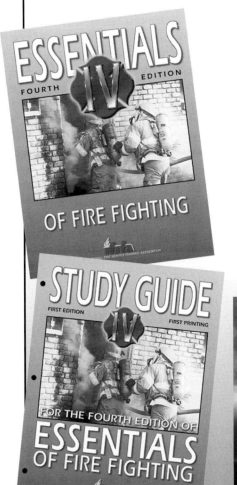

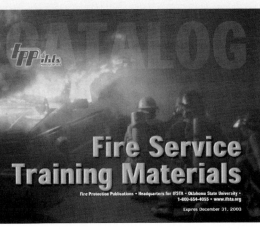

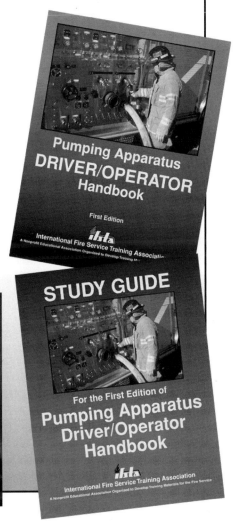